LASERS IN NEUROSURGERY

Foundations of Neurological Surgery

Robertson and Clark, Lasers in Neurosurgery. ISBN 0-89838-966-6.

LASERS IN NEUROSURGERY

Edited by

Jon H. Robertson, M.D.
University of Tennessee, Memphis

W. Craig Clark, M.D., Ph.D.
University of Tennessee, Memphis

Kluwer Academic Publishers

BOSTON DORDRECHT LANCASTER

DISTRIBUTORS

for the United States and Canada: Kluwer Academic Publishers, 101 Philip Drive, Assinippi Park, Norwell, MA, 02061, USA

for the UK and Ireland: Kluwer Academic Publishers, Falcon House, Queen Square, Lancaster LA1 1RN, UK

for all other countries: Kluwer Academic Publishers Group, Distribution Centre, P.O. Box 322, 3300 AH Dordrecht, The Netherlands

Library of Congress Cataloging in Publication Data

Lasers in neurosurgery.
(Foundations of neurological surgery; FONS 1)
Includes index.
1. Nervous system—Surgery. 2. Lasers in surgery.
I. Robertson, Jon H. II. Clark, W. Craig. III. Series.
[DNLM: 1. Laser Surgery. 2. Nervous System—surgery.
WL 368 L343]
RD593.L35 1988 617′.48 87-23953
ISBN 0-89838-966-6

PRINTED IN THE UNITED STATES.

CONTENTS

CONTRIBUTING AUTHORS

Robert E. Anderson, B. S., Department of Neurological Surgery, Mayo Clinic, Mayo Medical School, Rochester, Minnesota.

Michael L. J. Apuzzo, M.D., Professor, Department of Neurological Surgery, University of Southern California School of Medicine, Los Angeles, California.

James E. Boggan, M.D., Assistant Professor, Department of Neurological Surgery, University of California, Davis, Sacramento, California.

Robert E. Breeze, M.D., Clinical Instructor, Department of Neurological Surgery, University of Southern California School of Medicine, Los Angeles, California.

S. J. Goerss, B. S., Department of Neurological Surgery, Mayo Clinic and Mayo Foundation, Rochester, Minnesota.

Hector E. James, M.D., Professor of Neurosurgery and Pediatrics, University of California, San Diego, Medical Center, San Diego, California.

B. A. Kall, M.D., Department of Information Processing and Systems, Mayo Clinic and Mayo Foundation, Rochester, Minnesota.

Patrick J. Kelly, M.D., Professor, Department of Neurological Surgery, Mayo Clinic, Mayo Medical School, Rochester, Minnesota.

Walter J. Levy, M.D., Assistant Professor, Department of Surgery, Division of Neurosurgery, University of Missouri–Columbia, Health Sciences Center, Columbia, Missouri.

Michael Salcman, M.D., Professor and Head, Division of Neurological Surgery, University of Maryland School of Medicine, Baltimore, Maryland.

Thoralf M. Sundt, Jr., M.D., Professor and Chairman, Department of Neurological Surgery, Mayo Clinic, Mayo Medical School, Rochester, Minnesota.

John M. Tew, Jr., M.D., Professor and Chairman, Department of Neurosurgery, University of Cincinnati College of Medicine, Cincinnati, Ohio.

William D. Tobler, M.D., Assistant Professor, Department of Neurosurgery, University of Cincinnati College of Medicine, Cincinnati, Ohio.

Marion L. Walker, M.D., Pediatric Neurosurgeon, Children's Medical Center, Salt Lake City, Utah.

Robert E. Wharen, Jr., M.D., Department of Neurological Surgery, Montefiore Hospital, University of Pittsburgh, Pittsburgh, Pennsylvania

Clark Watts, Professor of Surgery (Neurosurgery), University of Missouri–Columbiar, Health Sciences Center, Columbia, Missouri

PREFACE

Developments in the field of instrumentation are among the major contributions to human advancement. The history of surgery has seen many revolutionary developments cause quantum leaps in progress. Electrocautery, the anesthesia machine, computed axial tomography, and the surgical microscope are all revolutionary instruments that have irrevocably changed the direction of neurological surgery.

In the early stages of application, there are always detractors and valid controversy concerning the value of a new instrument. Some will remember those who argued that the magnification and illumination provided by the microscope were not valuable to the skilled surgeon and would prolong the operative time and increase infection rates. Others may recall that Cushing was told to abandon the blood pressure recording device (Riva-Roca apparatus) because the recording of blood pressure during the course of an operative procedure was of no value.

In this book, Drs. Robertson and Clark evaluate the application of lasers in neurological surgery. Laser technology has probably attracted as much controversy as any other previous form of innovative instrumentation. Although laser applications have permeated nearly every aspect of surgical therapy, the expectations have frequently been unrealistic and the evaluation of technological development has always been painfully slow. The properties of vaporization, coagulation, and cutting unified in an invisible shaft of light have enabled the neurosurgeon to vaporize inaccessible tumors of brain and spinal cord, harness recalcitrant bleeding sites, and cut through the most formidable calcified tumors. The application of this new energy form in tandem with the surgical microscope has, in my opinion, extended the scope of all aspects of neurosurgery. We have much more work to do. It is necessary to document improved results and demand technological advances and safe innovations. This book and other recordings that will follow are necessary to chart the progress and enumerate the problems that will stimulate the more rapid development of this most incredible advance in instrumentation.

John M. Tew, Jr., M.D.

ACKNOWLEDGMENTS

We wish to express our gratitude to Mr. Carl Smith of Laser Technologies, Inc., Memphis, Tennessee, who first exposed us to surgical lasers early in their development as tools for neurological surgery. Also, this book could not have been completed without the expert secretarial assistance of Mrs. Louise Gates of the Department of Neurosurgery. She tirelessly completed the many drafts, correspondence, and other details necessary to bring this effort to fruition.

INTRODUCTION

What is the role of the laser in neurosurgery? This question first confronted the editors over 7 years ago and it is still not completely answered at the writing of this book. Early on, it was a less complicated issue because the question was—is there any place at all for laser technology in neurological surgery? The development of more sophisticated delivery systems and the demonstration of the utility of the device in the operating room have more or less made the use of the laser almost routine in many centers. Certainly the role of the laser has and will continue to evolve as we begin to understand more about the basic mechanisms by which the laser interacts with tissue. This volume makes an effort to describe the best known laser effect, i.e., thermal ablation of tissue, as well as specific neurosurgical applications of this technology. Also of importance is the effort to present a conservative, balanced view of this technology in describing situations where the laser does not impart any special advantage, as well as areas of current research and future development of interest to the neurosurgeon.

We have enlisted colleagues with a wide range of experience with the use of lasers in neurosurgery. Their views and experiences, coupled with our own, have hopefully been molded into an informative and readable monograph that will provide colleagues with a descriptive account of the various neurosurgical applications, as well as inspire continued investigation into new delivery systems, new applications, and the basic mechanisms of laser-tissue interaction.

Joh H. Robertson, M.D.
W. Craig Clark, M.D., Ph.D.

I. BACKGROUND

1. THE HISTORY OF LASERS IN NEUROSURGERY

John M. Tew, Jr.
William D. Tobler

The development of lasers and laser technology will be recognized as one of the major technological advancements of the twentieth century. Laser technology pervades all strata of society and impacts daily life from Star Wars technology to the grocery checkout line. The development of the quantum theory paved the way for Einstein's landmark paper in 1917 entitled "Zur Quantum Theorie der Strahlung," which detailed the principles for stimulated emission of photons [14]. Basov and Prokorhov further contributed to an understanding of stimulated emission. The first molecular oscillator or maser (microwave amplification by the stimulated emission of radiation) was produced by Gordon in 1954 [24]. The 1958 paper by Schawlow and Townes, "Infrared and Optical Masers," described the structure and function of a laser. They each received the Nobel Prize for these discoveries [47], Townes in 1964 and Schawlow in 1981. Theodore Maiman, of the Hughes Aircraft Company, is credited with producing the first laser light in July of 1960. He reported the production of stimulated emission at a wavelength of 6943A from the active medium of ruby (aluminum oxide crystal containing chromium atoms).

The unique characteristics (of optical purity and coherence) associated with laser light were immediately recognized. In 1961, Schawlow speculated about the potential infinite wavelengths available for lasers and the variety of applications. An immediate reaction to the potential for seminal developments was the formation of at least 500 research groups engaged in laser development in the United States by 1963 [46], and as many as 25 various active media had been used to produce laser light, including neodymium and carbon dioxide, the principal lasers used currently in neurosurgery.

Potential beneficial effects of laser radiation were recognized by clinical investigators in various medical fields. The retinal effects of laser radiation were recognized and defined. Because of the laser's coherence and small focal point, considerable effort had been spent to develop retinal photocoagulation for repairing and spot-welding of detached retinas in 1964 [35]. Dermatologists, led by Leon Goldman, studied the effects of pulsed ruby laser radiation upon skin and demonstrated both gross and microscopic effects. Fein and Klein studied the internal effects of laser radiation externally applied to laboratory animals [17]. They also studied the effects of ruby laser radiation on experimental tumors and documented that partial necrosis of the lesion occurred. In a 1964 review article in the *Journal of the American Medical Association*, Litwin reported that "because the focal point of

Robertson, J.H. and Clark, W.C. (eds), Lasers in Neurosurgery.

the laser is so fine, its use in the performance of microsurgery or the destruction of subcellular particles will be possible should such techniques ever be of use" [35].

Early Neurosurgical Applications

Most early efforts of pioneering neurosurgeons were directed toward describing the ablative effects of laser radiation [30, 44]. Focused and defocused ruby laser beams were pulsed and applied to the cranial vaults of experimental animals and were found to produce cerebral contusions, subdural hemorrhage, and often death, due to cerebral herniation from absorbed laser energy resulting in an intracranial explosion. Direct radiation of the cortical surfaces of cats with the ruby laser showed various degrees of tissue destruction, and in-depth reports of the histological detail were provided [18–20, 34]. Brown concluded that neurons have a greater sensitivity to the destructive effects of laser energy, and thus gray matter is more susceptible than white matter to the destructive effects of laser energy [10, 11].

More gross observations were unable to confirm the obvious: that focused energy caused greater apparent damage than defocused energy. Radiation of the cortex through an intact dura caused less damage than radiation of the brain directly. Arteries and veins larger than 0.5 mm bled regularly. And, lastly, it was noted that the laser created a wedge-shaped lesion when applied directly to the cortical surface [34].

In 1965, Rosomoff reported two human cases in which pulses of ruby laser were applied to carcinomatous lesions. Postmortem excision showed well-circumscribed areas of necrosis corresponding to the sites of laser application [43].

The intriguing concept of laser vascular anastomosis, which in recent years has been an area of concerted interest in laser applications, was first described in the germinal period of laser research by Yahr and Stulley [56]. In these experiments, a side-to-side anastomosis was made with cyanoacrylate glue, and then a hole was punched in the common wall with a ruby, neodymium, or carbon dioxide laser to achieve the anastomosis. This method never gained significant usage. Today, anastomoses are performed with laser welds, and their origination will be described later in this chapter.

The advent of the carbon dioxide laser, developed by Patel in 1964, ushered in a new era of laser surgery development [40]. Unlike the ruby laser, which operated only in a pulsed mode, the carbon dioxide laser operated in a continuous mode and was capable of achieving high powers.

Stellar and colleagues demonstrated the precise cutting and vaporization effects of the laser in 1968. In experimental melanomas and ependymoblastomas in mice, the carbon dioxide laser was shown to effectively vaporize entire masses of tumor. In addition, the laser demonstrated properties of coagulation and hemostasis. Experimentation with the production of minimal lesions and subsequent histological evaluation consistently showed the same pattern. A three-layer zone of injury was identifiable: (1) an inner charred layer; (2) a middle zone of dessication, and (3) an outer layer of edema. In 1969, Stellar reported the first human neurosurgical application of the carbon dioxide laser to partially vaporize a glioblastoma [48].

The Development of Clinical Application of laser Neurosurgery

THE CARBON DIOXIDE LASER

The present era of laser neurosurgery began in 1976. The development of portable laser units which could easily be transported into the operating room enabled surgeons to develop and apply laser technology to clinical practice. Ascher first used the laser in Austria in 1976 to remove a brain tumor, and since then he has used it in more than 1000 cases. Simultaneous reports of precise tissue effects and histological studies of laser effects began to appear [2–4].

Neurosurgeons began to use the carbon dioxide laser in the United States in 1979. In a few short years, their use has become widespread. Training programs to familiarize the surgeon with the features and advantages, as well as the safety aspects of laser surgery, have become requisite [9].

Encouraging reports of the efficacy of carbon dioxide laser techniques of vaporizing meningiomas, acoustic neuromas, and other tumors have appeared [5, 21, 23, 25, 28, 36, 41, 45, 49, 50, 51, 54]. The carbon dioxide laser is now a standard part of the armamentarium of the neurosurgeon. It is used primarily as an ablative tool, specially adapted to the microscope and used to vaporize extraaxial benign tumors of the brain or spinal cord.

Kelly has adapted the carbon dioxide laser for stereotactic procedures and precise laser vaporization of deep-seated tumors [29]. This technique, however, is highly specialized and has not become widely employed.

Others have used carbon dioxide lasers to vaporize discs but without great benefit. Microvascular anastomosis has been performed with a finely focused carbon dioxide laser beam, but the technique remains experimental at this time [39]. At present, fiberoptic cabels to transport the carbon dioxide laser energy are in developmental stages. Successful production of such a fiber may open the way for intravascular and percutaneous applications.

THE NEODYMIUM: YTTRIUM-ALUMINUM-GARNET (Nd:YAG)

Development of the Nd:YAG laser for medical applications began in the late 1960s and culminated in the first clinical neurosurgical application by Beck in 1976 [7]. The deeper tissue scatter effect and its preferential pigment absorption provided neurosurgeons with a potent coagulation laser [8]. The early years of experience by Beck and others have shown the Nd:YAG laser to be effective for vascularized tumors such as meningiomas, hemangioblastomas, and chordomas [6, 22]. More recently, attention has turned toward the application of the Nd:YAG laser for shrinking and coagulating arteriovenous malformations. Reports by Fasano [15, 16], Wharen, Anderson, and Sundt [55], and recently by Twe [52, 53], indicate that it may be useful, but they lack total consensus regarding its applicability to vascular malformations. Characteristics unique to Nd:YAG energy pose special risks to the patient, and great care must be exercised by the individual surgeon, as indicated in a report by Jain [26]. The recent lifting of restrictions by the Food and Drug Administration (FDA) now enables any trained neurosurgeon to use the Nd:YAG laser in the United States for coagulation of tumors.

Vascular anastomosis has been reported with the Nd:YAG laser and, theoretically, may be more sound than with the carbon dioxide laser because the Nd:YAG laser can penetrate through the entire depth of the vascular wall [27]. Little progress has emerged from the use of fiberoptic cables for endoscopic or percutaneous use.

THE ARGON LASER

The argon laser has a minor but interesting role in neurosurgery. Powers and Edwards have reported the only significant experience with the argon laser to date [13, 39]. It has not gained widespread use because of its relatively low powers, making it inefficient as an ablative instrument. The production of dorsal root entry zone (DREZ) lesions has been reported with argon as well as with carbon dioxide laser [32, 33, 37]. Unless a more powerful argon system is developed, widespread use of this laser in neurosurgery is not likely.

Argon-pumped dye lasers, which emit light in the visible portion of the spectrum at 630 nm, may be effective for photoradiation leading to tumor cell destruction [1, 31]. Hematoporphyrin derivatives are concentrated in rapidly dividing tissues, and when they are exposed to photons at 630 nm, superoxide radicals form, leading to cytotoxic effects [12].

Laws reported on a model for the treatment of gliomas with hematoporphyrins and a fiberoptic probe, which may be implanted stereotactically into the tumor for continuous-wave dye laser application [31]. Results of this technique in five patients with astrocytoma suggest that hematoporphyrin radiation therapy may be an adjunct to surgical tumor removal. This concept will require further investigative effort. The development of more effective photoactive substances has the potential for significant impact in this area.

In the decade since the present era of laser neurosurgery began, the carbon dioxide laser stands as the premier laser. It is used mainly as an ablative instrument in microsurgical procedures to remove benign extraaxial tumors in areas of difficult access. Little clinical use has been found for techniques other than ablation. The Nd:YAG laser is a coagulative instrument whose role is not as well defined. It will probably not be as widely employed as the carbon dioxide laser. The future of lasers, however, is assured in neurosurgery. The direction will likely be toward the implementation of technology to achieve percutaneous methods of tumor surgery, photoradiation techniques, and intravascular laser applications.

References

1. Apuzzo ML: Ionizing and non-ionizing radiotherapy in cerebral neoplasia: Specialized approaches. Presented at the 33rd Annual Meeting of the Congress of Neurological Surgeons, Chicago, IL., 1983.
2. Ascher PW: The CO_2 laser in neurosurgery. *Fortschr Med* 98:253–254, 1980.
3. Ascher PW: Newest ultrastructural findings after the use of CO_2 laser on CNS tissue. *Acta Neurochir* [Suppl] (Wien) 28:572–581, 1979.
4. Ascher PW, Heppner F: CO_2-laser in neurosurgery. *Neurosurg Rev* 7:123–133, 1984.
5. Bartal AD, Heilbronn VD, Avram J, et al: Carbon dioxide laser surgery of basal meningiomas. *Surg Neurol* 17:90–95, 1982.
6. Beck OJ: The use of the Nd:YAG and the CO_2 laser in neurosurgery. *Neurosurg Rev*, 3:261–266, 1980.
7. Beck OJ: Use of the Nd:YAG laser in neurosurgery. *Neurosurg Rev* 7:151–158, 1984.
8. Beck OJ, wilske J, Schoenberger J: Tissue changes following application to lasers of the rabbit brain. *Neurosurg Rev*, 1:31–36, 1979.
9. Brown JT, Cerullo LJ: Laser workshops in neurological surgery. *Lasers Surg Med* 4:241–246, 1984.
10. Brown TE, True C, McLaurin RL, et al: Laser radiation. I. Acute effect on cerebral cortex. *Neurology*, 16:730–737, 1966.
11. Brown TE, True C, McLaurin RL, et al: Laser radiation. II. Long-term effects of laser radiation on certain intracranial structures. Neurology 17:789–796, 1967.
12. Dougherty TJ, Kaufman JE, Goldfarb A, et al: Photoradiation therapy for the treatment of malignant tumors. *Cancer Res* 38:2628–2635, 1978.
13. Edwards MSB, Boggan JE: Argon laser surgery of pediatric neural neoplasms. *Childs Brain* 11:171–175, 1984.
14. Einstein A: Zur Quantum Theorie der Strahlung. *Physiol Zeitschr* 18:121–128, 1917.
15. Fasano VA: The treatment of vascular malformation of the brain with laser source. *Lasers Surg Med* 1:347–356, 1981.
16. Fasano VA, Urciuoli R, Ponzio M: Photocoagulation of cerebral arteriovenous malformations and arterial aneurysms with the neodymium: yttrium-aluminum-garnet or argon laser: Premliminary results in twelve patients. *Neurosurgery* 11:754–760, 1982.
17. Fine S, Klein E, Novak W, et al: Interaction of laser irradiation with biological system. *Fed Proc* (Suppl 14) 24:S35–S47, 1965.
18. Fox JL: The use of laser radiation as a surgical "light-knife." *J Surg Res* 9:199–205, 1969
19. Fox JL, Hayes JR, Stein MN, et al: Experimental cranial and vascular studies of the effects of pulsed and continuous wave laser radiation. *J Neurosurg*, 27:126–137, 1967.
20. Fox JL, et al: Lasers and their neurosurgical application. *Milit Med* 131:493–498, 1966
21. Gong-bai C: Laser vaporization on intracranial tumors. *Lasers Surg Med* 1:235–240, 1981.
22. Handa H, Takeuchi J, Yamagami T: Nd:YAG laser as a surgical tool. *Neurosurg Rev* 7:159–163, 1984.
23. Hara M, et al: Evaluation of laser surgery against brain tumor (Japan). *No Shinkei Geka* 8:363–369, 1980.
24. Hecht J, Teresi D: *Laser, Super Tool of the 1980s*. New York, Ticknor & Fields, 1982.
25. Hudgins R, Moody J, Sanders M, et al: Microsurgical laser vaporization of inaccessible

tumors of the central nervous system. *Dallas Med J* 76:245–250, 1981.
26. Jain KK: Complications of use of neodymium–yttrium-aluminum-garnet laser in neurosurgery. *Neurosurgery*, 16:759–762, 1985.
27. Jain KK: Sutureless microvascular anastomosis using a neodymium:YAG laser. *J Microsurg* 1:436–439, 1980.
28. James HE, Williams J, Brock W, et al: Radical removal of lipomas of the conus and cauda equina with laser microsurgery. *Neurosurgery* 15:340–343, 1984.
29. Kelly PJ, Kall BA, Goerss S, et al: Results of computer-assisted stereotactic laser resection of deep-seated intracranial lesions. *Mayo Clin Proc* 61:20–27, 1986.
30. Lambert PW, Fox JL, Earle KM: Cerebral edema after laser radiation: An electron microscopic study. *J Neuropathol Exp Neurol* 25:531–541, 1966.
31. Laws ER Jr, Cortese DA, Kinsey JH, et al: Photoradiation therapy in the treatment of malignant brain tumors: A phase I (feasibility) study. *J Neurosurg* 9:672–678, 1981.
32. Levy WJ, Gallo C, Watts C: Comparison of laser and radiofrequency dorsal root entry zone lesions in cats. *Neurosurgery* 16:327–330, 1985.
33. Levy WJ, Nutkiewicz A, Ditmore QM, et al: Laser-induced dorsal root entry zone lesions for pain control: Report of three cases. *J Neurosurg* 59:884–886, 1983.
34. Liss L, Roppel R: Histopathology of laser-produced lesions in cat brains. *Neurology* 16: 783–790, 1966.
35. Litwin MS, Glew DH: The biological effects of laser radiation. *JAMA* 187:842–847, 1964.
36. Mattos Pimenta LH, Mattos Pimenta A, Martins JL: The use of the CO_2 laser for the removal of awkwardly situated meningiomas. *Neurosurg Rev* 4:53–55, 1981.
37. Neblett C: Reconstructive vascular surgery with use of the CO_2 laser. Presented at the Congress on Laser Neurosurgery II, Chicago, IL, September 1982.
38. Patel CKN: Continuous wave laser action on vibrational-rotational transitions of CO_2 *Rhys Rev* 136:A1187–A1193, 1964.
39. Powers SK, Adams JE, Edwards MSB, et al: Pain relief from dorsal root entry zone lesions made with argon and carbon dioxide microsurgical lasers. *J Neurosurg* 61:841–847, 1984.
40. Powers SK, Edwards MSB, Boggan JE, et al: Use of the argon surgical laser in neurosurgery. *J Neurosurg* 60:523–530, 1984.
41. Robertson JH, Clark WC, Robertson JT, et al: Use of the carbon dioxide laser for acoustic tumor surgery. *Neurosurgery* 12:286–290, 1983.
42. Robertson JH, Clark WC: Carbon dioxide laser in neurosurgery. *Contemp Neurosurg* 5:1–6, 1983.
43. Rosomoff HL, Carroll F: Effect of laser on brain and neoplasm. *Surg Forum* 16:431–433, 1965.
44. Rosomoff HL, Carroll F: Reaction of neoplasm and brain to laser. *Arch Neurol* 14:143–148, 1966.
45. Sawaya R, Hawley DK, tobler WD, et al: Pineal and third ventricle tumors. In Youmans J (ed): *Neurological Surgery*, 3rd ed. In Press.
46. Schawlow AL: Advances in optical masers. *Sci Am* 209:34–45, 1963.
47. Schawlow AL, Townes CH: Infrared and optical masers. *Phys Rev* 112:1940–1949, 1958.
48. Stellar S, Polanyi TG, Bredemier HC: Experimental studies with the carbon dioxide laser as a neurosurgical instrument. *Med Biol Eng* 8:549–558, 1970.
49. Strait TA, Robertson JH, Clark WC: Use of the carbon dioxide laser in the operative management of intracranial meningiomas. *Neurosurgery* 10:464–467, 1982.
50. Takizawa T: The carbon dioxide laser surgical unit as an instrument for surgery of brain tumors—its advantages and disadvantages. *Neurosurg Rev* 7:135–144, 1984.
51. Tew JM Jr, Tobler WD: The laser: History, biophysics, and neurosurgical applications. *Clin Neurosurg* 31:506–549, 1984.
52. Tew JM Jr, Tobler WD: Present status of lasers in neurosurgery. *Advances and Technical Standards in Neurosurgery*, Vol 12. Wien, Springer-Verlag, in press.
53. Tew JW Jr, Tobler WD, Zuccarello M: The treatment of arteriovenous malformations of the brain with the neodymium:YAG laser. *Advances and Technical Standards in Neurosurgery*. In press.
54. Tobler WD, Sayaya R, Tew JM Jr: Successful laser-assisted excision of a metastatic midbrain tumor. *Neurosurgery* 18:795–797, 1986.
55. Wharen RE, Anderson RE, Sundt TM: The Nd:YAG laser in neurosurgery. Part 2, Clinical studies: an adjunctive measure of hemostasis in resection of arteriovenous malformations. *J Neurosurg* 60:540–547, 1984.
56. Yahr WZ, Stully KJ: Blood vessel anastomosis by laser and other biomedical applications. *J Assoc Adv Med Instrum* 1:28–31, 1966.

2. LASER TYPES

Robert E. Breeze,
Michael L. J. Apuzzo

Generally speaking, the lasers used in neurosurgery are continuous-wave devices with either gas or solid media. The devices most commonly used are the carbon dioxide and argon lasers (gas media) or the neodymium:yttrium-aluminum-garnet (Nd:YAG) (solid media) laser. The various types of lasers and delivery systems are in a constant state of development; new devices and applications are reported almost daily. This chapter will provide some perspective on the classification of lasers and acquaint the reader with those laser types commonly encountered in clinical research and practice. Before a system of classification is discussed, however, a few basic points must be reviewed.

Physical Principles

Briefly, laser light is produced by effecting a population inversion in a laser medium. Spontaneous emission in this quantum system leads to stimulated emission, a phenomenon that is exploited to produce coherent, collimated, and monochromatic light. The initial population inversion is brought about by the excitation of the laser medium by a process known as pumping. Each laser medium possesses a unique ensemble of energy levels in the form of electronic, vibrational, or rotational forces. These various energy levels are dynamically coupled, and decay from the higher levels is controlled by the laws of thermodynamics and quantum mechanics. The nature of the excitation, the nature of the decay, and the construction of the optical resonator determine the nominal operating wavelength(s), the spectral tuning range, the possible output waveforms, and the ultimate power output of the laser. Following is a discussion of classification schemes based on these physical principles.

Classification

The production of coherent light has been achieved in optical resonators utilizing literally thousands of different substances. Neutral and ionized gases, liquids, and solids have all been employed as laser media. The excitation of the laser medium has been effected with optical pumping, electrical discharges, gas-dynamic flow techniques, electron beams, chemical reactions, and nuclear decay. A given set-up is generally named for the predominant atomic or molecular species in the laser medium (i.e., a carbon dioxide laser is so named because a transition in the vibrational energy of the carbon dioxide molecule is responsible for the emission from that particular laser). Typically, the different laser types are divided into three main classes based on the phase of the laser medium (gas, liquid, or solid). These classes are further subdivided, again on the basis of the nature of the laser gain medium.

GAS LASERS

Gas lasers may be divided into two groups—atomic and molecular. The atomic group can be divided further into neutral and ionic varieties depending on the electronic configuration of the atomic species. In both cases, the population inversion is a function of electronic transitions. Molecular gas lasers are also divided into ionic and neutral varieties. As with atomic gases, the ionic molecular gases utilize electronic transitions. The neutral molecules may be divided into three groups, depending on whether the population inversion is based on electronic, vibrational, or rotational transitions.

Gaseous media can be pumped by a variety of methods. Typically, electrical discharges are employed, although electron beam excitation, optional pumping with a primary laser, and electrically or spontaneously induced chemical reactions are also employed. An interesting technique called gas-dynamic flow induces a population inversion by rapidly expanding a gas under very high pressure. This technique has been used to produce carbon dioxide lasers with very high energy outputs.

LIQUID LASERS

Liquid lasers are divided into three types: those utilizing an organic solvent with a dye chromophor, those utilizing an organic solvent with a rare earth chelate, and those utilizing an inorganic solvent, typically a trivalent rare earth ion. Liquid media are optically pumped with flashlamps, pulsed primary lasers, or continuous-wave primary lasers.

SOLID LASERS

Solid lasers utilize either a dielectric insulator or a semiconductor as their active medium. The dielectric insulators are divided into impurity-doped crystals, impurity-doped amorphous substances, and stoichiometric crystals (the active species is substituted into the crystal lattice in a reproducible manner). Semiconductors are classified on the basis of whether a p-n junction or an electron-hole plasma is involved in the energy transitions. Dielectric insulators are optically pumped with flashlamps, continuous-wave arc lamps, or other lasers. Semiconductors are excited by optical pumping, by electron beams, or by the injection of electrons.

FREE-ELECTRON LASERS

The lasers discussed up to this point all produce coherent electromagnetic radiation in the infrared, visible or ultraviolet range through stimulated emission in an excited medium. A laser beam of sorts can be produced also by passing a dilute electron beam through a periodic magnetic field and thereby inducing coherence. These devices are called free-electron lasers (FEL) and obviously fall outside the classification scheme outlined above.

CLASSIFICATION BY WAVELENGTH OF OUTPUT

An alternative to naming the laser gain medium is to refer to lasers by the type of light they produce. Historically the first coherent energy sources utilized microwave frequencies and were called *masers*. When the first device producing visible light was made, it was referred to as an *optical* maser. The term *laser* was subsequently applied to emphasize its operation in the visible spectrum. Today all devices producing coherent energy beams are commonly referred to as lasers, regardless of their wavelength. Modifiers such as infrared, blue-green, and red are applied to convey the laser's position along the electromagnetic spectrum. Along these lines it is interesting to note that lasers operating in the x-ray range are being developed, which will have tremendous applications in research.

CLASSIFICATION BY TEMPORAL FORM OF OUTPUT

Laser nomenclature often makes reference to the temporal form of the energy output. There are five basic temporal forms—continuous wave, pulsed, Q-switched, cavity-dumped, and mode-locked. The first two, continuous wave and pulsed, are conceptually quite simple. Continuous-wave lasers operate with a continuous excitation of the laser gain medium and a subsequent continuous output of laser light. Pulsed systems provide intermittent (pulsed) excitation with a subsequent noncontinuous output of energy. Pulse widths generally vary from 10^{-8} to 10^{-3} seconds, though longer pulses are sometimes utilized [24]. (Pulsed action should not be confused with gated delivery of power, a common feature of continuous-wave surgical lasers.)

In both continuous-wave and pulsed systems, the resonator cavity reflectivity of "Q" is held constant at a moderate value. Q-switched lasers operate with either a continuous or pulsed excitation mode. High bursts of power output are achieved by briefly holding the reflectivity at a very low level, thereby allowing a build-up of particles at the higher energy levels. The reflectivity is then rapidly raised to a moderate level, allowing for a burst of laser activity. Pulse widths on the order of 10^{-8} to 10^{-6} seconds are achieved [24]. Cavity-dumped systems also utilize continuous or pulsed excitation. Here, however, the pattern of reflectivity change is from a very high to a very low level. Pulse widths vary from 10^{-7} to 10^{-5} seconds [24]. Mode-locked lasers are excited by continuous or pulsed pumps. Extremely short bursts of energy (10^{-12} to 10^{-9} seconds) are produced by modulating the phase or loss of resonator modes at a rate related to the resonator transit time [24]. More will be said about Q-switched and mode-locked lasers when the Nd:YAG laser is discussed.

Surgical Lasers

Many different lasers are currently utilized in industrial, military and research applications. This section provides brief descriptions of those lasers commonly encountered in surgical applications, either clinical or research, at the time of this writing. No doubt the list will expand rapidly over the next decade.

In reviewing the different types, it should be kept in mind that surgical lasers are destructive devices. This destruction takes one of three forms—thermal, hydrodynamic, or photochemical. The mode of destruction is dependent on the wavelength, the power output, the temporal form of the output, the nature of the target, and the presence or absence of photosensitizers. These points will be amplified in the following discussions and in Chapter 4.

CARBON DIOXIDE LASER

The carbon dioxide laser was developed by Patel in 1964 [17]. It is a gas laser operating in the infrared range (nominal output at 10,600 nm), which utilizes vibrational transitions in a neutral molecule. Although a neutral carbon dioxide molecule is responsible for the infrared emission, the laser gain medium also consists of nitrogen and helium. The initial energy transfer is to an intermediary nitrogen molecule, which subsequently transfers its energy to a carbon dioxide molecule. The carbon dioxide molecule decays to the ground state first by emission of infrared radiation, then by collisions with helium atoms.

Pumping of the laser medium is typically carried out by a continuous electrical discharge, though many commercially available surgical carbon dioxide lasers can be operated in a pulsed mode, which allows for somewhat higher average energy outputs. Electrically pumped carbon dioxide lasers are capable of providing up to 240 W of continuous power, although surgical units generally range from around 50 mw to slightly over 100 W.

The efficiency of the carbon dioxide laser is quite high relative to other surgical lasers. Efficiency is expressed as the ratio of laser output energy to pumping energy. The efficiency of the carbon dioxide laser is approximately 13% [24]. The remainder of the energy is lost in the form of heat. From a practical point of view, this means that the carbon dixoide laser does not require a cumbersome external water bath for cooling, unlike the less efficient Nd:YAG and argon lasers, which have substantial amounts of wasted energy in the form of heat to dissipate.

At 10,600 nm, carbon dioxide laser light cannot be efficiently transmitted through standard quartz fiberoptic cables. Current carbon dioxide laser units utilize a system of articulated mirrors to transmit the light from the laser head to the handpiece or microslad. Several groups have developed fiberoptic bundles suitable for use with carbon dioxide lasers, though they are not widely available at the time of this writing.

Recently, low-power, solid-state carbon dioxide lasers utilizing radio frequency (RF) pumping have been introduced. These RF carbon dioxide lasers obviate the need for an external supply of laser medium, making the units smaller and more portable.

The carbon dioxide laser is used by several specialties, including general surgery, dermatology, plastic surgery, otolaryngology, and neurosurgery. Within the field of neurosurgery it is clearly the most widely used laser. Its surgical application is for incision and volume ablation, which it accomplishes by thermal destruction.

ARGON LASER

The argon laser was developed by Bennet and colleagues in 1962 [2]. It is a gas laser utilizing ionized argon atoms. Pumping is by a continuous direct current (dc) discharge. Power outputs up to 20 W are achieved with an efficiency of about 0.1% [5]. Surgical units are tuned for simultaneous output at 488 nm (blue) and 514 nm (green). Units are available with built-in filter systems allowing for both full range and green-only operation.

Argon laser light is delivered to tissues via a fiberoptic bundle. It is used for photocoagulation and vaporization. Its principal applications have been in ophthalmology, dermatology, and plastic surgery. Indeed, its frequent use for the photocoagulation of the retina in patients with diabetic retinopathy has made it the most widely used laser in medicine. Argon lasers have been used successfully on a variety of neurosurgical lesions [5, 19]. The University of Southern California school of Medicine for example, has a relatively large experience with the removal of skull base tumors utilizing the argon laser. Its use in general neurosurgery remains limited, however, partly because of the relatively low power output, coupled with the practical considerations related to cooling and power source requirements.

Nd: YAG LASERS

The Nd:YAG laser was developed by Johnson in 1961 [14]. It is an impurity-doped crystal laser which is usually pumped by either a xenon or krypton lamp. It can be operated in a continuous, pulsed, Q-switched, or mode-locked fashion. Its nominal output is at a wavelength of 1064 nm. Power outputs up to 300 watts with an efficiency of 2.6% are possible [24], though most continuous-wave surgical units provide power in the range of 100–150 W.

The Nd:YAG laser was initially introduced to the medical community as a device for endoscopic photocoagulation of gastrointestinal vessels. For this application, continuous-wave energy is utilized for its thermal effects. More recently, Q-switched and mode-locked YAG lasers have been introduced in the field of ophthalmology. These units provide hydrodynamic tissue effects with their extremely high pulse frequencies.

Because of its ability to coagulate tissues effectively while providing some degree of vaporization, the YAG laser has been considered a potentially useful instrument for neurosurgery. Several authors have reported considerable experience with the YAG laser in neurosurgery, particularly in Europe and Japan [2, 2]. Currently, the YAG laser is not approved for routine use in neurosurgery in the United States. Its major disadvantages relate to remote tissue affects and the need for extensive safety precautions.

Several recently introduced items may make the YAG laser more useful in the very near future. One is the coupling of a YAG laser to a carbon dioxide laser, providing the advantages of each in a single unit. Another is the YAG laser tuned to 1320 nm. This unit is said to have coagulation capabilities equal to the 1064 nm YAG laser, but to possess cutting qualities more like the carbon dioxide laser [9]. Finally, the report of sapphire scalpels coupled to a YAG laser raises the interesting possibility of thermal destruction coupled with gentle mechanical pressure to return a tactile sense to laser surgery [10].

HELIUM-NEON LASER

The helium-neon (HeNe) laser, the first of the gas lasers, was developed by Javan and associates in 1961 [13]. HeNe lasers utilize neutral atoms pumped by an electrical discharge. They operate at a wavelength of 633 nm (red) with an efficiency of 0.19% [24]. These lasers are small, solid-state units with relatively low outputs. Their principal application in medicine is to provide a visible, collimated light source, which can be used to aim infrared lasers and other devices. Their medical use in pain relief and the promotion of wound healing is unsubstantiated at present.

EXCIMER LASERS

An excimer is a substance that exists as a dimer in the excited state, but dissociates in the ground state. The most commonly used excimer laser sources are noble gas molecules, such as Xe_2. Unfortunately, these substances decay rapidly from the upper energy levels and require expensive electron-beam pumping devices. This problem can be circumvented by using a noble gas-halogen complex. Lasers utilizing these complexes operate in the ultraviolet range and can be operated in continuous or pulsed modes. Examples include KrF (249 nm), XeCl (380 nm), and XeF (351 nm). Because of their relatively short wavelengths, they may be focused to very small spot sizes. Their effect on tissue can be thermal or nonthermal (mechanical-vibrational) depending on the power and mode of operation. Considerable excitement has been generated by recent reports suggesting the use of excimer laser for laser angioplasty [4, 7].

DYE LASERS

Dye lasers are liquid (dye chromophor) lasers. They are of particular interest because they represent the phototype of the so-called tunable laser. The exact wave length emitted by a given optical resonator is a function of several parameters. All lasers can be "tuned" over at least a narrow range. Liquid dye lasers, however, have a very high gain-bandwidth product per unit length, allowing broad tunability.

Numerous organic dyes are used in commercially available lasers. The rhodamine dyes are among the most familiar within the medical community. Several rhodamine dyes are routinely used, and they are classified under a number of different names. One simple system of naming them utilizes the approximate wavelength at which they operate. The five readily available rhodamine dyes are rhodamine 560, 575, 590, 610, and 640. Rhodamine 610, also known as rhodamine B, has a maximal output at 630 nm, with a tunable range from 601 to 675, when pumped with a primary argon laser [24]. The rhodamine-B dye laser is used extensively by researchers in the field of photoradiation therapy.

KTP/532 LASER

The KTP/532 laser or frequency-doubled Nd: YAG laser represents an interesting concept in laser construction. This laser consists of a standard 1064 nm Nd:YAG laser whose output is passed through a potassium titanyl phosphate (KTP) crystal. Nonlinear scattering within the crystal results in frequency doubling, thereby producing a laser beam with a wavelength of 532 nm. Units of this type with outputs up to 12 W have been used experimentally within the field of dermatology [1].

RUBY LASERS

The ruby laser was developed by Maiman in 1960, making it the first laser to operate in the visible spectrum [15]. It utilizes chromium ions in an aluminum oxide crystal and is, therefore, a solid laser of the impurity-doped crystal variety.

TABLE 2-1. Comparison of Surgical Lasers Used in Neurosurgery

Type	Class	Wavelength (nm)	Maximum Power (w)	Efficiency (%)	Delivery System	Tissue Interaction	Use in Neurosurgery
CO_2	Neutral gas	10,600 (infrared)	100–200	13	Mirrors experimental fiberiptics	Ablation and incision; surface effect	Extensive
YAG	Impurity-doped crystal	1,060 (near infrared)	100–150	2.6	Fiberoptics	Coagulation and vaporization; significant remote effect	Experimental in U.S.A.
Argon	Ionized gas	488 (blue); 514 (green)	10–15	0.1	Fiberoptics	Coagulation and vaporization; pigment-dependent absorption	Limited

The nominal output wavelength is 690 nm (red). The industrial applications of the ruby laser have been supplanted, for the most part, by neodymium-based crystal lasers. It is interesting to note, however, that the ruby laser was the first laser to be used in the field of neurosurgery. Rosomoff and Carroll reported irradiating human brain tumors with a ruby laser in 1966 [20]. Today, the ruby laser is not employed in the field of neurosurgery. Its use in other fields is anecdotal at this time.

KRYTON LASER

The element krypton is used as a laser gain medium in certain neutral gas lasers. Its electronic transitions are, for the most part, in the infrared range. There are, however, readily available krypton lasers that operate at 647 nm (red). These lasers have been used in Europe in the field of ophthalmology since 1975, and, more recently, in the United States as an alternative to the more commonly used argon laser [16, 18, 21].

COPPER VAPOR LASERS

Copper exhibits electronic transitions at 0.5106, 0.5700, 0.5782, 1.820, and 1.823 μ. The 511 nm (green) and 578 nm (yellow) wavelengths have been exploited in the commercial production of pulsed neutral gas lasers with relatively high power outputs and good efficiency. Peak power outputs around 40 and average power outputs in the range of 40 W with an efficiency of approximately 1.2% have been reported [12, 23]. Copper vapor lasers have been used experimentally in the field of ophthalmology [9].

GOLD VAPOR LASER

Pulsed lasers utilizing gold vapor as the laser gain medium are commercially available. The nominal output wavelength of these units is 628 nm (red). They have become particularly popular with medical researchers in the field of photoradiation therapy because their wavelength corresponds closely to one of the absorption peaks of hematoporphorin derivative, a photosensitizing dye used extensively by investigators in that field.

DIODE LASERS (SEMICONDUCTOR)

Numerous reports have appeared in the literature describing the relief of pain and the promotion of wound healing with low-energy lasers. Many of these studies have utilized HeNe lasers. Some reports mention the use of semiconductor lasers. Most of the semiconductor lasers mentioned are injection lasers utilizing either GaAs diodes or AlGaAs diodes. GaAs diode lasers have output wavelengths ranging from 830 to 920 nm. AlGaAs diode lasers range from 620 to 900 nm. Many other types of diode lasers are commercially available.

Conclusion

A variety of laser types is available to the clinician researcher. The utility of any given unit is determined by the physical properties of the light it produces. The different laser types are classified on the basis of their laser gain medium, their output wavelength, and their temporal mode of action. Within the field of neurosurgery, carbon dioxide lasers are used most commonly. YAG lasers and argon lasers are employed much less frequently. Selected characteristics of these three laser types are outlined in Table 2-1. The ideal neurosurgical laser has not yet been developed.

References

1. Apfelberg DB, Bailin P, Rosenberg H: Preliminary investigation of KTP/532 laser light in the treatment of hemangiomas and tattoos. *Lasers Surg Med* 6:33–42, 1986.
2. Beck OJ: Use of the Nd:YAG laser in neurosurgery. *Lasers Surg Med* 5:345–356, 1985.
3. Bennett WR Jr, Faust WL, McFarlane RA: Dissociative excitation transfer and optical maser oscillation in NeO_2 and Ar_2O rf discharges (letter). *Physiol Rev* 8:470–473, 1972.
4. Cabrini GP, Ferrari C, Villani R, et al: Effects of argon and excimer laser radiation on carotid artery atheromatous plaques. Presented at the

Sixth Congress of the International Society For Laser Surgery and Medicine, Jerusalem, 1985.

5. Edwards MSB, Bogan JE, Fuller TA: The laser in neurological surgery. *J Neurosurg* 59:555–566, 1983.
6. Einstein A: Zur QuantumTheorie der Strahlung. *Physiol Zeitschr* 18:121–128, 1917.
7. Farrell EM, Higginson LAJ, Walley VM, et al: Excimer laser ablation of atherosclerotic plaque. Presented at the Sixth Congress of the international Society for Laser Surgery and Medicine, Jerusalem, 1985.
8. Frank F, Beck OJ, Hessel S, Keiditsch E: Comparative investigations of the effects of the Nd: YAG laser at 1.06 micron and 1.32 micron on tissue. Presented at the Sixth Congress of the International Society for Laser Surgery and Medicine, Jerusalem, 1985.
9. Gabay S, Ben-Siar I, Cohen S: Copper vapour laser—Possible clinical applications. Presented at the Sixth Congress of the International Society for Laser Surgery and Medicine, Jerusalem, 1985.
10. Gordon JP, Zeigler HJ, Townes CH: The maser—new type of amplifier, frequency standard and spectrometer. *Physiol Rev* 99:1264–1274, 1955.
11. Hira N: Contact laser surgical scalpel using low power Nd:YAG Laser. Presented at the Sixth Congress of the International Society for Laser Surgery and Medicine, Jerusalem, 1985.
12. Iseau AA, Lemmerman GY: Investigation of a copper vapor pulsed laser at elevated powers. *Sov J Quantum Electron* 7:799–801, 1977.
13. Javan A, Bennett WR Jr, Herriott DR: Population inversion and continuous optical maser oscillation in a gas discharge containing a HeNe mixture. Letter. *Physiol Rev* 6:196–110, 1961.
14. Johnson H: Optical maser characteristics of rare-earth ions in crystals. *J Appl Physiol* 34:897–909, 1961.
15. Maiman TH: Stimulated optical radiation in ruby. *Nature* 187:493:494, 1960.
16. Olk RJ, Burgess DB: Krypton red laser photocoagulation in the treatment of juxtafoveal subretinal neovascular membranes. *Ophthalmology* 101:130–131, 1986.
17. Patel CKN, McFarlane RA, Faust WL: Selective excitation through vibration energy transfer and optical maser action in N_2-CO_2. *Physiol Rev* 13:617–619, 1964.
18. Peyman GA, Li M, Yoneya S, et al: Fundus photocoagulation with the argon and krypton lasers: A comparative study. *Ophthalmic Surg* 12:481–490, 1981.
19. Powers SK, Edwards MSB, Bogan JE, et al: Use of the argon surgical laser in neurosurgery. *Neurosurg* 60:523–530, 1984.
20. Rosomoff HL, Carroll F: Reaction of neoplasm and brain to laser. *Arch Neurol* 14:143–148, 1966.
21. Shakin JL, Yannuzzi LA, Shakin EP, Fisher YL: Krypton red laser photocoagulation for subretinal neovascularization. *Ophthalmology* 92: 1387–1395, 1985.
22. Takeuchi J, Handa H, Taki W, et al: The Nd: YAG laser in neurological surgery. *Surg Neurol* 18:140–142, 1982.
23. Walter WJ: 40 KW pulsed copper laser. *Bull Am Phys Soc* 12:90, 1967.
24. Weber MJ (ed): *CRC Handbook of Laser Science and Technology*. Boca Raton, FL, CRC Press, 1982.

3. FUNDAMENTALS OF LASER PHYSICS

W. Craig Clark

The purpose of this chapter is to provide a discussion of the basic physical principles involved in the operation of the laser. Although an in-depth discussion of the physical principles involved in the generation and control of a laser beam can involve complicated mathematical and theoretical physics, the inclusion of complicated concepts is not requisite to an understanding of these principles sufficient for the surgeon. Only those principles necessary to maximize the effectiveness of the laser in various neurosurgical applications will be presented in this discussion. Several recent reviews on the subject are available, which may provide additional information [2–5, 7, 8].

The basic laws of thermodynamics tell us that energy can neither be created nor destroyed. This holds true for the laser as well as other sources of energy. The disorganized energy of excited atomic systems is emitted as photons; these controlled emissions are then organized into a concentrated beam of energy or light known as a laser beam. The basic physical principles that govern the generation and control of this concentrated beam can basically be divided into three major categories: (1) wave mechanics; (2) atomic physics; and (3) light. An understanding of these basic physical principles will serve as a foundation for a more detailed discussion concerning how these basic physical principles may be applied in the manipulation and control of a laser beam.

Basic Physical Principles

WAVE MECHANICS

Certain terms are used to describe a wave. Those that will prove important to our discussion include:

1. Wavelength (λ)—the distance between any two successive wave crests.
2. Frequency (f)—the number of waves passing a given point per second, usually expressed as cycles per second or Hertz.
3. Velocity (1/T)—the velocity at which the wave profile moves forward.
4. Amplitude (a)—the magnitude of the oscillations defined as the height of the wave crest (Figure 3-1).

It is important to understand this terminology so that the actions and reactions within the laser tube can be discussed which a common nomenclature.

Earlier we described the basic reaction as one of converting a disorganized energy source into an organized energy source, with the creation of a concentrated beam of light. When discussing lasers as a source of light, it is important that we differentiate their electromagnetic radiation from the visible spectrum of light with which we are all more familiar [7]. One way of doing this is by depicting the electromagnetic spectrum in a chart (Figure 3-2). This chart simply organizes the various sources of electromagnetic radiation according to their respective wavelengths and illustrates two major points. First, the energy that we normally refer to as "light" in everyday usage actually makes up a very small portion of the electromagnetic spectrum. Second, an examination of the electromagnetic spectrum shows the respective locations of the various surgical lasers along this continuum of electromagnetic radiation. For instance, the argon laser at 488–514 nm lies within the visible light spectrum and, as a result, does not require a separate aiming or pilot beam in order to direct the surgical laser. In contrast, both the neodymium:yttrium-aluminum-garnet (Nd:YAG) and carbon dioxide lasers are both within the infrared region of the spectrum and require a separate, visible pilot or aiming beam in order to direct the surgical laser.

The majority of the effects seen with the use of the various lasers in neurosurgery are basically thermal effects. Although there are some "cold" lasers now in the research stage that achieve their effects by interrupting molecular bonds, the tissue effects for which lasers are known are predominately thermal effects, which occur only as the result of the absorption of the laser photon by a biological tissue. Until the laser photons or light is absorbed and converted to thermal effects, the laser beam is subject to all of the vagaries of any other source of light, and any number of things may happen [4]. Of course, the laser light may be absorbed by the tissue in question and converted to heat. However, depending on the wavelength of the laser and the optical absorption characteristics of the tissue being irradiated, the laser light may be reflected totally, transmitted completely through the medium, or scattered within the tissue in question (Figure 3-3).

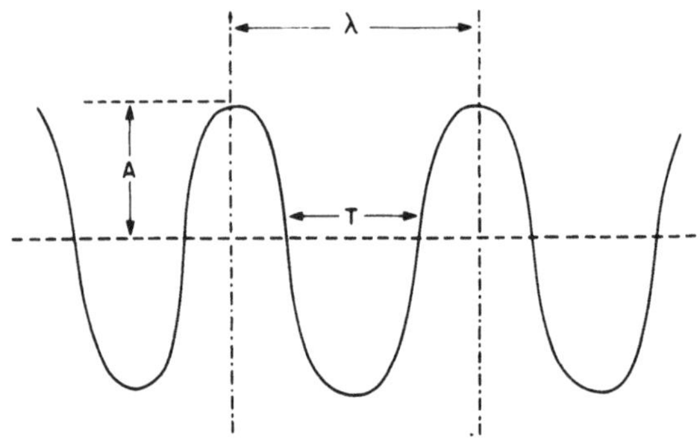

FIGURE 3-1. Waveform specification. A wave is depicted using the terms wavelength (λ) frequency (f), amplitude (A), and velocity (1-T).

FIGURE 3-2. Electromagnetic spectrum. Sources of electromagnetic irradiation arranged according to wavelength.

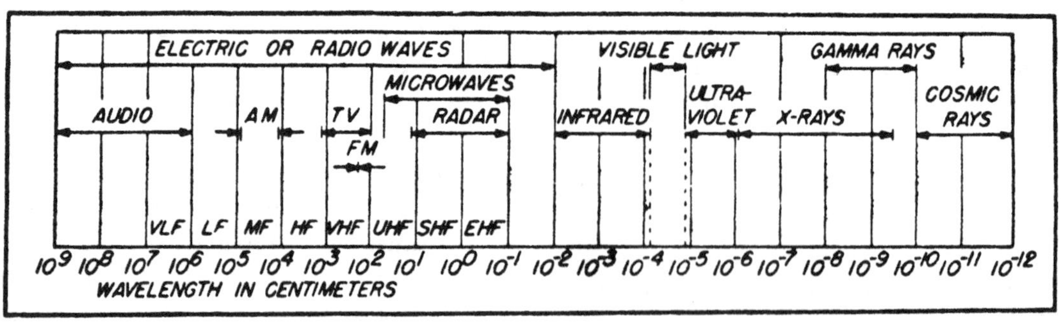

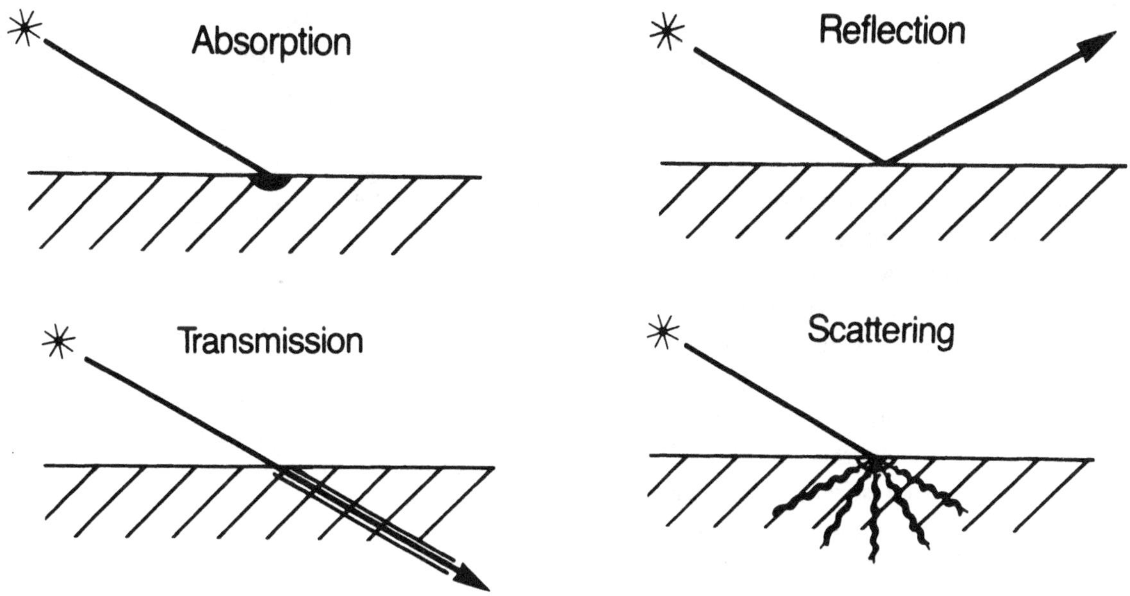

FIGURE 3-3. The laser beam may be reflected, scattered, or transmitted like any other light source until it is absorbed and converted to heat.

ATOMIC PHYSICS

The atom is composed of a positively charged nucleus surrounded by negatively charged electrons. The electrons of a given atom may orbit close to the nucleus or far away from it. The farther away from the nucleus the electron orbits, the more reactive the atom becomes. Thus, an electron in the outer shell of an atom is potentially more reactive than one that orbits close to the nucleus. When an atom is in its most stable or ground state, its electrons orbit closest about the nucleus, and it can only absorb outside energy. As photons are absorbed, they increase the internal energy of the atomic system, moving the orbiting electrons further from the nucleus and making the atom more reactive or excited (Figure 3-4). Conversely, when an excited or reactive atom gives up energy, its electrons fall from a higher energy level to a lower one, emitting a quantity of energy or photons equal to the "energy gap" or difference in energy between the electron orbits (Figure 3-5). This loss of energy or decay toward a lower energy state that results in the spontaneous, random emission of photons is called *spontaneous emission*.

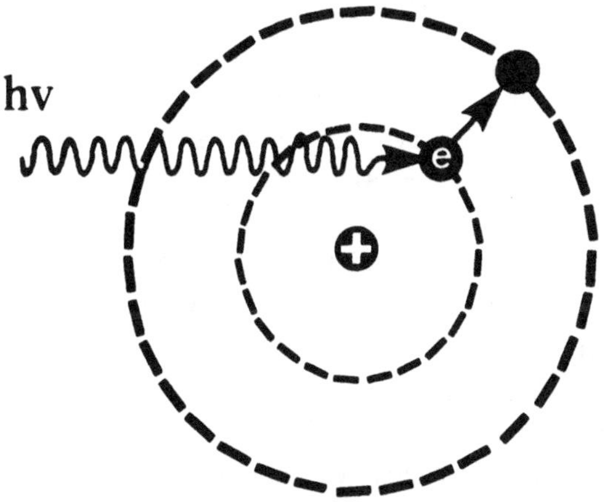

FIGURE 3-4. When exogenous energy is added to an atomic system in the ground state, it absorbs the energy and becomes more reactive.

Transitions between the various subatomic energy levels may take place not only spontaneously but also as a result of stimulation of excited atomic systems by photons of an appropriate frequency. Stimulated emission, which is the basis of laser operation, occurs when an excited atom is bombarded with photons of the same frequency that would ordinarily be emitted spontaneously with a complete decay to the ground state. The result of this stimulated emission is the emission of not only the photons that represent the energy gap between the excited and ground states, but also the photons used to incite the reaction (Figure 3-6). These photons are unique in that they are in phase with respect to both space and time (coherent), are of a single wavelength (monochromatic), and travel parallel to one another (collimated). The photons thus emitted stimulate further emissions, resulting in an exponential cascade of photons in a very short period of time. Thus, for purposes of our discussion, there are only a limited number of types of reactions with which we must be concerned. First, if the atomic system is in a relaxed or ground state and energy is added from an outside source, the system must absorb this energy, resulting in the movement of electrons further from the nucleus and the conversion of the atomic system to an excited or reactive state. On the other hand, if the atomic system is already in an excited or reactive state, the process that takes place is a function of attempts at active intervention and control. Second if nothing is done, the excited or reactive atomic systems will naturally decay as they seek their original most stable state. To get back to this original most stable or ground state, the system must emit or give up the energy that it had originally absorbed. The system emits energy proportional to the energy gap between the reactive and nonreactive or ground states in the form of photons in a spontaneous, random fashion. On the other hand, one does not have to simply wait for the disorganized, spontaneous, random emissions to occur. Instead, if photons at the specific frequency and wavelength desired are added to the excited atomic system, the emission of photons is stimulated. The photons that are added in order to cause or incite this reaction act like a catalyst, in that they are

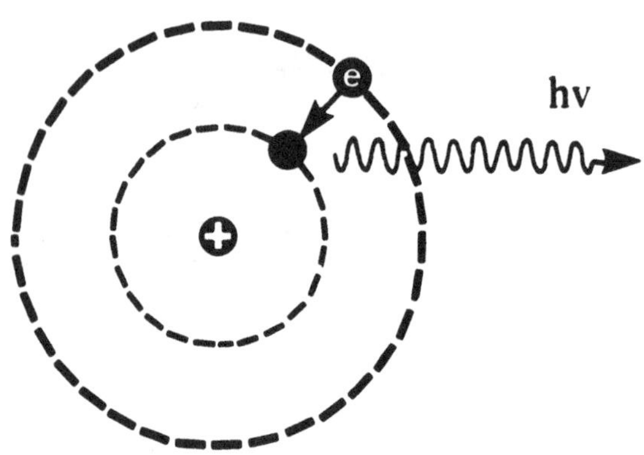

FIGURE 3-5. An atomic system that is reactive will tend to decay back to a more stable state in a spontaneous, random fashion.

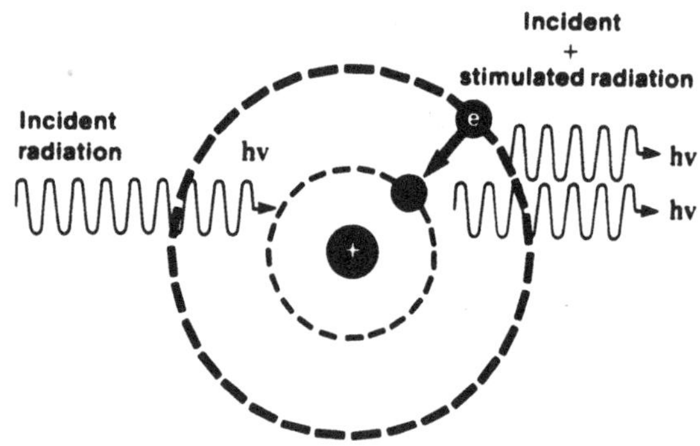

FIGURE 3-6. An atomic system may be stimulated to emit the energy it had originally absorbed by adding energy at the same frequency and wavelength of the photons desired to be emitted.

completely preserved, and may incite additional reactions to occur [8].

GENERATION OF THE LASER BEAM

A laser consists of a tube or resonance cavity with mirrors at either end. At each end of the tube is a reflective mirror. One of these mirrors not only reflects, but also partially transmits, the specific wavelength of light generated by the emission of photons within the laser tube. A source of electrons, or medium, is contained within the tube. The problem in designing a laser is to select a medium in which most of the atoms can become excited so that photons of the appropriate frequency passing through them will generate a cascade of photons. For example, the medium in a carbon dioxide laser is a mixture of carbon dioxide, nitrogen, and helium gases.

In order for stimulated emission to predominate over absorption, there must be a great excess of atoms in the excited state. Atoms are raised to an excited state by providing some outside source of energy. An electric current is often used as this energy source, but other alternatives include radio frequency diodes and other lasers. This stimulation of the electrons in the medium to raise them to an excited state is called *pumping*.

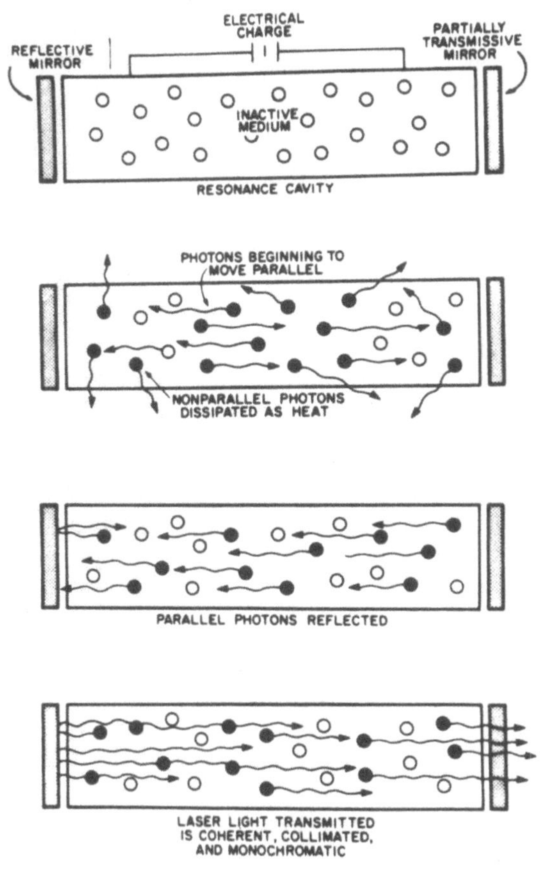

FIGURE 3-7. Generation of a laser beam. See text for description.

As more and more of the atoms reach an excited state, photons are emitted. Those that travel in an axis parallel to the resonance cavity are reflected from the mirrors. Those photons that are not parallel to the axis of the tube are lost as heat. At the instant in time when there are more atoms in the excited state than in the ground state, a population inversion occurs (i.e., the population of electrons is excited rather than in the ground state). The photons resulting from the process of stimulated emission are reflected back and forth between the mirrors until they increase exponentially in activity and intensity. This steadily increasing activity is called the *photon cascade*. The photon cascade continues to increase until a shutter is opened at the end of the tube, allowing the coherent, collimated, and monochromatic laser light to pass through the partially transmissive mirror (Figure 3-7).

The concepts of both temporal and spatial coherence are very important from the standpoint of increasing the efficiency of the lasing reaction within the resonance cavity. Quite simply, temporal coherence refers to the wave profiles of the various photons emitted within the laser tube. If these wave profiles are in phase with respect to time (temporal coherence), there is a summation of the amplitude of these various wave profiles, resulting in an overall increase in the amplitude of the oscillations within the laser tube. If the wave profiles are not in phase with respect to time, one can expect feedback effects with no resulting increase in the amplitude of the oscillations of the wave profile within the laser tube. The same principles apply to spatial coherence and the benefits of the wave profile being in phase with respect to space. Once again, if the wave profiles are not in phase with respect to space there is a feedback, or cancelling effect and no overall incrase in the amplitude of the wave profile within the laser tube or resonance cavity. This achieves practical significance when one considers that the efficiency of the lasing reaction within the laser tube will be a function of the number of effective collisions and resulting stimulated emissions of photons that occur with coherent versus incoherent wave profiles.

Laser beams are essentially monochromatic in that the photons within the beam are of a single wavelength. The concept of monochromicity achieves practical significance when it is viewed in the context of simple optical systems. Because most of our information regarding simple optical systems and lenses is derived from the interaction between simple lens systems and incandescent light sources, the most useful comparison is between a laser light source versus an incandescent light source, and their respective interactions with simple optical systems. An incandescent light source is not collimated (nonparallel), and at the focal point of the lens system, spot or area images are formed. Further, incandescent light is composed of light at a variety of wavelengths (heterochromatic), with each wavelength of light focusing at a different point, resulting in an area or spot image at the focal point of the simple lens system. In contrast to the above example, a laser has photons of a single wavelength. When focused through a simple lens system these photons are concentrated and form a point image at the focal point of the lens system. This interaction with a simple optical system imparts two very important characteristics to the laser: (1) high concentrations of energy may be focused into very small spaces, resulting in very high energy concentrations per unit area; and (2) the ability to focus a laser to a point image imparts a level of precision that cannot be achieved with an incandescent light source [7] (Figure 3-8).

Earlier we discussed the necessity for the absorption of the laser light by tissues in order to create the thermal effects that are characteristic of surgical laser use. We will now turn our attention to the control of these thermal effects.

Control of Thermal Effects

The thermal effects of all types of surgical lasers are the result of the absorption of the laser beam

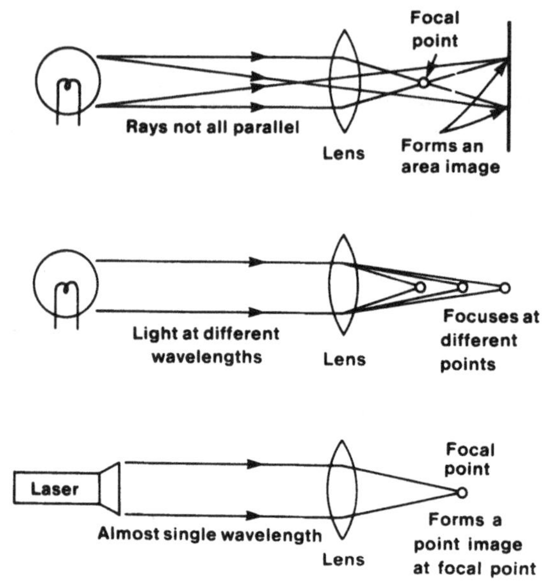

FIGURE 3-8. Comparison of incandescent and laser light sources and their interactions with simple lens systems.

by tissue. Thus, the laser may cause hemostasis, coagulation, cutting, or vaporization as the light energy is transferred to the tissue and becomes thermal energy. The effects of a laser on any given biological tissue are determined by the power density and radiant exposure of the laser beam and by the coefficient of absorption of the tissue for the specific wavelength of the laser in question [1].

Power density is an operating parameter of great importance in the operation of the surgical laser. It is defined as the concentration of power (watts) per unit area (cm^2) and is expressed as:

$$\frac{\text{Power setting}}{\pi(\text{spot size in mm})^2} \times 400 = \text{power density (watts/cm}^2\text{)}$$

Because the power density is greatly influenced by variations in the spot size, and the spot size is likewise influenced by the transverse electromagnetic mode (TEM) of the beam and the focal length of the laser lens system and its relationship to the operating microscope, both determinants of spot size are important variables.

Because of the increased control and precision inherent in the use of the operating microscope, we have not advocated the use of the laser as a freehand instrument in neurosurgery. Rather, it is our opinion that the laser should be used exclusively with the operating microscope to take advantage of this increased precision and control. The operating microscope is attached to the laser by a coupling device called a microslad. This device allows the laser arm or optical fiber to be coupled to the operating microscope. It consists of a track-mounted lens, which allows continuously variable focusing/defocusing to achieve a variety of surgical effects. The laser beam is transmitted through this track-mounted lens system to a small mirror that is connected to a joystick micromanipulator. Movement of the micromanipulator changes the angle of incidence between the small mirror and the laser beam that has passed through the lens system, and directs the laser beam into the operating field. A simple table can be constructed to show the minimal spot sizes that can be achieved with various combinations of operating microscope objectives and laser lenses of different focal lengths (Table 3-1). Examination of this table reveals two important points. First, as we would expect from our experience with the operating microscope, as the objective working distance increases, the precision decreases. Second, regardless of the objective focal length chosen for the operating microscope, maximal precision and the ability to focus the laser beam to its minimal spot size is achieved only when the focal length of the laser lens system matches the focal length of the operating microscope objective lens. It is important to understand these relationships between the laser beam and its optical system because the ability to vary the focal point causes a change in the spot size and resultant surface area irradiated, which results in the production of a continuum of power densities and effects ranging from coagulation to cutting or tissue vaporization. Thus, with the focal point on the tissue surface, the laser is focused, resulting in maximum power densities, cutting or vaporization, and more precision. Conversely, with the focal point at some distance above the tissue surface, a divergent or unfocused beam strikes the tissue resulting in lower power densities, coagulation, and less precision (Figure 3-9). One should recall from the earlier discussion of the power density equation that higher power densities can be achieved with larger spot sizes, but because of the squaring of the spot size in the denominator,

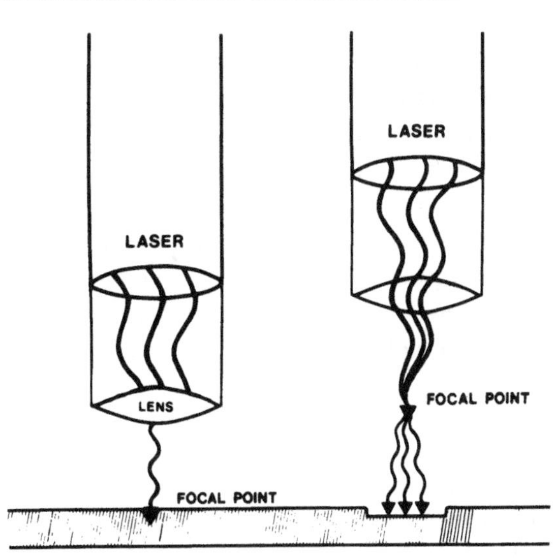

FIGURE 3-9. Focused and defocused laser beams. The beam is focused when the focal point is at the tissue surface. It is defocused when the focal point is above (divergent beam) or below (convergent beam) the tissue surface.

TABLE 3-1. Effect of Matching Focal Lengths on Spot Size

Laser Lens	Objective	Spot Size (mm) 200	300	400
	200	0.45	2.9	5.8
	300	2.1	0.6	2.1
	400	3.3	1.6	0.8

Note: Maximal precision is achieved only when the laser and operating microscope have the same focal length.

large amounts of power are required to compensate for relatively small increases in spot size. In fact, when the laser is used for tumor debulking, it is our preference to use a defocused beam with a large amount of power.

The TEM of any laser system is a parameter incorporated into the design of the system—the radial distribution of power across the laser beam. It is usually shown as TEM_{nm}, with the n and m representing the modes in various axes of a three-dimensional coordinate system.

Although an infinite number of TEM's are theoretically possible, we will discuss only those commonly seen in surgical lasers. A TEM_{00}, or fundamental mode, configuration has its maximal power distribution along the axis of the laser, with a rapid gradual decrease of power as the outer edges of the laser tube are approached. This creates a gaussian or normal distribution of power along the axis of the laser tube and provides a good approximation of the type of lesion created with a TEM_{00} device (Figure 3-10A). A TEM_{01}, or doughnut mode, configuration, has its minimal power concentration along the axis of the laser tube. Rather, it achieves its maximal power at the outer edges of the laser tube, with a resultant bimodal distribution of power. The tissue lesion created with this type of device shows a characteristic residual spicule of tissue in the middle of the crater (Figure 3-10B). The final mode of laser commonly used in surgery is a TEM_{10}, or multimode, configuration. This mode is like the TEM_{00} device in that it is able to achieve high levels of power along the axis of the laser tube. It is like the TEM_{01} device in that it continues to maintain these high levels of power at the outer edges of the laser tube, which permits only larger minimal spot sizes to be achieved. Because this particular type of laser beam is comprised of many different modes of laser energy, the tissue lesion created with this device closely resembles a "hobnail" print (Figure 3-10C). For our purposes, it is sufficient to say that lasers in the TEM_{00} or fundamental mode are capable of achieving smaller spot sizes and the increases in precision and power density that result. For example, the smallest spot size that may be achieved with a TEM_{01} laser at a working distance of 400 mm is 2.0 mm, compared to a minimum spot size of 0.8 mm achievable with a TEM_{00} device. At a power setting of 10 W, this results in a power density of about 300 W/cm^2 for the TEM_{01} device and a power density of almost 2000 W/cm^2 for the TEM_{00} device (Table 3-2).

The next parameter important in the control of the thermal effects of surgical laser systems is radiant exposure. Radiant exposure is simply defined as the exposure in seconds of a tissue to a laser beam at a specified power density. It is expressed as:

$$\text{Power density } (W/cm^2) \times \text{duration of exposure (sec)} = \text{radiant exposure } (W/cm^2)$$

The major significance of this parameter is that the majority of the damage that occurs in tissue adjacent to tissue irradiated with the laser is caused by the conduction of heat from the sides of the crater. The amount of heat conducted to contiguous structures is largely a function of the time of exposure of the tissue to the laser beam. The amount of tissue damage subsequently seen will also depend upon the local blood flow to the surrounding tissue, tissue density, and other factors subject to little or no manipulation by the surgeon. Thus, the surgeon should attempt to minimize the amount of heat conducted by decreasing the exposure variable. This is accomplished by delivering the laser radiation in very short, pulsed bursts rather than in a continuous

FIGURE 3-10 (A) Distribution of power from a TEM_{00} laser and cross-section of a typical lesion created with this distribution of power. (B) Distribution of power from a TEM_{01} laser. Note the bimodal distribution of power and resultant spicule of tissue in the crater created with this device. (C) Distribution of power from a TEM_{10} laser. Note the multimodal (hobnail) distribution of power and multiple indentations in the floor of the crater created with this device.

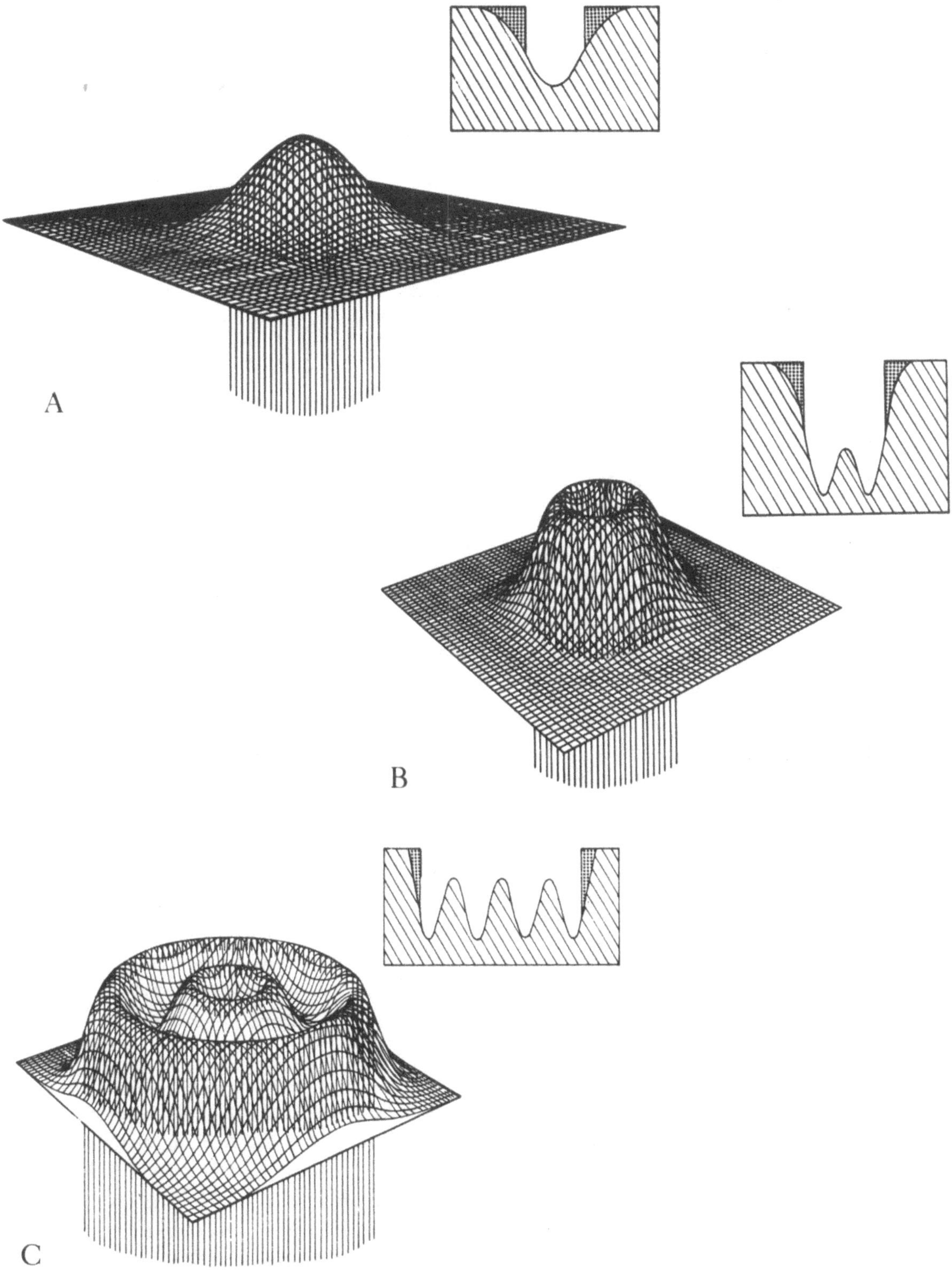
A
B
C

TABLE 3-2. Effect of Spot Size on Power Densities*

Spot size (mm)	0.45 (TEM_{00})	0.80 (TEM_{00})	2.0 (TEM_{01})
Working distance	200	400	400
	POWER DENSITY (W/cm^2)		
Power (W)			
20	12,582	3,984	637
10	6,291	1,992	318

Because spot size is squared in the denominator of the power density equation, power levels must be greatly increased to compensate for small changes in spot size.

fashion. This allows for the dissipation of the small amounts of heat that may be conducted and decreases the damage to the surrounding normal tissues. Also, by understanding this relationship, the surgeon may choose to use a continuous laser beam when debulking a large tumor, because maximal tissue destruction and coagulation necrosis in surrounding tumor tissue are desired.

Superpulse is another method of minimizing the spread of heat to contiguous structures; it imparts increased precision to the use of the laser [6]. Unfortunately, this term has become a major focus of several commercial marketing strategies, and this unbridled enthusiasm would appear to have resulted in some confusion regarding just what the capabilities of superpulse really are. The term *superpulse* connotes large amounts of power; a superpulse of 500 W is advertised as achievable with various surgical lasers. In reality, superpulse has little to do with the rate of tissue removal. The rate of tissue removal is controlled by the average power available and the spot size. Instead, superpulse can increase the precision of a surgical laser dissection by delivering the beam at intense powers in short, repetitive bursts. The brief "off" period following each short burst serves to minimize the spread of heat to surrounding tissues (Figure 3-11).

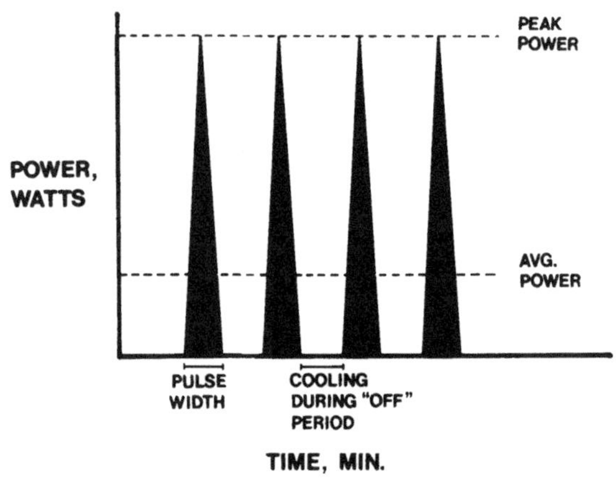

FIGURE 3-11. Superpulse waveform. Note that average power determines speed of tissue evaporation and that cooling occurs during "off" periods or the duty cycle.

The final parameter for the control of laser thermal effects is the coefficient of absorption. This parameter is also inherent in a given surgical laser system because it is wavelength-dependent and is not subject to any intraoperative control by the surgeon. However, since only that laser radiation that is absorbed is converted to useful surgical effects, this parameter should be carefully studied before any laser is selected for a specific application.

The coefficient of absorption is dependent on wavelength because maximal levels of absorption of certain types of laser light occur when the wavelength of the laser closely approximates the wavelength of the coloring or pigmentation of tissue. These pigment-dependent lasers rely on the coloring of tissue for their absorption and subsequent conversion to thermal energy. This phenomenon is known as *selective absorption* and will be discussed in more detail.

The concept of selective photothermolysis

describes the pigment-dependent absorption of specific wavelengths of laser light [1]. It is based on the fact that certain wavelengths of light will be absorbed more readily by tissues with pigmentation of a compatible wavelength. For instance, the naturally occurring pigments hemoglobin and melanin are highly absorptive of light around 550 nm. Therefore, we would expect that a laser with a wavelength in this general area would be highly and selectively absorbed by both blood and darkly pigmented tissue. The argon laser produces a beam with a wavelength between 488 and 514 nm, which is highly absorbed by these tissue pigments. Also, such a beam is reflected, scattered, or transmitted by nonpigmented or clear tissues or fluids, because there is no pigment source that causes the beam to be absorbed and transformed to thermal energy [4]. Since nonpigmented tissues do not transmit the beam completely, some heat is generated within the tissue from scattering of the beam. However, in clear fluids the beam is completely transmitted for a considerable distance, as is shown by the transmission of the argon beam through the various structures of the eye to the retina in several ophthalmologic procedures. Other lasers, such as the carbon dioxide laser, do not possess the characteristic of selective photothermolysis. On the contrary, they are absorbed on the basis of the water content of tissue rather than the pigmentation of the tissue to be irradiated. Because biological tissue is approximately 80% water, virtually all soft tissues absorb the carbon dioxide beam quite well. As the intracellular water absorbs the laser beam, it boils and is vaporized, and a purely thermal effect results [6].

A comparison of the surgical laser devices available on the basis of the coefficient of absorption results in advantages and disadvantages for each of the respective beams, depending on the application for which the device is being evaluated.

The absorption of the various beams should be viewed with regard to measurable physical parameters, the coefficient of absorption, and the penetration of the beam in clear liquids. Although the heterogeneous nature of the pigmentation present in biological tissue is generally accepted, these parameters are useful for the comparison of the various beams. The former is important because it provides a quantitative assessment of the conversion of the laser's light to thermal energy and the latter because it provides information regarding the depth of penetration of the beam into tissue, the transmissibility of the beam, and the potential for irrigants and naturally occurring fluids, such as cerebrospinal fluid, to act as insulators against unwanted thermal damage in surrounding tissue.

A comparison of the relative coefficients of absorption (Table 3-3) shows that the carbon dioxide beam has a much higher coefficient, and as a result it would be expected to be absorbed much more efficiently. This results in less effect on deeper tissue and less scatter of the beam [7]. The argon beam is more poorly absorbed because of its inherent pigment selectivity. Therefore, it causes more of a photocoagulation effect than vaporation, but vaporization may be achieved at the maximum power densities. As a further result of this selective absorption, there are more deep heating effects below the surface of the tissue, as well as an enhanced level of hemostasis.

The comparison of the affinity of the devices for water and their subsequent depth of penetration in water (Table 3-4) shows that the carbon dioxide beam is almost completely absorbed at the surface, with no penetration, whereas the argon beam is completely transmitted to a depth

TABLE 3-3. Coefficient of Absorption of Various Surgical Lasers in Soft Tissue

Laser	Absorption Coefficient
Argon	0.30
Nd-YAG	0.18
Carbon dioxide	80

TABLE 3-4. Depth of Penetration of Various Lasers in Water

Laser	λ(nm)	Penetration (mm)
Argon	488	67.00
Nd:YAG	1,060	27.00
Carbon dioxide*	10,600	0.01

* Note that the carbon dioxide laser is absorbed at the surface with no penetration.

of greater than 60 mm. It would then be expected that the presence of any fluid in the operative field could potentially be very helpful or disastrous if the carbon dioxide beam were being utilized. Any fluid in the field will act as an insulator against the transmission of thermal effects created by the carbon dioxide beam, because its wavelength is so completely absorbed at the surface of the fluid. On the other hand, any tissue the operator wishes to cut, coagulate, or evaporate must be kept relatively dry to effect the absorption of the beam by the intracellular water of the tissues. This is not the case with the argon beam because of its selective absorption by certain pigmented tissues. Clear fluids transmit the argon beam, and this is exactly the characteristic that makes the device so ideal for photocoagulation in the retina. Nonpigmented tissues do not absorb this wavelength very well, and this allows the beam to pass to deeper pigmented structures. This is the characteristic that makes the argon beam so well suited for the photocoagulation of port wine hemangioma.

On the basis of this examination of the basic physical principles involved in the generation of a laser beam and an understanding of the control of the thermal effects generated by these devices, it is clear that there is no one best type of laser for all potential applications. However, an understanding of the physical basis of the generation and control of the various laser beams and their respective thermal effects should aid the neurosurgeon in the evaluation of current and proposed applications of this technology.

References

1. Clark WC, Robertson JH, Gardner G: Selective absorption and control of thermal effects: A comparison of the laser systems used in otology and neurotology. *Otolaryngol Head Neck Surg* 92:73–79, 1984.
2. Dixon JA: Lasers in surgery. *Curr Prob Surg* 21: 1–65, 1984.
3. Fuller TA: The physics of surgical lasers. *Lasers Surg Med* 1:5–14, 1981.
4. Glover JL, Bendick PJ, Link WJ: The use of thermal knives in surgery: Electrosurgery, lasers, plasma scalpel. *Curr Prob Surg* 15:34–42, 1978.
5. Hudgins WR, Jacques D: The laser in neurosurgery. In Rand RW (ed): *Microneurosurgery*. St. Louis, 1985, pp 49–61.
6. Jain KK: Incision of the brain with the varipulse carbon dioxide laser: A preliminary study for potential application in neurosurgery. *Neurosurgery* 18:762–765, 1986.
7. Polanyi TG: Physics of surgery with lasers. *Clin Chest Med* 6:179–202, 1985.
8. Robertson JH, Clark WC: Carbon dioxide laser in neurosurgery. *Contemp Neurosurgery* 5:1–6, 1984.

4. THE INTERACTION OF LASER LIGHT WITH NEURAL TISSUE

James E. Boggan

In this chapter I will attempt to clarify the role various factors play in determining the tissue response to irradiation with laser energy.

Distribution of Light in Tissue

Laser light incident on tissue can be reflected, transmitted, scattered, or absorbed (Figure 4-1A). The relative importance of each of these optical phenomena varies with the wavelength of the incident light and the type of tissue involved. The distribution of light in tissue is governed by wavelength-dependent optical properties of the target tissue, primarily absorption and scattering, as well as by the physical parameters of the incident laser beam (e.g., energy, power density, exposure time, spot size, etc.). Tissue is a heterogeneous and highly structured medium consisting of multiple cellular and subcellular interfaces and particles that are made up of complex biomolecules whose absorption characteristics vary. Tissue components such as stroma, blood vessels, and different cell types have very different optical properties. As a consequence, light propagating through tissue is subject to countless reflections, variations in refraction, diffraction, absorptions, changes in optical polarization and assorted scattering [22, 53]. In addition, the optical properties of tissue may be altered by exposure to laser light, such that the distribution of light during or after an initial exposure may be completely different [23].

In general, light that is reflected from the tissue surface has no effect; however, as a consequence of reflection, the amount of light that actually enters the tissue, and is thus available to interact with tissue chromophores, is decreased. Measurements of reflected light at the tissue surface also include light that is backscattered out of the target tissue. Unlike light that is reflected from the tissue surface (regular and diffuse reflection), light that is backscattered within the target tissue may, as I shall discuss below, contribute to the effect incident laser light will have on the target tissue. Although transmitted light and reflected light generally have no effect on the target tissue, consideration of these two aspects of the laser-tissue interaction are pertinent to the safe use of lasers. For example, laser users may become secondary targets as a consequence of laser light reflected from tissue, and tissue components deep to the target tissue may be damaged unintentionally if their optical characteristics are such that transmitted light is absorbed.

Scattering has the effect of increasing the volume of tissue in which the photons of the incident laser beam are distributed and may eventually be absorbed (Figure 4-1B). This effect actually increases the spot size of the laser beam within the target tissue and thus decreases the concentration of photons per unit volume

Robertson, J.H. and Clark, W.C. (eds), Lasers in Neurosurgery.

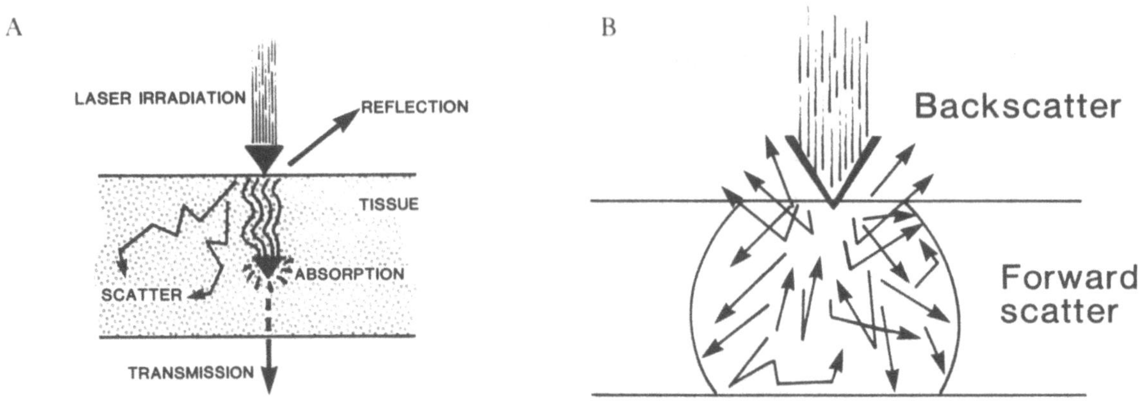

FIGURE 4-1.(A) The laser-tissue interaction. Factors that determine the distribution of light within tissue. As a rule absorption is necessary for light to have an effect on tissue. (B) Effect of scattering. Scattering of light by tissue causes a random redistribution of the path-incident photons taken through tissue. This causes the spot size of the incident laser beam to increase within the target tissue.

tissue (i.e., decreases power density) [23]. Because scattering increases the path length traveled by light within the target tissue, and thus the probability of eventual absorption by tissue chromophores, scattering results in increased absorption of the incident light [1]. If the incident light is propagated a few tenths of a millimeter into tissue, it may become almost uniformly scattered so that beyond this region the light distribution is relatively isotropic [53, 60]. Although there is no energy loss in the scattering process itself, scattering, particularly backscattering, along with absorption contributes to the exponential decrease in light intensity with increasing depth in the target tissue [1]. Backscattering along the axis of the incident laser beam, however, may actually result in a light intensity within the tissue that is significantly greater than that of the incident beam. Conceptually this phenomenon can be thought of as exposure of a subsurface portion of the target tissue to the incoming laser beam as well as to laser light that has been backscattered from tissue deep to this site. At the visible and near infrared wavelengths where light may penetrate several millimeters into some tissues, scattering is a major factor in determining the distribution of light within tissue. In general, the longer the wavelength, the less light is scattered by tissue, so that deeper penetration into tissue is possible, provided absorption does not change along with the increase in wavelength [1]. Of course, the amount of scattered light reflected from or transmitted through tissue depends not only on internal reflectances, but also on the absorption properties of the tissue [60]. In the case of a highly absorbed laser beam (e.g., carbon dioxide laser), where scattered light cannot propagate far anyway, scattering has a negligible effect on the distribution of light within the target tissue [22].

Chromophores (in a broad sense, any substance that absorbs light) mediate absorption in tissue; different chromophores have different absorption spectra. The amount of light that a tissue will absorb at a given wavelength depends on the structure, concentration, and absorption characteristics of the tissue chromophores. Absorption characteristics of proteins, nucleic acids, pigments, water, and other intracellular molecules additively determine the absorption characteristics of the tissue as a whole. At wavelengths above 2000 nm, tissue water is the primary chromophore responsible for absorption of laser energy; whereas at the visible wavelengths (450–700 nm) pigments such as hemoglobin, cytochromes, and melanin are the primary absorbers. As a rule, photons traverse tissue without effect until they are absorbed. Upon absorption their energy is invested in the absorbing molecule or chromophore. The excited molecule then dissipates the acquired energy by remission of photons (fluorescence or phosphorescence), chemical reactions or rearrangements (photochemistry), by nonradiative deexcitation (heating), or (rarely) by the ejection of electrons (ionization). Ultraviolet and visible light can cause electronic excitation of chromophore molecules leading to specific chemical reactions that can be precisely confined to target molecules. The low photon energy of infrared light excites specific vibrational or rotational modes of target chromophore molecules and primarily results in heating. These thermal effects are relatively nonspecific. However, the coherence of laser beams allows for spatial confinement of the thermal effects to very fine volumes of tissue. X-rays, gamma radiation, and other high-energy photons affect tissue by relatively indiscriminate ionization of biomolecules, depending on their electron density; thus, the ability to select target molecules is limited [15]. Corresponding photon energies from the commonly used surgical lasers are: 2.4 electron volts (eV) and 2.6 eV for argon laser at 514 nm and 488 nm, respectively, 1.17 eV for the neodymium:yttrium-aluminum-garnet (Nd:YAG) laser at 1060 nm, and 0.12 eV for the carbon dioxide laser at 10,600 nm. Photon energies for the ultraviolet laser wavelengths are: argon fluoride at 193 nm = 6.4 eV; krypton fluoride at 248 nm = 5 eV; xenon chloride at 308 nm = 4 eV; and the fourth harmonic of the Nd:YAG at 266 nm = 4.7 eV. X-rays and gamma rays have photon energies in the range between 10^5 and 10^8 eV, penetrate long distances through tissue, and do not need to be absorbed in order to affect tissue molecules.

The depth of laser light transmission is governed by the wavelength-dependent optical density (OD) of the tissue, which is defined as: $OD = \log_{10}(1/T)$, where T is the ratio of transmitted light power to incident light power. Since the optical density is directly proportional to the concentration of light-absorbing chromophores (C) and the tissue thickness or light path length (X), a further derivation of Beer's law is: $OD = a/2.3\ CX$ (a is the absorption coefficient, which is an indicator of the degree of light absorption by the tissue). Any laser beam with a high absorption coefficient in the target tissue will be transmitted only a very short distance before being completely absorbed by tissue chromophores. The depth at which 63% of incident light has been absorbed (i.e., the 1/e depth) is called the penetration depth [49, 53]. The depth at which 90% of incident light has been absorbed is usually called the extinction length, and is equal to 2.3 times the penetration depth. Because some of the decrease in light intensity may not be due to real absorption, but to light scattering, the attenuation coefficient, which combines the absorption coefficient and scattering coefficient, is a better predictor of the laser beam penetration depth [23, 60]. As a result of scattering, the actual penetration depth is somewhat longer than the reciprocal of the attenuation coefficient, but shorter than the reciprocal of the absorption coefficient [23]. The higher the attenuation coefficient, the less the incident laser beam will penetrate into or spread within the tissue, and the more confined will be the volume of tissue affected by laser light. In general, accurate absorption coefficients, scattering coefficients, and penetration depths are not known for the various laser wavelengths in all body tissues. However, Table 4-1 gives representative values for some important laser wavelengths.

Characteristics of the incident laser beam that also have an effect on the distribution of light within tissue are pulse energy, power density, the degree of focus, and the spot size. Laser beams of high irradiances 10^{10}–10^{12} W/cm^2, delivered in short pulses (< nanoseconds), induce nonlinear effects, which result in optical breakdown of the target tissue (see text following). In such beams the high density of photons

TABLE 4-1.

Wavelength (nm)	Laser	Tissue	Penetration Depth	Absorption Coefficient (cm^{-1})	Scattering Coefficient (cm^{-1})	Reference
193–248	Excimer		0.01–1μm	~10^4		40,9
400		Fat		0.7		—
418	Argon	Membranous Tissue		30		2
		Blood and intact microvessels		2760		2
488	Argon	Brain	0.4–0.5 mm			53,54
488–514	Argon	Whole Blood Water	0.2 mm meters	144		50,41,30
500		Fat		0.4		—
		Cat Brain (in vivo)	0.7 mm	13.3		53
514	Argon	Brain Neonatal	0.4–0.6 mm			53,52
		Brain and tumors	<1.5 mm			52,54
		Blood vessel wall		11.1	11.0	60
		Atherosclerotic plaque		18.0	19.0	60
		Retinal pigment		1500		—
577	Dye, yellow	Membranous tissue		8		2
		Blood and intact microvessels		322		2
		Cat brain	0.39 mm	26		53
600		Fat		0.2		—
630	Dye, red	Brain	3–5 mm			64
		Brain	1–3 mm			53,52
		Atherosclerotic plaque		2.0	12.0	60
		Blood		6.2		—
660		Brain	1.6 mm			53
700		Membranous tissue		5		2
800		Blood		6		—
1060	Nd:YAG	Kidney and liver		15.5		—
		Brain	3–8 mm			52
		Cat Brain (in vivo)	5.5 mm	1.8		62
		Cat Blood		3.8		62
		Bladder wall		0.11	9.89	23
		Whole Blood		34.4		50

TABLE 4-1. (Continued)

Wavelength (nm)	Laser	Tissue	Penetration Depth	Absorption Coefficient (cm^{-1})	Scattering Coefficient (cm^{-1})	Reference
		Atherosclerotic plaque		1.4	2.3	60
		Blood vessel wall		0.9	2.8	60
		Water	60 mm			41
1320	Nd:YAG	Whole Blood		12.7		50
2500–3000	Hydrogen fluoride	Wet Tissue	1μm			65
10,600	CO_2	Wet Tissue	25μm	>500	0	65
		Bladder + H_2O	0.03–0.02 mm	200	0	23,22

(—) Indicates calculated

creates local electrical fields that induce ionization, the formation of plasma and shock waves that each perturb the expected distribution of light in complex ways. Optical breakdown can occur in completely transparent media such as air, where the threshold for this phenomenon is between 10^{12} and 10^{14} W/cm^2 [3, 45]. Similarly, high power density, continuous-wave laser beams incident on tissue may instantaneously affect the target tissue, changing its physical or chemical state and thus the optical properties. On the other hand, low power density beams, which are used to evaluate the optical properties of tissue, have no effect on the target tissue, so that light is distributed within the tissue as predicted by measured absorption and scattering parameters. The state of beam focus, i.e., whether the laser beam is precisely focused on the target, divergent, or convergent, determines the initial direction or path the laser beam photons will take in the tissue and, in part, determines the location of maximal beam intensity within the tissue (Figure 4-2). For example, a convergent beam incident on tissue will potentially result in the maximal beam intensity being located at a point below the surface of the tissue. In the case of a laser beam that can propagate some distance into tissue because of low absorption and minimal to moderate scattering, the maximal effect on the target tissue will be at a submerged location. When a highly absorbed convergent laser beam is used to vaporize tissue, the surgeon would note that the speed of tissue removal would rapidly increase as the depth of tissue ablation progressed; a consequence of the increase in beam power density due to convergence. In contrast, a divergent beam entering tissue will, with propagation, continue to decrease in intensity with increasing depth to an extent greater than would be predicted by the known wavelength-dependent optical properties of the tissue. The effect on tissue deep to the site of beam incidence will be much less or negligible. For highly absorbed laser beams, the effect of beam focus is not a significant factor in determining the distribution of light within the target tissue, but affects the laser-tissue interaction primarily by altering or determining the power density of the incident beam. For highly absorbed and/or minimally scattered laser beams, the transverse electromagnetic mode (TEM) structure of the incident beam (that is, the distribution of energy intensity in a cross-section of the beam), determines the location of maximal effect of the laser beam and the shape of the laser lesion [41]. For example, laser beams in the fundamental mode TEM_{00} will have the maximal intensity in the center of the laser beam spot and a rapid decline in beam intensity lateral to the central axis of the beam. As a consequence, the depth of the laser lesion in

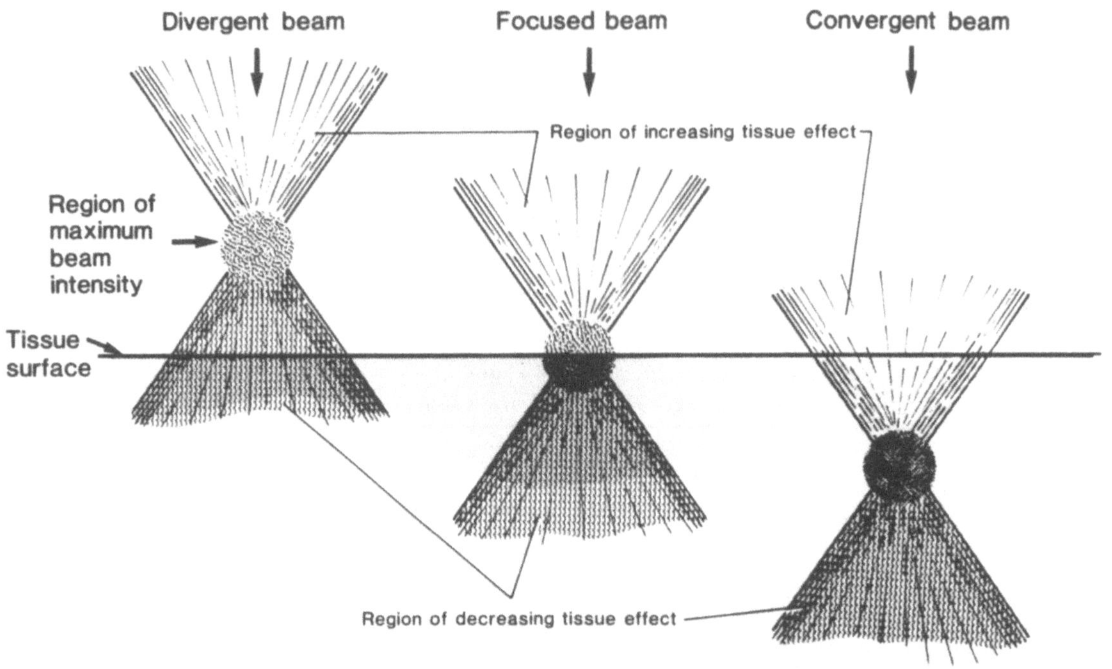

FIGURE 4-2. Effect of beam focus. Divergent beams should be used for coagulation so that tissue deep to the surface will be heated less than tissue at the surface. This decreases the depth of tissue damage that can occur with long laser exposures and avoids the risk of subsurface explosions that can occur when poorly absorbed laser beams are used.

tissue will be greatest in the center of the target area, and the lesion will be conical in shape (Figure 4-3) (see Chapter 3).

Photothermal Interactions

The primary applications of surgical lasers are photovaporization (to make incisions and vaporize tissue) and photocoagulation (to control bleeding and thermally devitalize tissue) (Table 4-2). In these photothermal applications, tissue damage is determined by the magnitude, time duration, and extent (i.e., tissue volume) of heat deposited in the tissue. The conversion of laser energy to heat within tissue is primarily governed by the dose rate (i.e., power density) and optical penetration depth of the laser beam [60]. If the amount of laser energy converted to heat is low because energy delivery is slow (low power density) or absorption minimal (as in the scattering-dominated interaction), tissue heating may not occur or occurs slowly; heat can thus be conducted to surrounding tissue and

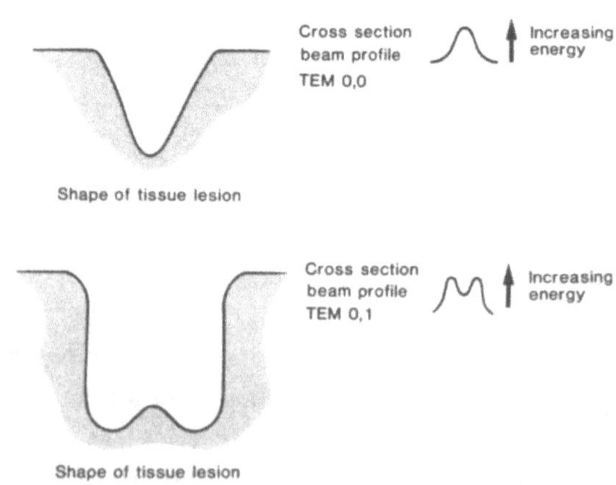

FIGURE 4-3. Effect of laser beam mode structured.

TABLE 4-2.

Surgical Function	Laser	Beam Focus	Power Density (w/cm^2)	Total Length of Exposure	Comments
INCISION	CO_2	Focused	>2,500	<0.5 sec	
	Argon	Focused	>7,500	short	
	Nd:YAG*	Finely Focus (<0.5 nm dia.)	>25,000	↓	
COAGULATION	CO_2	Defocused	<500	0.5 sec	Beam spot size should be only slightly larger than vessel to be coagulated
	Argon	Divergent	~500	long	
	Nd:YAG	↓	350–2,000	↓	
VAPORIZATION	CO_2	Defocused	>2,500	Continuous	Laser powers usually inadequate to achieve*
	Argon	Divergent	>5,000		
	Nd:YAG*	↓	?		
TISSUE WELDING	CO_2	Focused	<1,000	<1 sec	
	Argon		<1,000		
	Nd:YAG	↓	>15,000		

* Not recommended for this application

dissipated without any effect on tissue or can cause a more generalized, but controlled, slow dessication and photocoagulation of the target tissue [15]. In coagulation, the gradual loss of tissue water leaves dehydrated tissue components that have a very high heat of vaporization so that more laser energy can be absorbed and reirradiated or conducted as heat to surrounding tissue without vaporizaion. In dehydrated or relatively water-free tissue such as bone, temperatures greater than 100°C are easily reached [39]. Increasing the power density or coefficient of tissue absorption will increase the rate of heat delivery to the target tissue. If the rate of energy delivery is rapid (exceeds the capacity of the tissue to dissipate heat and exceeds the sublimation threshold), tissue water rapidly converts to steam. Verschueren [58] calls this vaporization process "explosive tissue evaporation," in that the vaporization of water is accompanied by a >1000-fold increase in volume. The high energy required for the vaporization of tissue water and the sudden ejection of heated tissue and steam has a thermostatic effect (water jacket) that limits the heating of surrounding nontarget tissue [21, 39, 65]. At high temperatures, phase transitions and loss of water occur, which drastically change the absorption and scattering coefficients of the target tissue as well as the thermal conductivity and specific heat [22, 60]. Unfortunately, a single thermal model is not available for predicting temperature fields in laser-irradiated tissue that incorporates light scattering, temperature-dependent changes in thermal properties, vaporization of water, modification of thermal properties as a function of water content, and changes in absorption coefficients due to tissue damage [60].

The greater the penetration depth of the incident laser beam, the greater will be the volume of thermally affected tissue [52, 65]. Internal scattering increases the volume of tissue in which the laser beam is distributed and thus increases the amount of tissue that will be heated; however, it also decreases the rate of heating because the power density of the beam is less as a consequence of beam spread. Laser beams incident on tissue that have minimal penetration depths because of high absorption (e.g. carbon dioxide laser) or induced changes in the tissue optical properties (e.g., charring) will cause very confined superficial heating of the target tissue. In a simple case of unidirectional high absorption, the heat deposited in tissue will be approximately equal to the product of the absorption coefficient and the light intensity [60]. Because of the significantly smaller volume of tissue in which the laser light is distributed, a highly absorbed beam, such as the carbon dioxide laser, will deliver energy to the target tissue (i.e., the tissue volume in which the light is distributed) that is orders of magnitude higher than that delivered by a poorly absorbed highly scattered beam, such as the Nd:YAG laser, despite using incident laser beams of equal spot size, power, and exposure duration [41]. A practical consequence is that the carbon dioxide laser is particularly well suited for vaporization of tissue, whereas the Nd:YAG laser requires extremely high power densities for tissue vaporization. Another consequence however, is that because tissue heating by the Nd:YAG laser is slow and simultaneously affects a larger volume, coagulation and hemostasis are better than that seen with the carbon dioxide laser.

Thermal damage to any tissue derives from kinetic excitations and follows a common mechanistic pathway, regardless of the wavelength used to cause the heating [1]. Most enzymes are heat-labile, and at 60°C to 70°C collagen and other structural proteins are denatured. Nucleic acids and membranes are damaged at temperatures above 80°C. Tissue heated above 70°C undergoes coagulation necrosis, which is useful for causing hemostasis due to denaturation of plasma proteins and tissue contraction. Above 100°C, vaporization of tissue water with rapid volume expansion occurs, which is useful for physically separating (incising) or ablating tissues. By determining the distribution and penetration depth of laser light, the wavelength-dependent optical properties of tissue influence the interplay between tissue removal and hemostasis [9].

Although thermal effects are nonspecific, precise tissue damage with lasers is achieved by spatial confinement of optically induced heating [1]. Because of coherence, laser light can be focused into microbeams that are small enough to target subcellular organelles [5]. Focusing the laser beam into submillimeter spot sizes of high power density is the primary technique used to produce spatially confined tissue heating to incise tissue in surgical applications. Because heating of tissue is initiated only at sites of optical absorption, another technique of producing specific thermal damage is *selective photothermolysis* [2]. In selective photothermolysis, a wavelength is chosen such that optical absorption in the target chromophore is, ideally, 10 times or greater than that of absorption occurring in the surrounding tissue. Using this technique, many endogenously pigmented or dye-labeled structures can be selectively and simultaneously damaged in vivo without precisely aiming the laser beam [1, 2, 34]. Similarly, in surgical applications of argon lasers, the high absorption of this laser in blood can be used to selectively target blood vessels when low power densities are employed, providing blood vessel occlusion without damaging surrounding or underlying neural tissue [42].

Whether one uses lasers in a focused or nonfocused application, another parameter of extreme importance in determining the specificity of thermal damage is the duration of target exposure to the laser beam. If laser exposures of duration shorter than the time required for heat to conduct away from the target (thermal relaxation time) are used, selective thermal damage is maximized [2, 52, 65]. If the duration of laser exposure is long compared with the time required for first-order diffusion of a significant quantity of heat to structures that are some distance away from the target, thermal damage will be more extensive and less specific. For example, incisions made with a slowly moving laser beam or long-duration laser exposure will have wider craters with more surrounding heat-damaged tissue than will those of similar depth made by short-duration pulses or a higher power density beam moved rapidly across the tissue [2, 13, 15, 37, 41]. In selective photothermolysis, the incident energy is delivered in short laser pulses, the time duration of which corresponds to retention of heat within the target structures [1, 2]. As a consequence, a maximum transient temperature differential between the target structure and its surroundings will be achieved, damaging the target structures only. In this case, heat localized in the target can easily surpass that required for thermal denaturation, but as heat diffuses to surrounding structures (after the laser exposure), in the process being dissipated over a greater volume, the macroscopic temperature rise of surrounding tissues will be much less and below the level at which thermal damage occurs. For macroscopic thermal damage, the boundaries between normal and damaged tissue represent points of threshold thermal injury [60]. The time associated with retention of heat within a finite volume of tissue depends on the size and thermal properties of the target structure and its surroundings and on the spot size of the laser beam. Another determinant of the thermal relaxation time of laser-heated tissue is the wavelength-dependent penetration depth [9, 65]. Small focal spots on tissue less than 0.1 mm in diameter can cool within milliseconds, wheras larger focal spot sizes may require seconds [49]. Selective photothermolysis uses pulse durations in the nanosecond range to confine thermal damage to organelles, whereas pulses less than milliseconds are used to damage small vessels [2] or dye-labeled neurons [34].

The current "superpulse" options offered on surgical carbon dioxide lasers may decrease, but do not eliminate thermal damage to tissue surrounding the laser incision [13]. As a rule, the pulse energies are not high enough to ablate tissue nonthermally, and the pulse repetition rates are too high to allow thermal relaxation of the target in between pulses. It is interesting that Deckelbaum and colleagues [13, 14] have been able to produce tissue incisions that do not demonstrate lateral thermal injury using pulsed lasers emitting at 532 nm, 1064 nm, and 10,600 nm. These wavelengths, of course, are those of the argon, Nd:YAG, and carbon dioxide lasers, although the lasers used were high-peak-power pulsed units with low repetition rates. Thermal injury was observed when continuous-wave exposures or pulse repetition rates were used (e.g., >2 kHz) that did not allow thermal relaxation of the target tissue in between pulses. To eliminate thermal injury, pulse energies greater than 60 mJ/pulse (pulse duration 20 ns and peak power in the megawatt range) were necessary at 532 and at 1060 nm; pulse energies greater than 10 mJ/pulse were required at the excimer laser wavelengths; and greater than 80 mJ, pulse duration less than 1 μsec and a beam power density of 6×10^6 W/cm^2 was necessary with the carbon dioxide laser. Certainly, at these pulse energies (and power densities in the megawatt range) one cannot be absolutely sure that tissue injury did not occur as a consequence of nonthermal processes. Considering the low photon energy (0.1 eV) at the carbon dioxide laser wavelength, a nonthermal process is highly unlikely. Although much discussion is made on limiting thermal damage surrounding laser incisions, it is this coagulation consequent to thermal effects that makes the incision of tissue by laser inherently hemostatic.

The photothermal laser-tissue interaction observed in the most frequently used continuous-wave surgical lasers (argon, carbon dioxide, and Nd:YAG) will now be reviewed in order to provide an overview and basis for predicting the phothermal interaction at other wavelengths.

The histological appearance of tissue changes induced by the thermal effects of continuous-wave surgical lasers is very similar regardless of laser type [4, 7]. Typically, four zones are observed (Figure 4-4): (1) a vaporization seam where tissue has been removed; (2) a zone of carbonization and dense hypereosinophilic coagulation necrosis where tissue morphology is lost and which may have areas of honeycombing; (3) a pale zone of homogeneous coagulation necrosis with preservation of tissue morphology and edema; and (4) slightly edematous normal tissue. The relative thickness of each of these zones of tissue damage varies with the laser wavelength, duration of laser exposure, and power density of the laser beam. For example, short exposures (<second) to low-power-density laser beams (<200 W/cm^2) may not induce histological changes in the target tissue. In lesions made by the Nd:YAG laser, there tends to be minimal vaporization, surrounded by coagulation and heat-damaged tissue that increases and becomes most evident some hours after the exposure to laser [16]. Damage to neurological tissues by lasers induces an inflammatory response that is typical for injury to this type of tissue by heat, infarction, etc [7]. Usually, however, disruption of the blood-brain barrier is minimal and short-lived; the area of injury is sharply demarcated from the surrounding normal tissues; and the volume of tissue damage can be precisely controlled.

The interaction of the carbon dioxide laser with tissue is an example of an absorption-dominated case. The carbon dioxide laser is highly absorbed by tissue water; tissue penetration is minimal and pigment-independent. The conversion to heat occurs rapidly within a very small volume of tissue. Vaporization is achieved at a lower laser power than with the argon or Nd:YAG lasers. Because the beam is confined to a small volume of tissue and heating occurs so rapidly, the thermal effects on surrounding tissue are minimal. As a consequence, lateral tissue coagulation is limited as is the hemostatic effect. However, at low power densities the carbon dioxide laser will effectively coagulate arterioles 0.3 to 0.5 mm in diameter [59]. Figure 4-5 shows a typical carbon dioxide laser lesion in brain. Depending on the irradiation parameters, the zone of carbonization surrounding an incision made with the carbon dioxide laser may be as narrow as 20 to 30 μm, the zone of photocoagulated tissue 100 μm, and the zone of edema 100 μm thick [15, 59]. Damage to the cerebral microcirculation may extend up to 3 mm in diameter [7, 56]. Beck and associates [4] found that the damage zone surrounding brain incisions made with the carbon dioxide laser was dependent on the time exposure, varying from 0.45 mm thick for exposures of 0.5 second to 0.98 mm thick for exposures of 8 seconds duration in focused applications. The depth of the lesion directly correlated with the total energy whether a series of short exposures or a single long exposure was used [4, 37]. For example a 1 second, 6 W exposure 7000 W/cm^2 power density beam (spot size 0.6 mm in diameter) caused a lesion 4.7 mm deep with a fissure width of 0.6 mm [4].

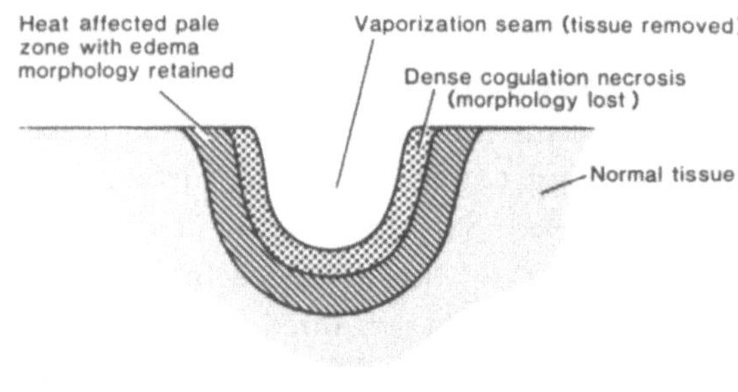

FIGURE 4-4. Diagram of tissue injury zones caused by laser.

Comparing the effects of bipolar coagulators and the carbon dioxide laser on neural tissue, Cozzens and Cerullo [12] found that the laser caused less tissue injury on histological evaluation and by assessment of blood-brain barrier integrity using Evans blue. Affirming the common mechanistic pathway of injury—tissue heating—both types of lesions produced similar zones of tissue injury. The bipolar coagulator was more effective in causing coaptive coagulation of high-flow or thick-walled vessels, but the laser had the advantage of not requiring mechanical manipulation of tissue. In a similar study comparing neural tissue injury by carbon dioxide lasers and unipolar cautery-cutting current, Walter and coworkers, [59] and Takizawa [55] also found that the zones of tissue injury were similar for the two techniques. On electron microscopic and routine histological evaluation, the laser-made incisions had smooth walls and less heat-damaged tissue surrounding the zones

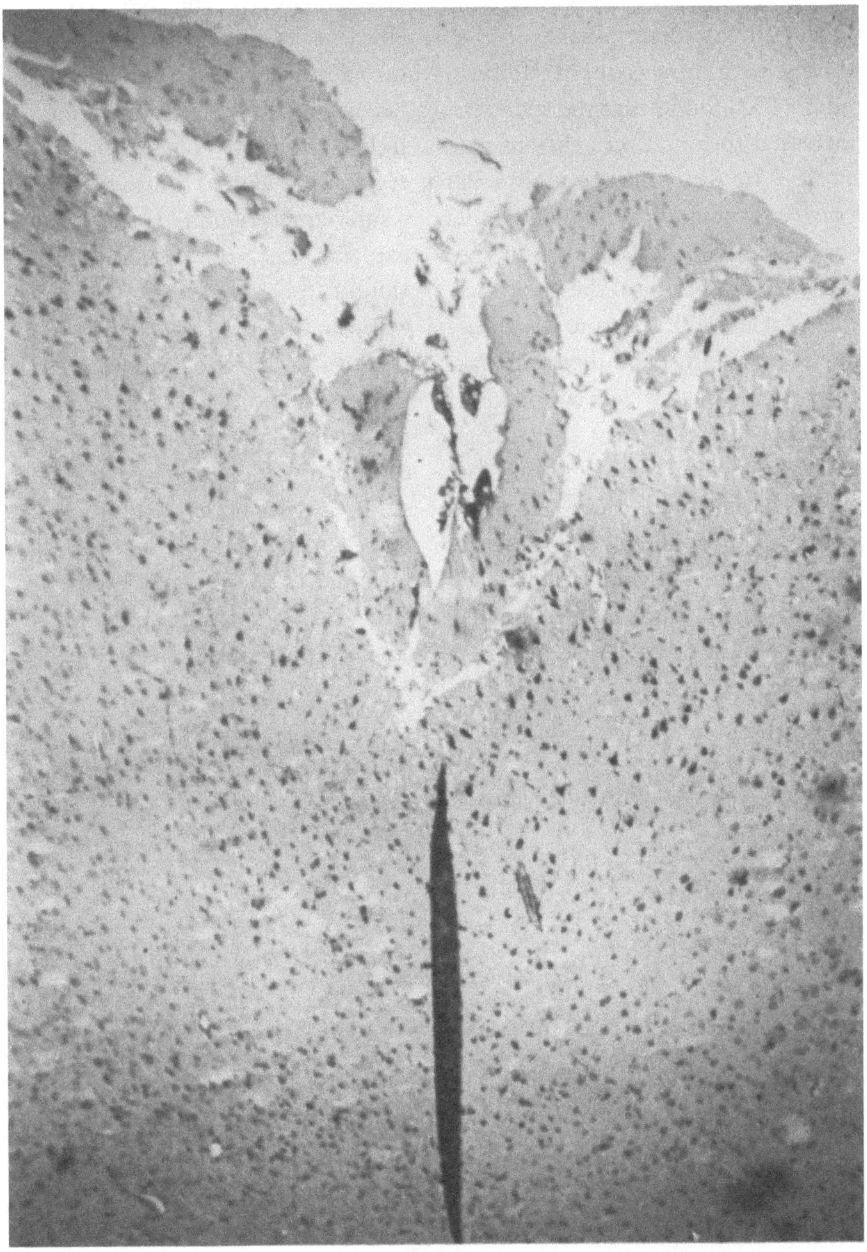

FIGURE 4-5. Carbon dioxide laser lesion in rat brain. Lesion in rat brain made with a focused carbon dioxide laser beam of spot size 0.4 mm, power density of 12,500 W/cm^2, and exposure duration of 0.4 second. The damaged tissue extends approximately 1 mm deep and 0.86 mm wide at the tissue surface.

of vaporization; whereas the electrocautery incisions were irregular and filled with red blood cells and tissue debris.

The thermal interaction of the Nd:YAG laser light with tissue is an example of a scattering-dominated case. At the primary Nd:YAG laser wavelengths (1060–1340 nm), there is no major tissue chromophore to absorb the light, although Nd:YAG absorption in blood is approximately 100 times greater than is the absorption in brain tissue alone [62]. Because absorption is minimal, scattering is the primary determinant of the distribution of light within the tissue. Halldorsson and Langerholc [22] found that the spot size of this laser increased to four times that of the incident beam after transmission through a 2-mm-thick section of stomach in vitro and that backscattering caused a two-fold increase in the spot size of the incident beam at the proximal tissue surface. The relatively isotropic distribution of light due to scattering, and the comparatively deep penetration due to low absorption within the tissue, enable this laser to cause a slow deep heating of tissue that is useful for producing hemostasis or deep tumor necrosis. The tissue-heating effect of the Nd:YAG laser is more pronounced in pigmented and vascularized areas, and the laser may be effective in coagulating arteries up to 2 mm in diameter [4, 16, 59, 62]. However, the Nd:YAG laser is not as effective as the carbon dioxide or argon lasers for vaporization. If the incident Nd:YAG laser beam is collimated, a subsurface increase in light intensity consequent to backscattering results in maximal heating of the target tissue in a submerged region [10, 35]. This phenomenon explains the Nd:YAG laser–induced decrepitation or "popcorn effect," in which a subsurface explosion occurs because this tissue is heated to the boiling point of water faster than is the surface tissue [26, 32]. Although this scattering-induced phenomenon is also present with the carbon dioxide laser, the site is so near to the surface that it is insignificant [32]. Acute, lesions made with the Nd:YAG laser may reveal minimal macroscopic evidence of tissue damage with only blanching and some swelling at the tissue surface (Figure 4-6); however, the delayed

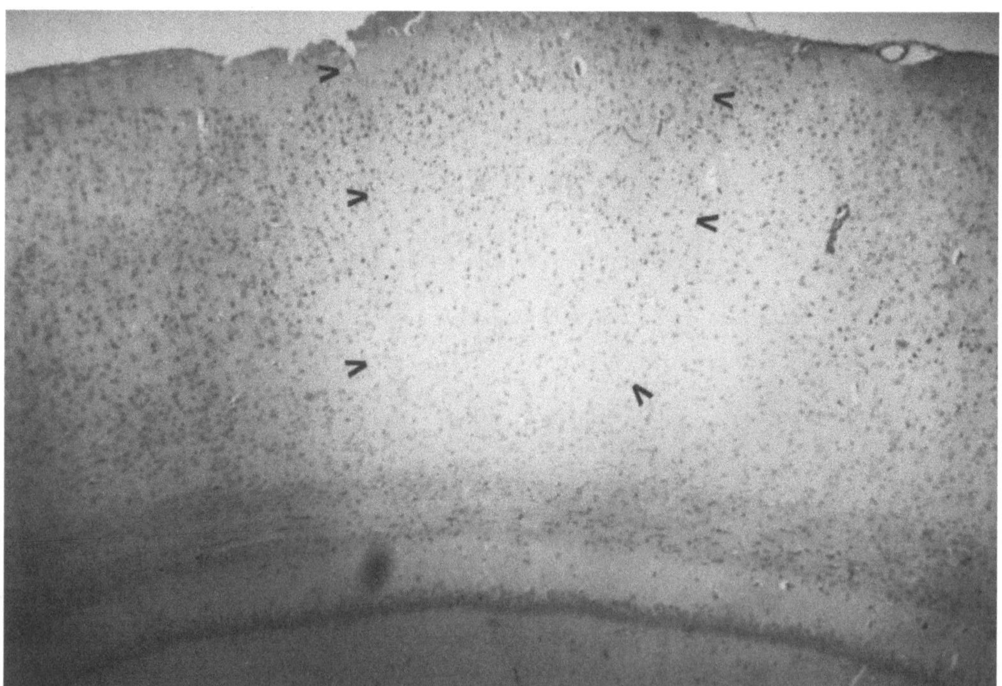

A

FIGURE 4-6. (A) Acute Nd:YAG laser in rat Brain. Lesion in rat brain made with a focused Nd:YAG laser beam of spot size 1 mm, power density of 10,000 W/cm^2, and exposure duration 0.4 second. The area of histologically damaged tissue (outlined with arrowheads) extends approximately 2 mm into the tissue. (B) Nd:YAG Laser lesion in rat brain at 1 week. The extent of tissue injury is now clearly demarcated by the inflammatory response. (C) Nd:YAG laser lesion in rat brain at 1 month.

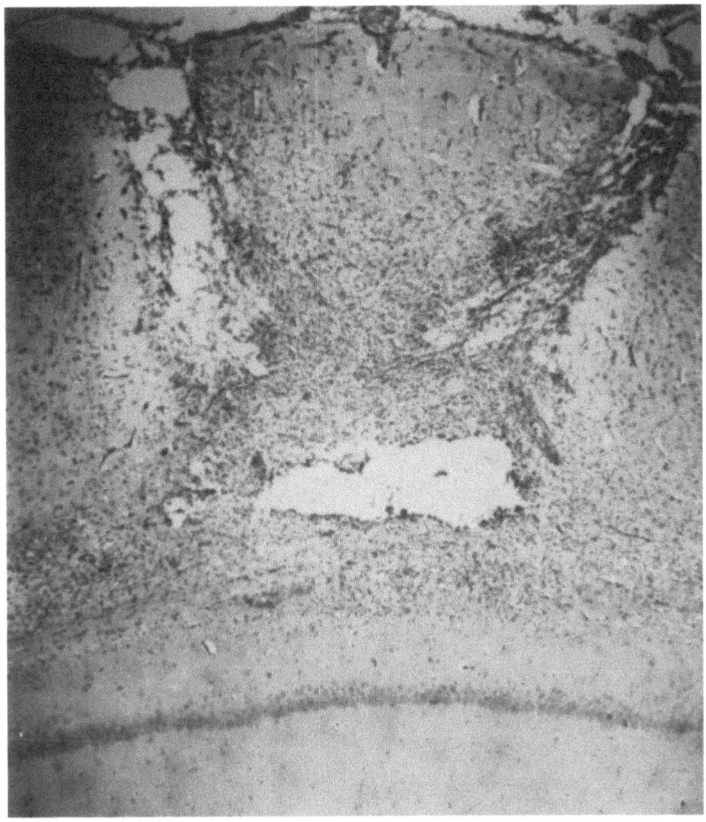

B

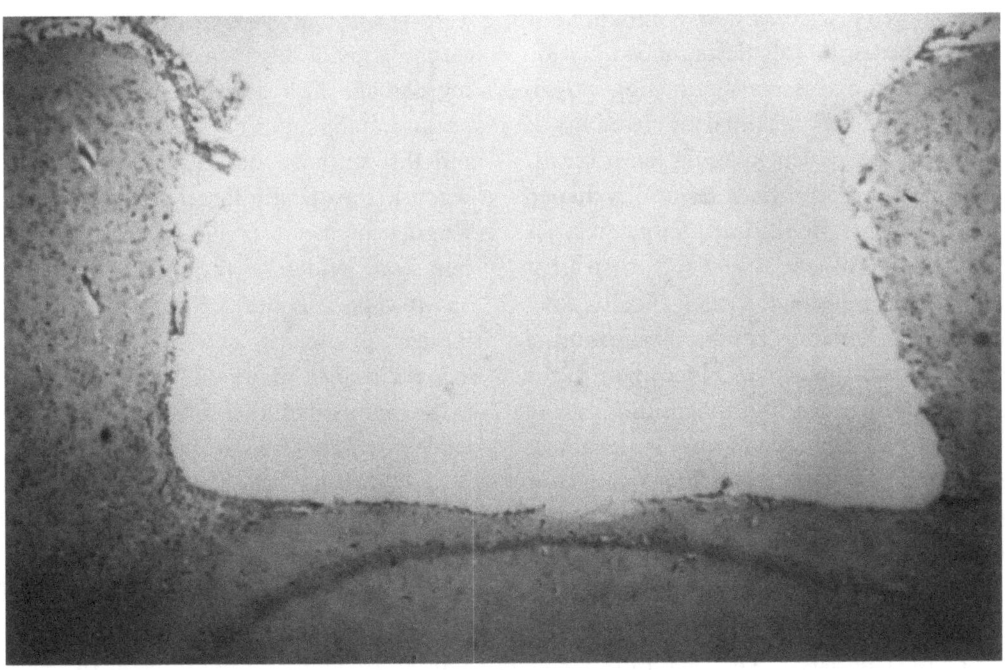

C

breakdown of necrotic tissue reveals the distant thermal effects of this laser and its tendency to cause maximal tissue injury below the tissue surface [4, 16, 59, 63]. Eggert and associates [16], using power densities between 200 and 700 W/cm^2 in exposures 1 to 4 seconds in duration, created brain lesions between 1.3 and 3.1 mm in depth and 1.3 to 5.8 mm in diameter acutely. At energy densities less than 200 J/cm^2, the lesions were usually not evident macroscopically. Beck and coworkers [4] caused brain lesions 3.78 mm in depth and up to 6.8 mm in diameter using power densities between 22 W/cm^2 and 1000 W/cm^2 in a defocused mode (spot size = 2.4 mm) and 0.5- to 4-second exposures; the lesions made with a focused beam (1.2 mm spot size) of power density 1900 to 4000 W/cm^2 and less than 1-second exposure produced lesions 2.6 mm in depth with a diameter at the tissue surface of 2.8 mm. Tissue charring, at the higher power densities, and the resulting high absorption of the laser beam, probably decreased laser penetration [16]. This may also explain why Wharen, and colleagues [63] found that brain lesions made with power densities up to 3000 W/cm^2 at exposures lasting seconds were approximately 2 mm in depth despite calculating a penetration depth of 5.5 mm in avascular brain. Eggert [16] found that edema was maximal by 16 hours as was the increase in evident coagulation necrosis. Edema surrounding the laser lesions evaluated by Evans blue were significantly larger relative to lesion size with the Nd:YAG than that reported around argon and carbon dioxide laser lesions [6, 63]. Probably because absorption of the laser beam was greater in blood than in the surrounding brain tissue and maximum heating occurred more rapidly, blood vessels distant to the focus point of the laser were affected despite grossly normal intervening brain [16, 63]. Kuroiwa and associates [31] also observed that many blood vessels in the edema zone surrounding Nd:YAG coagulation brain injury were shrunken and coagulated. The blood-brain barrier defect was maximal in the depths of the lesion in contrast to carbon dioxide, laser–made lesions in which the defect was maximal at the tissue surface. Histologically one has difficulty distinguishing whether Nd:YAG laser lesions are made with a focused or nonfocused laser beam, and the volume of tissue damage is similar to that seen with bipolar coagulation [16]. Nonetheless, this laser is particularly useful for nontouch coagulation of arteriovenous malformations and highly vascular tumors or for ablating tissue without vaporization [59]. The 1320-nm wavelength of the Nd:YAG laser is being evaluated for photothermal applications because this wavelength is more highly absorbed in tissue water than is the 1060-nm wavelength [48, 50]. Unfortunately, decreased absorption in tissue pigments may actually allow greater tissue penetration than at 1060 nm. The 1320-nm wavelength may be useful for inducing regional tissue hyperthermia for the local treatment of tumors.

The interaction of the argon laser with tissue represents an intermediate case where scattering and direct absorption by tissue chromophores are important determinants [7]. In a comparative study on brain, lesions made by argon laser were similar in depth to equal power density carbon dioxide laser–made lesions, causing tissue damage to a depth of 1 mm when focused beams having a power density of 12,500 W/cm^2 and 0.4 seconds' duration were used [7]. The argon lesions have a larger zone of homogeneous coagulation necrosis surrounding the vaporization seam, which result in improved hemostasis, but it vaporizes tissue less efficiently than does the carbon dioxide laser (Figure 4-7). Acutely, focused lesions made with the argon laser tend to be hemispheroidal in shape, whereas those made with the carbon dioxide laser are conical [7]. In addition, the argon interaction depends on tissue pigmentation because it is highly absorbed in cytochromes, hemoglobin, and melanin. Over 95% of the argon laser is absorbed within 0.21 mm of blood [30]. Similar to neural lesions made by the carbon dioxide laser and unlike those made by the

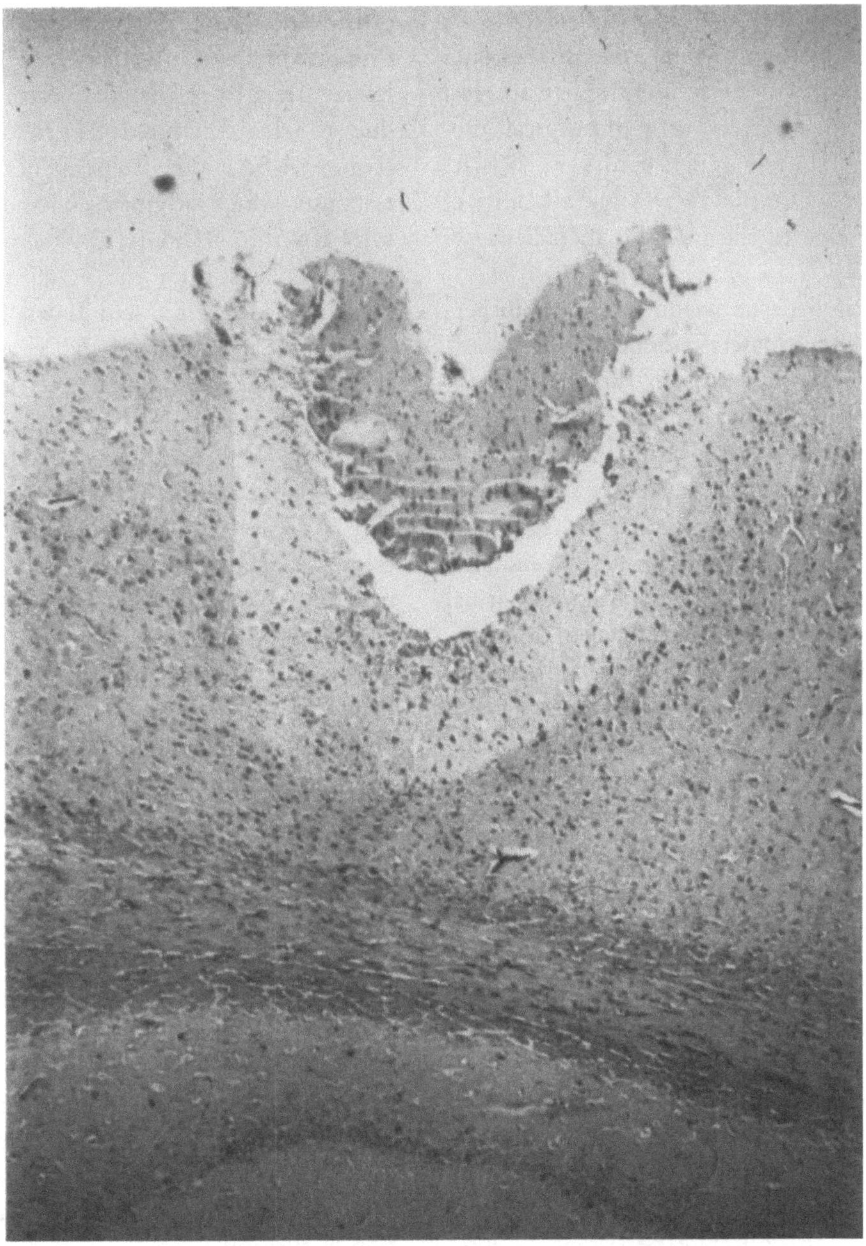

FIGURE 4-7. Acute argon laser lesion in rat brain made with a focused argon laser beam of spot size 0.2 mm, power density, 12,500 W/cm^2, and exposure duration of 0.4 second. The lesion is approximately 0.65 mm wide at the tissue surface and 1 mm deep.

Nd:YAG laser, focused argon laser lesions increase in size minimally as a consequence of occult tissue injury and the inflammatory response caused by thermal damage [7]. Because the wavelengths produced by argon and Nd:YAG lasers are poorly absorbed in saline, irrigation fluids and cerebrospinal fluid do not impair transmission or the tissue effect of these lasers, except to cool the target tissue surface and decrease heating of surrounding tissues.

Since the first demonstration by Fox and colleagues [18] that the argon laser could be effective in vaporizing neural tissues, this laser has been shown to be a useful microsurgical instrument in a variety of neurosurgical procedures on brain and spinal cord [15, 42]. Its use, however, is limited by the unavailability of high power due to the inherent inefficiency of this laser.

Laser-assisted tissue welding is a photothermal application of lasers currently under investigation (see Chapter 14). In this application, laser-induced tissue heating appears to cause a denaturation and solubilization of tissue collagens and proteins. In the temperature range between 70° and 90°C, the collagen triple helix unwinds, but with cooling appears to randomly recross-link and interdigitate, losing its normal periodicity [44, 48]. This collagen relinking during cooling, along with protein denaturation, may be mechanism by which severed tissue ends can be welded during exposure to lasers. Although the initial studies investigating tissue welding involved use of the 1060-nm-wavelength Nd:YAG laser in small vessel anastomoses [26], subsequent studies have revealed that these anastomoses may be performed using the argon [20, 30, 44], 1320-nm-wavelength Nd:YAG [48], and carbon dioxide lasers [19, 36, 38, 46]. Similar studies welding severed nerve ends also indicate that various laser wavelengths may be effective [17, 30, 48]. Neblett [38, personal communication] has also been using a low-power carbon dioxide laser to weld dural edges and grafts together in selected clinical cases to obliterate persistent cerebrospinal fluid leaks. In tissue welding, the tissue edges to be bonded are reapproximated in most cases with stay sutures, then exposed to low-power-density, intermittent laser beams (200–2000 W/cm^2) for periods of 0.1 to 2 seconds. Successive adjacent regions along the anastomotic site are treated with the laser until the full circumference has been spot-welded together. In reports using the Nd:YAG laser, much higher power density beams (>15,000 W/cm^2) have been required than might be expected because of the penetration depth of this wavelength in thin membranous avascular tissue [28, 48]. The initial strength of the anastomosis seems to be due to the denatured protein and collagen (Figure 4-8A). The subsequent inflammatory response, which originates on the extraluminal surface within 48 hours, and the proliferation of myofibroblasts from the vessel wall result in fibrous tissue being laid down that provides long-term strength to the anastomotic site (Figure 4-8B). Although the normal elastic lamellar morphology is lost, there is evidence that new elastin fibrils are produced [20]. Reendothelialization seems to begin by day 3 and is complete by 2 weeks. In laser-assisted microvascular anastomosis, patency rates between 70% and 100% have been reported. Advantages seem to include increased speed in performing the anastomosis, decreased foreign body and scar formation, and excellent growth of the anastomotic site. Disadvantages reported are a significant incidence of aneurysms and stenoses. Although clinical use has been reported [27], the procedure is still experimental, and results largely depend on experience. Knowing whether the weld is adequate depends on subjective assessment of tissue blanching (increased light scattering) as an indicator of appropriate tissue heating by the laser beam. With increased experience and the development of more objective techniques to ensure the adequacy of the welds for different tissues and lasers, laser-assisted tissue welding is likely to become another routine photothermal application of surgical lasers.

Photochemical Interactions

Photochemical interactions depend on the matching of laser wavelengths with specific excitation bands of endogenous or exogenous chromophores (photosensitizers) to initiate specific chemical reactions within the target tissue [9]. The magnitude of the photochemical reaction depends on a variety of factors, primarily

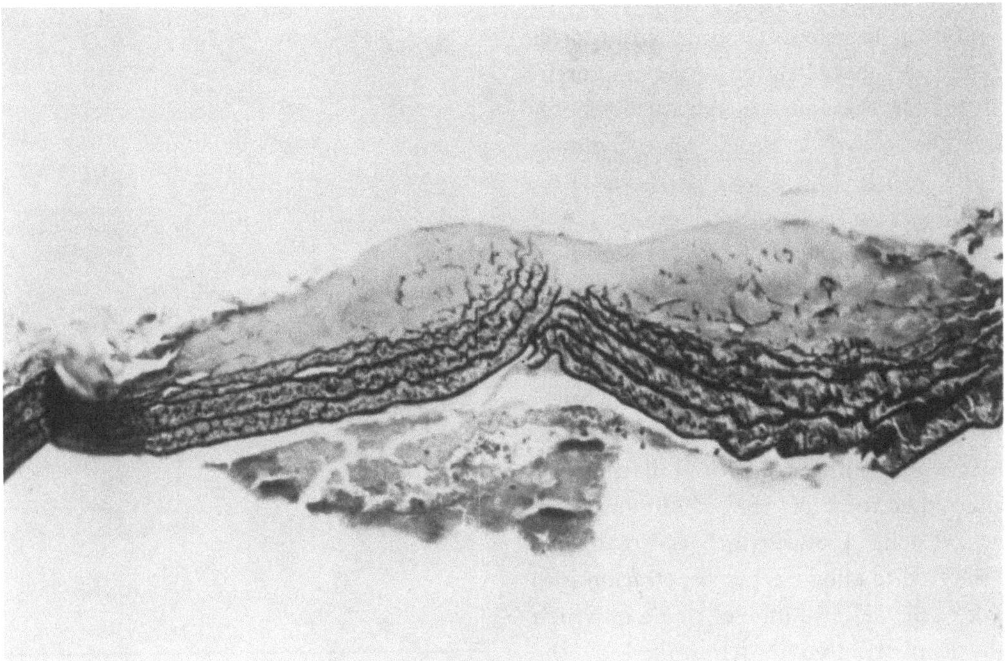

A

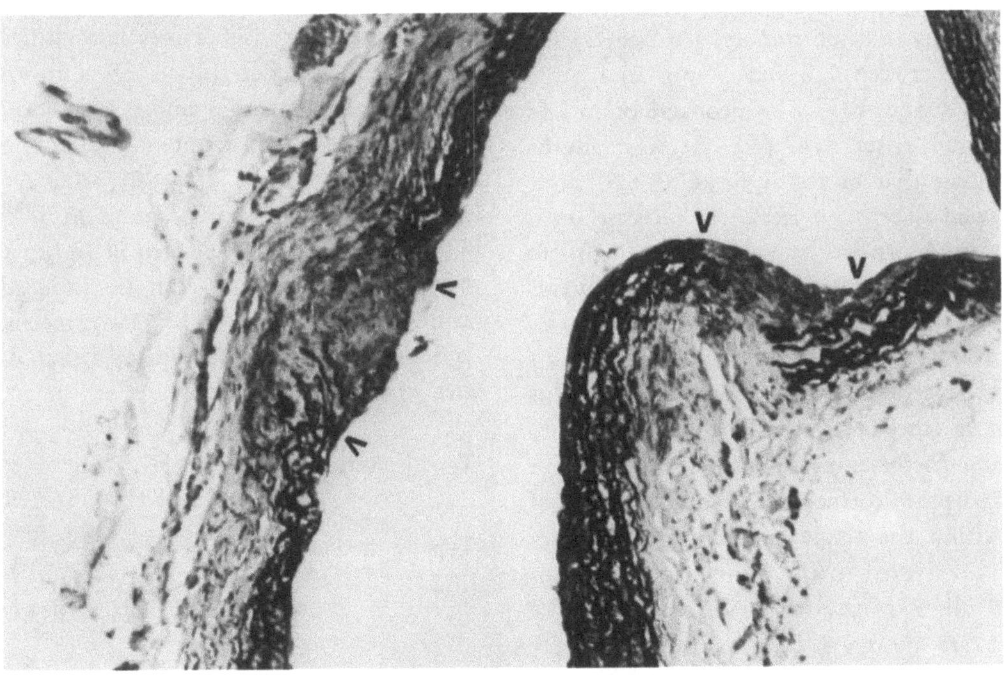

B

FIGURE 4-8. (A) Acute histology of laser-assisted vascular anastomosis. High-power photomicrograph of an end-to-end anastomosis in a rat carotid artery wall made with argon laser, Elastin van Geison stain. (B) Histology of laser-assisted vascular anastomosis at 1 month. High-power photomicrograph of an end-to-end anastomosis in rat carotid artery made with carbon dioxide laser at 1 month. Arrowheads denote luminal sites of anastomotic region. (From C. B. Moon, J. E. Boggan, et al., unpublished.)

the total light dose (i.e., energy density, which is the product of exposure time and power density) and the concentration of the photosensitizer in the target tissue. In contrast to photothermal applications for lasers, photochemical applications utilize low power densities (i.e., <1 W/cm^2) and long exposure times (i.e., >10 minutes). Light dose rates (i.e., power densities) less than 200 mw/cm^2 are used to avoid thermal effects. As a rule, only photons in the visible and ultraviolet portions of the spectrum are energetic enough to initiate photochemical reactions. The wavelength of light used to excite the target chromophore must fall within the absorption spectrum of the photosensitizer. However, as long a wavelength as possible is usually selected to allow deeper penetration into the target tissue. The volume of tissue in which the light is distributed is determined by the penetration depth and the mode of light delivery [53, 54, 64]. Light in the red portion of the spectrum, which has been used in the photochemotherapy of brain tumors, has penetration depths of between 1.2 and 5 mm in normal brain and longer depths in neonatal brain and brain tumor tissue [54, 64]. At wavelengths longer than that of red light (600–670 nm), penetration depths progressively increase until significant absorption by tissue water begins to occur (approximately 1350 nm). Laser wavelengths between 600 and 1200 nm seem to be most promising for photochemical interactions because penetration depths are longest in this portion of the optical spectrum, and, since scattering coefficients are usually much larger than absorption coefficients, the distribution of light within the tissue is relatively isotropic. Light is delivered to the target tissue via implanted fibers or external irradiation. Delivery systems are designed to provide a relatively uniform light flow throughout the target tissue [43, 54, 64]. Of interest, the distribution of light within tissue containing a high concentration of a highly absorbing photosensitizer can be significantly attenuated consequent to light absorption by the photosensitizer itself.

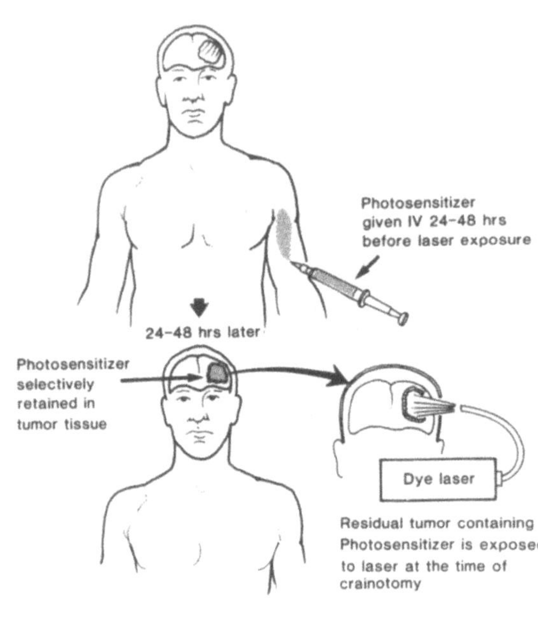

FIGURE 4-9. Photochemotherapy of brain tumors.

In neurosurgery, laboratory and clinical studies are underway in which lasers are used to excite exogenous chromophores that localize to or are retained within tumor tissue [6, 8, 11, 29, 33, 40, 43, 47, 51, 61, 62, 64] (see Chapter). When the chromophore is excited by an appropriate wavelength of light, a cytotoxic chemical reaction can be induced that results in tumor necrosis. Two mechanisms appear to be involved in causing tissue damage with photosensitizers:

Type I mechanisms:

$$S + hv > S^*$$
$$S^* + RH > (S) + RH^*$$

Type II mechanisms:

$$S + hv > S^*$$
$$S^* + 0_2 > (S) + 1_{0_2}^*$$
$$1_{0_2}^* + RH > RH(0)$$

In the above equations, S is the photosensitizer, S* is the light-activated, excited state of the photosensitizer, and (S) is the deexcited photosensitizer, which may or may not have been altered by the interactions. The activating wavelength of light is represented by hv, RH represents any tissue component that may be damaged by the interaction, RH* is the excited radical state or damaged tissue component, RH(0) is the oxidized tissue component, and 1_{0_2} is singlet oxygen. Type II reactions involve singlet oxygen as an intermediate, are called photodynamic, and are dependent on the state of tissue oxygenation. In either type of photosensitization, excited radicals may be produced that can also damage tissue. The selectivity of tissue damage is determined by the localization of the photosensitizer as well as the area targeted with the light.

Most photosensitizers are fluorescent organic dyes that have relatively stable singlet and triplet states and can thus efficiently transfer absorbed energy to surrounding molecules [9]. Photosensitizers currently under investigation for use in brain tumor therapy are hematoporphyrin derivatives (HPD's), phthalocyanines, chlorine derivatives, or rhodamine derivatives. Rhodamine-123 is a cationic lipophilic dye that is taken up by and retained within mitochondria [43]. It seems to be retained for long periods in tumor cells, is nontoxic at very low tissue concentrations, and can photosensitize human and animal tumor cells exposed to blue-green light [43]. The mechanism of tissue injury by light-activated rhodamine has not been determined and the requirement of blue light for activation limits the volume of tissue that can be targeted because of the limited penetration of these wavelengths into tissue. However, the synthesis of similar lipophilic dyes that absorb light at longer wavelengths is in progress.

The photosensitizer currently receiving the most attention clinically is HPD. It is actually a mixture of multiple porphyrins that are highly aggregated, hydrophobic compounds that cross the intact blood-brain barrier only minimally. After intravenous injection, maximal tumor uptake seems to occur between 4 and 24 hours [8, 29, 62]. In most studies, the drug is activated by red light at 630 nm. Although killing of human [33, 40, 61, 64] and animal [6, 11, 29] brain tumor cells has been demonstrated in vitro and in vivo, the mechanism of tumor damage in vivo depends, at least partly, on damage to the tumor bed vasculature [8, 24, 47]. Damage on the cellular level primarily involves membrane and mitochondrial injury [11, 47]. HPD, particularly the dihematoporphyrin either and ester form, is being evaluated in clinical trials and preliminary results have been promising [29, 33, 40, 47, 64]. However, issues regarding the pharmacokinetics, tumor tissue distribution and uptake, and treatment fractionation have not been resolved [6, 8, 11, 29, 61]. Toxicity has been minimal, although some studies have suggested that normal brain may also be damaged [11]. The majority of laboratory and clinical studies have not found significant uptake of HPD by normal brain, and damage to normal brain has not been significant [6, 8, 29, 62]. The possibility of intratumor drug administration to overcome drug delivery problems and decrease the risk of toxicity to normal tissue is being studied in animal models [51] and some human tumors [E. Laws, personal communication].

Photosensitizers that absorb in the near infrared wavelengths so that larger tumor volumes can be targeted by more deeply penetrating light or that can specifically target glioma cells are needed. In addition, the possibility of potentiating the photochemical cytotoxicity with laser-induced tissue hyperthermia that can be delivered via the same fiberoptic system is also being investigated [24, 52].

Nonlinear Interactions

In the electromechanical mode of interaction, the combination of temporal coherence in the generation of ultrashort pulses (e.g., picosecond or nanosecond regimes) of high peak power and the ability to precisely focus laser radiation (spatial coherence) is used to produce laser beams whose interaction with tissue is dominated by radiant field effects [3, 9]. When tissues are exposed to focused high-peak-power laser beam pulses on the order of 30 ps for mode-locked Nd:YAG lasers and 10 ns for Q-switched Nd:YAG lasers, the laser-tissue interaction process is not maintained by linear absorption and tissue damage is not determined by thermal effects [9, 45]. Rather, the high-peaked-power laser pulse creates high irradiances (approximately 10^{10} W/cm^2 for nanosecond pulses and 10^{12} W/cm^2 for picosecond pulses) that locally generate high electric fields [9, 45]. These large fields induce a dielectric breakdown of the target tissue, resulting in the formation of a microplasma (i.e., an ionized volume with a very large free electron density). The subsequent photoproduction of extraneous free electrons, called electron avalanche or inverse Bremstrahlung effect, causes rapid growth of the plasma. The acoustic and shock waves produced by the plasma expansion generate a localized mechanical disruption of the target tissue. This process is initiated by thermionic emission when the Q-switched lasers and a multiphoton absorption process with mode-locked lasers. Interestingly, the plasma produced so strongly absorbs the incoming photons during electron avalanche that it can actually shield distal structures from damage by the laser beam. In addition, the wide cone angle of the focused beam also protects structures distal to the zone of focus by causing a rapid drop in the power density of the incident beam due to rapid divergence past the point of focus. The primary application for this type of laser tissue interaction is in ophthalmology, where semitransparent structures in the eye can be disintegrated with a pulsed Nd:YAG laser beam. The volume of affected tissue can be confined to a radius of less than 200 μm [3]. In studies investigating the effect of high-peak-power pulsed lasers on the myocardium, thermal injury was not observed; however, this may have been due to the short pulse durations as opposed to nonlinear effects [13].

The ultraviolet (UV) laser photoablative process is believed to consist of photodissociation (i.e., the direct breaking of intramolecular bonds, caused by absorption of incoming photons), followed by effluent desorption [9, 57]. Individual photon energies at excimer laser wavelengths (193–351 nm) are quite high, actually on the order of the energy required to break chemical bonds. UV light is extremely strongly absorbed by most biological molecules in the band between 193 and 260 nm, with absorption coefficients as large as 10^4 cm^{-1} common and penetration depths of a few micrometers [9]. UV photoablation can produce very precise cuts in tissue without evidence of thermal injury to surrounding tissues [25, 57]. Similarly, sharp cuts (2–3 μm) with precise control of the ablation depth can be made using the fourth harmonic of the pulsed Nd:YAG laser. Pulsed excimer lasers produce pulses of duration on the order of 10 ns and peak power densities around 10^8 W/cm^2. At these wavelengths, which have minimal penetration depths, pulse durations are shorter than the thermal relaxation time of water (30 μs), so that the lack of evidence for thermal injury may be due to extreme spatial confinement of heating. Long UV exposures at low power densities might be associated with a large thermal component to the tissue injury [25, 40]. There are currently no neurosurgical applications for these nonlinear laser-tissue interactions. However, such precise nonthermal tissue damage certainly has appeal in surgery on the central and peripheral nervous systems.

Conclusion

The use of lasers has had a significant impact on the delivery of neurosurgical care. An understanding of the laser-tissue interaction is essential for the appropriate and safe use of lasers in surgical applications, and for the development of new applications that can improve our managment and understanding of problems affecting the nervous system.

References

1. Anderson RR, Parrish JA: Microvasculature can be selectively damaged using dye lasers: A basic theory and experimental evidence in human skin. *Lasers Surg Med* 1:263–276, 1981.

2. Anderson RR, Parrish JA: Selective photothermalysis: Precise microsurgery by selective absorption of pulsed radiation. *Science* 220:524–527, 1983.
3. Aron-Rosa D: Use of a pulsed neodymium-YAG laser for anterior capsulotomy before extracapsular extraction. *Am Intra-ocular Implant Soc J* 7: 332–333, 1981.
4. Beck OJ, Wilske J, Schonberger JL, Gorisch W: Tissue changes following application of lasers to the rabbit brain. *Neurosurg Rev* 1:31–36, 1979.
5. Berns MW, Aist J, Edwards J, et al: Laser microsurgery in cell and developmental biology. *Science* 213:505–513, 1981.
6. Boggan JE, Bolger C, Edwards MSB: The effect of hematoporphyrin derivative photoradiation therapy on survival in the rat 9L gliosarcoma brain tumor model. *J Neurosurg* 63:917–921, 1985.
7. Boggan JE, Edwards MSB, Davis RL, et al: Comparison of the brain tissue response in rats to injury by argon and carbon dioxide lasers. *Neurosurgery* 11:609–616, 1982.
8. Boggan JE, Walter R, Edwards MSB, et al: Distribution of hematoporphyrin derivative in the rat 9L gliosarcoma brain tumor analyzed by digital video fluorescence microscopy. *J Neurosurg* 61:1113–1119, 1984.
9. Boulnois JL: Photophysical processes in recent medical laser developments: A review. *Lasers Med Sci* 1:47–66, 1986.
10. Burke L, Rovin RA, Cerullo LJ, Brown JT: Thermal effects of the Nd:YAG and carbon dioxide lasers on the central nervous system. *Lasers Surg Med* 5:67–71, 1985.
11. Cheng MK, McKean J, Boisvert D, Tulip J: Photoradiation therapy: Current status and applications in the treatment of brain tumors. *Surg Neurol* 25:423–435, 1986.
12. Cozzens JW, Cerullo LJ: Comparison of the effect of the carbon dioxide laser and the bipolar coagulator on the cat brain. *Neurosurgery* 16: 449–453, 1985.
13. Deckelbaum LI, Isner JM, Donaldson RF, et al: Reduction of laser-induced pathologic tissue injury using pulsed energy delivery. *Am J Cardiol* 56:662–667, 1985.
14. Deckelbaum LI, Isner JM, Donaldson RF, et al: Use of pulsed energy to minimize tissue injury resulting from carbon dioxide laser irradiation of cardiovascular tissue. *J Am Coll Cardiol* 7:898–908, 1986.
15. Edwards MSB, Boggan JE, Fuller TA: The laser in neurological surgery. *J Neurosurg* 59:555–566, 1983.
16. Eggert HR, Kiessling M, Kleihues P: Time course and spatial distribution of neodymium: yttrium-aluminum-garnet (Nd:YAG) laser-induced lesion in the rat brain. *Neurosurgery* 16: 443–448, 1985.
17. Fischer DW, Beggs JL, Kensato DL, Shetter AG: Comparative study of microepineurial anastomoses with the use of CO_2 laser and suture techniques in rat sciatic nerves: Part 1. *Neurosurgery* 17:300–308, 1985.
18. Fox JL, Hayes JR, Stein MN, et al: Experimental cranial and vascular studies of the effects of pulsed and continuous wave laser radiation. *J Neurosurg* 27:126–137, 1967.
19. Frazier OH, Painvin GA, Morris JR, et al: Laser-assisted microvascular anastomoses: Angiographic and anatomopathologic studies on growing microvascular anastomoses: preliminary report. *Surgery* 97:585–589, 1985.
20. Godlewski G, Rouy S, Dauzat M: Ultrastructural study of the arterial wall repair after argon laser micro-anastomosis. *Lasers Surg Med* (in press).
21. Hall RR, Beach AD, Baker E, Morison PCA: Incision of tissue by carbon dioxide laser. *Nature* 232:131–132, 1971.
22. Halldorsson T, Langerholc J: Thermodynamic analysis of laser irradiation of biological tissue. *Appl Optics* 17:3948–3958, 1978.
23. Halldorsson T, Rother W, Langerholc J, Frank F: Theoretical and experimental investigations prove Nd:YAG laser treatment to be safe. *Lasers Surg Med* 1:253–262, 1981.
24. Henderson BW, Waldow SM, Potter WR, Dougherty TJ: Interaction of photodynamic therapy and hyperthermia: Tumor response and cell survival studies after treatment of mice in vivo. *Cancer Res* 45:6071–6077, 1985.
25. Isner JM, Donaldson RF, Deckelbaum LI, et al: The excimer laser: Gross, light microscopic and ultranstructural analysis of potential advantages for use in laser therapy of cardiovascular disease. *J Am Coll Cardiol* 6:1102–1109, 1985.
26. Jain KK: Complications of use of the neodymium:yttrium-aluminum-garnet laser in neurosurgery. *Neurosurgery* 16:759–762, 1985.
27. Jain KK: Sutureless extra-intracranial anastomosis by laser (letter). *Lancet* 2:816–817, 1984.
28. Jain KK: Sutureless microvascular anastomosis using a neodymium-YAG laser. *J Microsurg* 1:436:439, 1980.
29. Kaye AH, Morstyn G, Ashcroft RG: Uptake

and retention of hematoporphyrin derivative in an in vivo/in vitro model of cerebral glioma. *Neurosurgery* 17:883–890, 1985.

30. Krueger RR, Almquist EE: Argon laser coagulation of blood for the anastomosis of small blood vessels. *Lasers Surg Med* 5:55–60, 1985.
31. Kuroiwa T, Tsuyumu M, Takei H, Inaba Y: Effects of Nd:YAG and CO_2 lasers on cerebral microvasculature. *J Neurosurg* 64:128–133, 1986.
32. Langerholc J: Moving phase transitions in laser-irradiated tissue. *Appl Optics* 18:2286:2293, 1979.
33. Laws ER, Cortese DA, Kinsey JH, et al: Photoradiation therapy in the treatment of malignant brain tumors: A phase 1 (feasibility) study. *Neurosurgery* 9:672–678, 1981.
34. Macklis JD, Madison R: Unfocused laser illumination kills dye-treated mouse neurons by selective photothermolysis. *Brain Res* 359:158–165, 1985.
35. Marchesini R, Andreola S, Emanuelli H, et al: Temperature rise in biological tissue during Nd:YAG irradiation. *Lasers Surg Med* 5:75–82, 1985.
36. McCarthy WJ, Hartz RS, Yao JST, et al: Vascular anastomoses with laser energy. *J Vasc Surg* 3:32–41, 1986.
37. Mihashi S, Jako GJ, Incze J, et al: Laser surgery in otolaryngology: Interaction of CO_2 laser and soft tissue. *Ann NY Acad Sci* 267:263–294, 1976.
38. Neblett CR, Morris JR, Thomsen S: Laser-assisted microsurgical anastomosis. *Neurosurgery* 19:914–934, 1986.
39. Parrish JA, Deutsch TF: Laser photomedicine. *IEEE J Quantum Electronics* QE-20:1386–1396, 1984.
40. Perria C, Capuzzo T, Cavagnaro G, et al: First attempts at the photodynamic treatment of human gliomas. *J Neurosurg Sci* 24:119–129, 1980.
41. Polanyi TG: Laser physics: Medical applications. *Otolaryngo Clin North Am* 16:753–774, 1983.
42. Powers SK, Edwards MSB, Boggan JE, et al: Use of the argon surgical laser in neurosurgery. *J Neurosurg* 63:523–530, 1984.
43. Powers SK, Pribil S, Gillespie GY, Watkins PJ: Laser photochemotherapy of rhodamine-123 sensitized human glioma cells in vitro. *J Neurosurg* 64:918–923, 1986.
44. Pribil S, Powers SK: Carotid artery end-to-end anastomosis in the rat using the argon laser. *J Neurosurg* 63:771–775, 1985.
45. Puliafito CA, Steinert RF: Short-pulsed Nd: YAG laser microsurgery of the eye: Biophysical considerations. *IEEE J Quantum Electronics* QE-20:1442–1448, 1984.
46. Quigley M, Bailes J, Kwaan H, et al: Aneurysm formation after low power CO_2 laser assisted vascular anastomosis. *Neurosurgery* 18:292–298, 1986.
47. Sandeman DR: Photodynamic therapy in the management of malignant glioma: A review. *Lasers Med Sci* 1:163–174, 1986.
48. Schober R, Ulrich F, Sander T, et al: Laser-induced alteration of collagen substructure allows microsurgical tissue welding. *Science* 232:1421–1422, 1986.
49. Sliney DH: Laser-tissue interactions. *Clin Chest Med* 6:203–208, 1985.
50. Steichen JD, Dashner K, Martuza RL: Distribution of hematoporphyrin derivative in canine glioma following intraneoplastic and intraperitoneal injection. *J Neurosurg* 65:364–369, 1986.
51. Stokes LF, Auth DC, Tanaka D, et al: Biomedical utility of 1.34 μm Nd:YAG laser radiation. *IEEE Trans Biomed Eng* BME-28:297–299, 1981.
52. Svaasand LO, Boerslid T, Oeveraasen M: Thermal and optical properties of living tissue: Application to laser-induced hyperthermia. *Lasers Surg Med* 5:589–602, 1985.
53. Svaasand LO, Ellingsen R: Optical penetration in human brain. *Photochem Photobiol* 38:293–299, 1983.
54. Svaasand LO, Ellingsen R: Optical penetration in human intracranial tumors. *Photochem Photobiol* 40:73–76, 1985.
55. Takizawa T: Comparison between the laser surgical unit and the electrosurgical unit. *Neurol Med Chin* 17:95–105, 1977.
56. Toya S, Kawase T, Iisaka Y, et al: Acute effect of the carbon dioxide laser on the epicerebral microcirculation. *J Neurosurg* 53:193–197, 1980.
57. Trokel SL, Srinivasan R, Braren B: Excimer laser surgery of the cornea. *Am J Ophthalmol* 96: 710–715, 1983.
58. Verschueren RCJ: Tissue reaction to the CO_2 laser in general. In Andrews AH, Polanyi TG (eds): *Microscopic and Endoscopic Surgery with the CO_2 Laser.* Bristol, England, John Wright PSG, 1982, pp 85–93.
59. Walter GF, Ascher PW, Ingolitsch E: The effects of carbon dioxide and neodymium-YAG lasers on the central and peripheral nervous

systems, and cerebral blood vessels. *J Neurol Neurosurg Psychiatry* 47:745–749, 1984.
60. Welch AJ: The thermal response of laser irradiated tissue. *IEEE J Quantum Electronics* QE-20: 1471–1481.
61. Wharen RE, So S, Anderson RE, Laws ER: Hematoporphyrin derivative photocytotoxicity of human glioblastoma in cell culture. *Neurosurgery* 19:495–501, 1986.
62. Wharen RE, Anderson RE, Laws ER: Quantitation of hematoporphyrin derivative in human gliomas, experimental central nervous system tumors, and normal tissue. *Neurosurgery* 12: 446–450, 1983.
63. Wharen RE, Anderson RE, Scheithauer B, Sundt TM: The Nd:YAG laser in neurosurgery. Part 1. Laboratory investigations: dose-related biological response of neural tissue. *J Neurosurg* 60:531–539, 1984.
64. Wilson BC, Muller PJ, Yanche JC: Instrumentation and light dosimetry for intraoperative photodynamic therapy (PDT) of malignant brain tumors. *Phys Med Biol* 31:125–133, 1986.
65. Wolbarsht ML: Laser Surgery: CO_2 or HF. *IEEE J Quantum Electronics* QE-20:1427–1431, 1984.

II. INTRACRANIAL APPLICATIONS

5. BENIGN SUPRATENTORIAL TUMORS

W. Craig Clark
Jon H. Robertson

In adults, 60% of brain tumors are supratentorial. A little less than half of these are benign tumors. Meningiomas and pituitary adenomas are the most common, but since the majority of pituitary tumors are removed with suction and the laser is not routinely used, this discussion will concentrate on the meningiomas. A few other interesting entities are included, but these occur far more infrequently than the meningiomas.

Meningiomas constitute from 13% to 19% of all intracranial tumors [4, 9, 15, 31, 39], with 80% to 90% of all intracranial meningiomas found above the level of the tentorium [26, 31]. Like other extraaxial intracranial tumors, meningiomas cause symptoms and signs primarily due to compression of adjacent brain and cranial nerves, and in this sense there is no specificity to the presenting clinical pattern that indicates the tumor type with certainty [26]. However, the sites of intracranial meningiomas bear a general relationship to the areas of most abundant arachnoid granulations, and the clinical presentation of each tumor is best described in reference to its anatomical location [31].

Parasagittal and Falx Meningiomas

Tumors in these locations constitute about one-third to one-fourth of all intracranial meningiomas [9, 26, 31]. The parasagittal tumor is attached to the superior sagittal sinus and occupies the space between the falx and the convexity dura, indenting the medial surface of the hemisphere [30, 31].

The falx meningioma is not visible on the surface of the brain. It arises from the falx or inferior sagittal sinus, depresses the pericallosal artery and corpus callosum, and indents the medial hemisphere. When the tumor is large, it is difficult to differentiate from the parasagittal meningioma. Charateristics that may aid in this differentiation include the tendency for the falcine meningiomas to extend through the falx to become bilateral, and the usual absence of hyperostosis as compared to parasagittal tumors [31] (Figure 5-1).

The importance of dividing the sagittal sinus into thirds for descriptive purposes has long been recognized [9, 25]. Each of these locations tends to present with particular features and determines (1) the methods used to manage the sinus when it is involved with tumor; (2) the relative importance of the sagittal veins at differing locations; and (3) the presenting and postoperative neurological manifestations of lesions that occur [25].

The anterior one-third of the sinus extends from the crista galli to the coronal suture. Meningiomas arising in this portion of the sagittal sinus may give little clinical evidence of their location [31]. Although they produce headache, seizures, and an insidious deteriora-

Robertson, J.H. and Clark, W.C. (eds), Lasers in Neurosurgery.

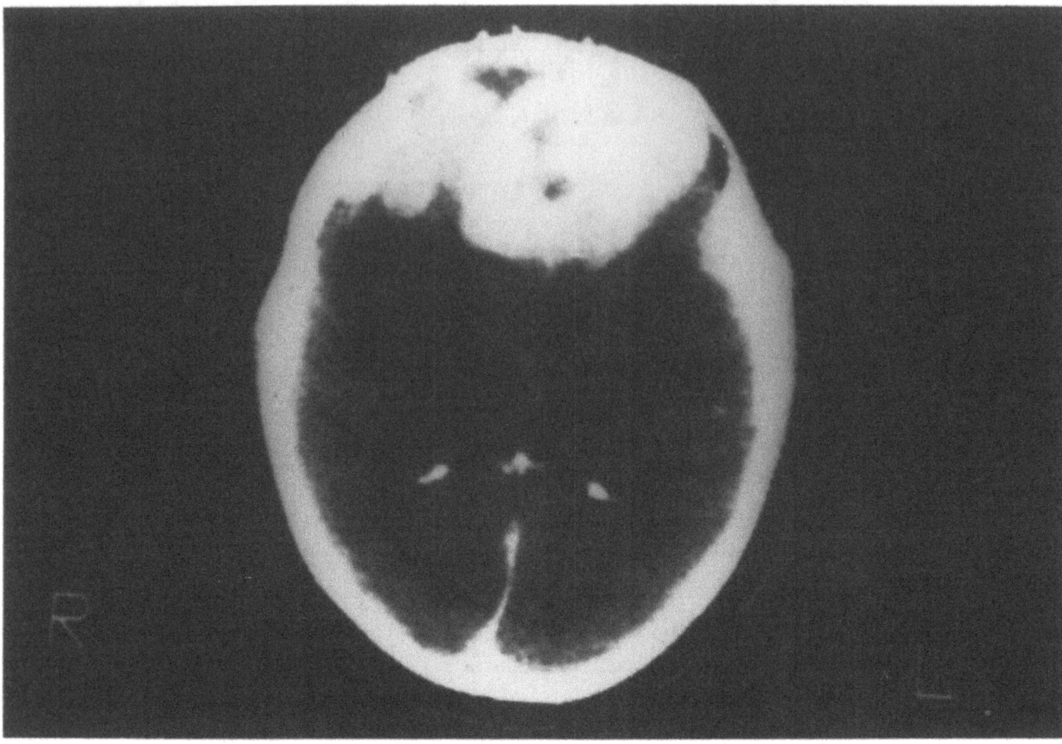

FIGURE 5-1. CT scan of a falx meningioma. Note the bilateral extent of the tumor.

tion of personality and intellect leading to progressive dementia, a complete discussion of the presenting symptomatology is beyond the scope of this chapter, and one of the excellent reviews of this topic should be consulted [25, 30] (Figure 5-2).

The patient is pretreated with dexamethasone, 4 mg orally every 6 hours for at least 48 hours prior to surgery, and adequate serum levels of phenytoin are achieved in order to ensure anticonvulsant prophylaxis. The patient is positioned to minimize intracranial pressure. The head is fixed in the Mayfield pin headrest, rotated no more than about 30 degrees to the contralateral side in order to avoid any obstruction of the neck veins, and elevated about 25 to 30 degrees to promote venous drainage. It is important at this time to be sure the head can be further elevated if excessive bleeding should occur from the sagittal sinus. For tumors in the anterior third of the sinus, the head is slightly extended.

A modified Souttar skin flap is fashioned to provide wide exposure of the cranium and allow removal of a free bone flap that crosses the midline and the underlying superior sagittal sinus and provide wide exposure of the tumor to be resected. Some surgeons prefer a bone flap that does not cross the sagittal sinus because accidental laceration of the sinus wall with a saw may provoke considerable blood loss before the flap can be turned and the bleeding controlled [25]. We have not found this to be an insoluble problem and prefer burr holes one-third over the sinus and two-thirds over dura on either side of the sinus. The sinus is then stripped from the calvarium before the power saw is used, and the cuts over the sinus are made last. The dural flap is hinged medially on the sinus and is outlined over the tumor as it is lightly palpated with forceps. If the dura is adherent to the tumor, internal decompression may be performed through the involved dura. If not, the free dural flap is hinged medially and secured with dural retrac-

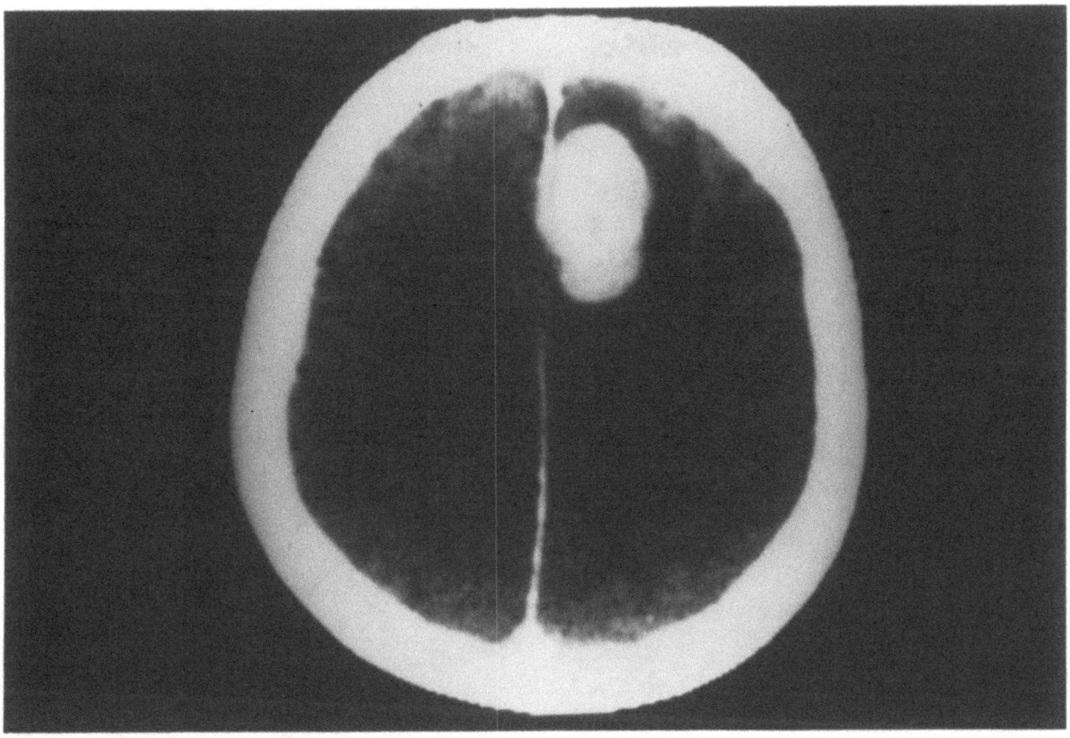

FIGURE 5-2. CT scan of a parasagittal meningioma attached to the anterior third of the sagittal sinus.

tion sutures. Any exposed normal cortex and the sinus are protected by wet cottonoid strips or Gelfoam. The operating microscope and laser are brought into position. Suction-irrigation is used during the internal decompression to further decrease the spread of heat to surrounding tissues. It is usually necessary to rely upon bipolar coagulation for hemostasis because the laser cannot deal with vessels much larger than 1.0 to 1.5 mm in diameter. The internal decompression is performed using about 60 W of continuous, defocused laser power. If there is calcification within the tumor, larger amounts of power may be necessary (80–100 W range). By using larger amounts of power and abundant irrigation, we have found that tumor tissue is evaporated more cleanly with less carbonization and that the internal decompression proceeds much more rapidly.

Once the tumor bulk is reduced, the capsule becomes more pliable and may be folded inward on itself. The capsule is pulled medially and either cut off in segments with miroscissors or evaporated piecemeal with the laser. The gap created by retracting the tumor capsule inward allows separation of the arachnoid from it. Any arteries attached to the capsule are carefully dissected free until it can be confirmed that they are actually running into and supplying the tumor. Only then are they coagulated or clipped. The capsule is then removed bit by bit until all that remains is the portion that is attached to the falx or sinus. In cases where the attachment is in the anterior one-third of the sinus, the sinus may be sacrificed without risking serious sequelae.

The middle third of the sagittal sinus extends from the coronal suture to the lambdoid suture and incorporates the motor and sensory areas and the Rolandic veins. Middle-third tumors classically present with focal epilepsy that usually first affects the foot. Progressive hemiparesis or sensory loss usually starts in the leg, but as the tumor extends laterally the arm

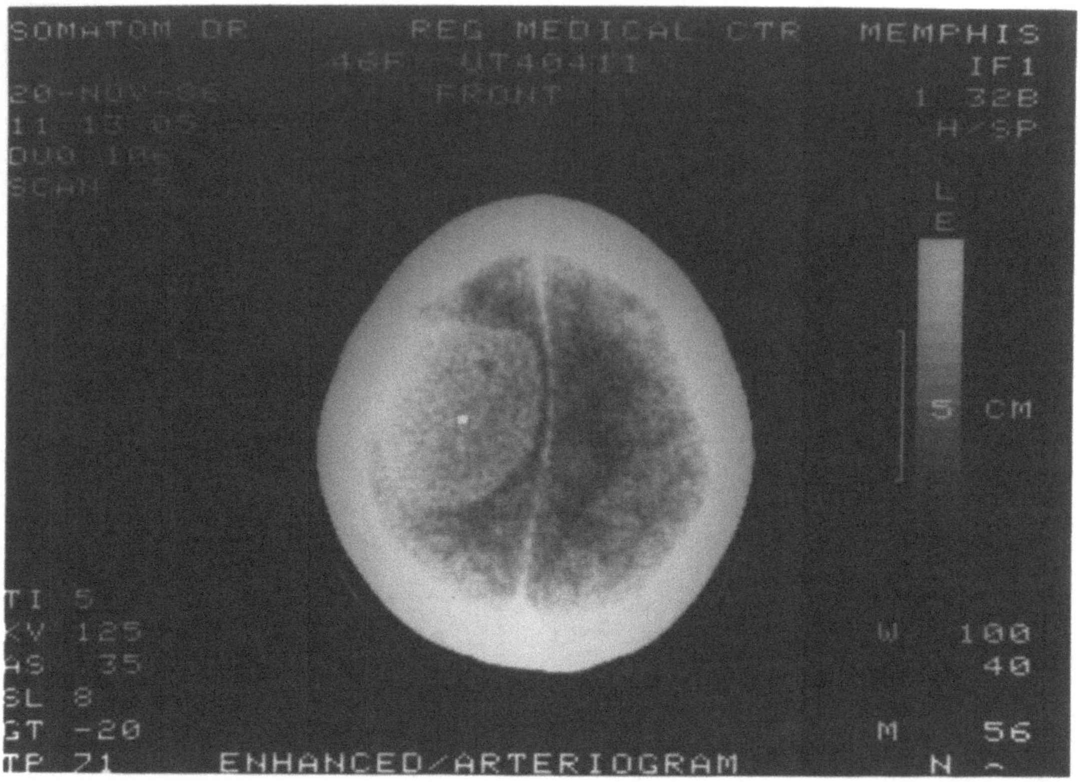

FIGURE 5-3. CT scan of a parasagittal meningioma with middle-third sagittal sinus attachment.

becomes involved and may become the most severely affected limb [31]. Preoperative digital subtraction angiography is of critical importance in the assessment of the patency of the sinus (Figure 5-3).

Preoperative steroids and anticonvulsants are used in the routine fashion. Positioning is the same as for the anterior-third tumors except that the head is slightly flexed.

Either a biparietal or temporal skin flap is fashioned, with the midline and at least an additional 2 to 3 cm beyond exposed. A free bone flap that crosses the midline is removed as described earlier. The opening of the dura and the initial debulking of the tumor are carried out in the same manner as with anterior-third tumors. Once the capsule is removed except for the portion that is attached to the sinus, the next step is determined by the extent of sinus involvement.

A classification of the level of sinus involvement has been proposed by Bonnal [5], and a variety of authors have proposed different methods of repairing the sinus after removal of a parasagittal meningioma [6, 16, 17, 25, 29]. Schmidek and Kapp [34] discuss a variety of these repairs in detail. If the tumor is attached only to the wall of the sinus, the site of attachment may be coagulated with the bipolar forceps or carefully evaporated with low wattage laser energy until a clean, shiny, dural surface is obtained. In cases where a portion of the tumor lies in a dural reflection of the lateral wall or roof of the sinus, the external layer of the sinus is usually all that is involved, and this may be removed, leaving the internal layer and the venous sinus intact. If the tumor invades only the lateral angle of the sinus, the sinus is opened, the tumor is evaporated or removed with microsurgical technique, and the sinus is then closed with nonabsorbable sutures. In cases where the preoperative arteriogram has shown that the sinus is completely occluded, preservation of the neighboring cortical veins is even

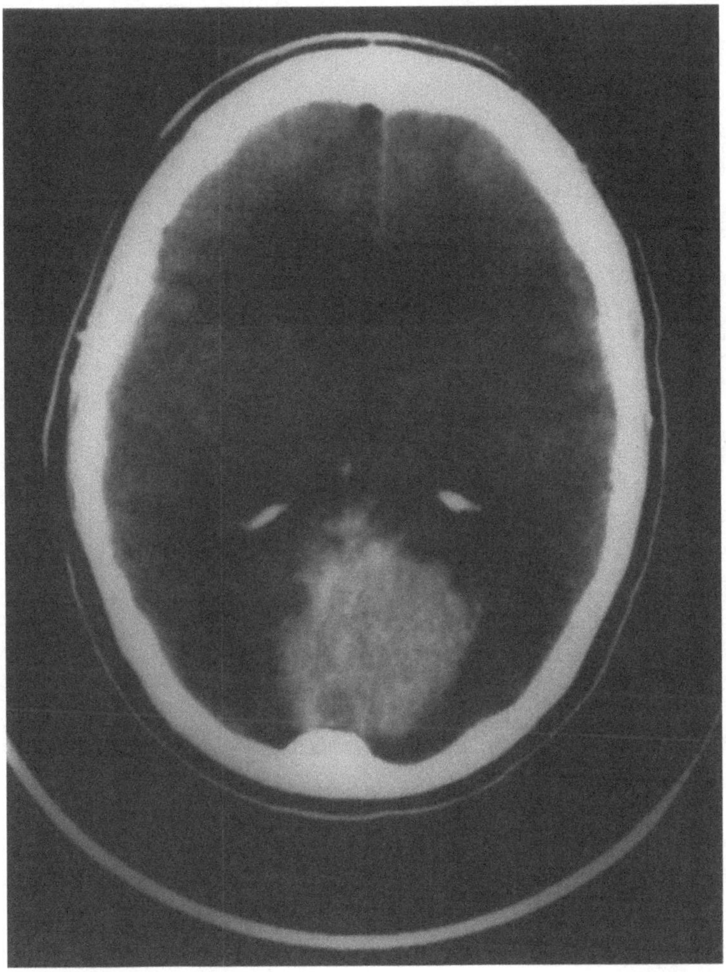

FIGURE 5-4. CT scan of torcular meningioma.

more critical because it is assumed that they constitute at least a portion of the collateral circulation that has prevented venous infarction and serious preoperative neurological deficits. A clinical decision must then be made whether to attempt resection of the sinus. In the event the operator decides to attack the occluded sinus, various authors have recommended use of a total autogenous vein graft repair [6, 7], pericranial graft repair [25], lyophilized dura [16], or other means of reconstituting the sagittal sinus.

Once the tumor has been removed, the sinus appropriately managed, and adequate hemostasis secured, the dural defect is repaired, the bone flap replaced, and the scalp closed in the customary fashion.

The posterior third of the sagittal sinus extends from the level of the lambdoid suture to the torcular Herophili. The major signs and symptoms of meningiomas in this area are slowly progressive, visual field defects and often present as a homonymous hemianopia or visual hallucinations of the occipital lobe type. Because of the contiguous lateral sinuses at the level of the torcular, preoperative digital subtraction angiography becomes even more important in the assessment of the venous drainage consisting of demonstration of the patency of the sinus, dominance of one or the other lateral sinuses, and the presence of venous collaterals (Figure 5-4).

Patients with posterior-third tumors are operated on in the prone position, with the head

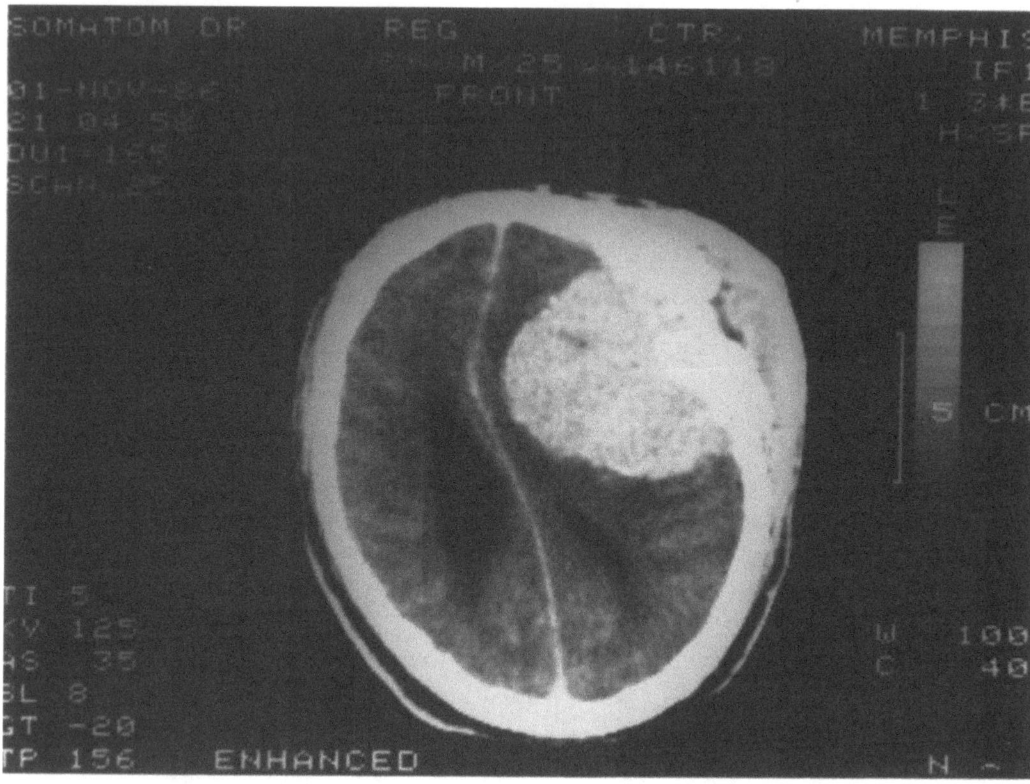

FIGURE 5-5. CT scan of a large convexity meningioma with skull erosion.

fixed in a pin headrest and rotated toward the side of the tumor to provide maximal exposure. Most venous drainage in this area is from the lateral and inferior aspects of the occipital lobe into the lateral sinus, the superior petrosal sinus, and the adjacent tentorial veins. The scalp and free bone flaps are fashioned in the customary manner. The approach down to the tumor and its exenteration is completed in the usual fashion, followed by retraction of the tumor capsule medially, away from the cortex, and its evaporation or excision so as to leave only the basal attachment. At this point the extent of sinus involvement is assessed. If there is only adherence to the sinus, the tumor is removed and the dura coagulated with low-power, defocused laser energy. On the other hand, sinus involvement presents a much more difficult problem. The sinus in this area is not easily obliterated with finger pressure to control hemorrhage while excising a portion of the sinus without causing severe venous distention and edema. As a result, the surgeon usually has to be content with coagulation of the tumor on the sinus wall unless the sinus is completely occluded. If the sinus is occluded and there are no large sagittal veins on either side, the sinus may be excised as previously described.

Convexity Meningiomas

These tumors are free of attachment to the dural sinuses and tend to be concentrated in the region adjacent to the coronal suture [14]. Various reports have placed their incidence varying from about 13% to 34% of intracranial meningiomas [9, 26, 31] (Figure 5-5).

The vascular supply to these tumors is often via the middle meningeal artery or one of its branches. Once this supply is interrupted and the dura opened, the pulsations of the brain often tend to aid in the delivery of the tumor mass.

The techniques of surgical removal vary little from those previously described and primarily consist of an internal decompression using high-wattage, defocused, continuous laser energy. Once the capsule becomes pliable, it is retracted inward on itself and evaporated or excised. Decompression and capsule removal continue in a stepwise fashion until total removal is achieved.

Depending on the size of these tumors and their level of adherence to brain, alternatives to removal include the cutting loop and the ultrasonic surgical aspirator.

Sphenoidal Ridge Meningiomas

The sphenoid ridge is the boundary between the anterior and middle fossae. From the anterior clinoid process medially, the lesser wing of the sphenoid bone comprises the inner two-thirds of the ridge and the greater wing makes up the outer third, which terminates laterally at the pterion. Meningiomas in this area may encroach upon the anterior fossa, middle fossa, sylvian fissure, orbit, and cavernous sinus [31]. These tumors usually make up about 18% to 20% of series of meningiomas [9, 26, 31].

The presentation of these tumors is primarily determined by the site of origin of these tumors along the sphenoid wing [26], which Cushing divided into the inner (clinoidal), middle (alar), and outer (pterional) portions [9].

Tumors that arise at the anterior clinoid process typically cause unilateral loss of vision and primary optic atrophy as a result of optic nerve compression. If the optic tract or chiasm is also involved, there may be an incongruous homonymous-type field defect, but the visual loss is more pronounced in the ipsilateral eye [18]. Cranial nerve involvement may occur at the superior orbital fissure and most often is the abducens nerve [26]. Hypoesthesia in the distribution of the first division of the trigeminal nerve may also occur [1], and is most often associated with cavernous sinus involvement [26].

Medial sphenoid ridge meningiomas continue to present a challenge to the neurosurgeon. In the past, the major problems associated with the removal of these tumors occurred as a result of the tumor's intimate attachments to major neurovascular structures deep within the cranial cavity, and these structures still occasionally cause difficulties. However, the limits of resectability of these tumors must now be considered carotid artery involvement (rather than encasement) and significant cavernous sinus invasion and involvement without occlusion, which is fortunately rare (Figure 5-6).

Scalp and bone flaps are reflected so as to expose the sphenoid ridge and allow removal of the squamous portion of the temporal bone to the floor of the middle fossa. The sphenoid wing is removed with rongeurs and a high speed drill to the level of the orbitomeningeal artery. This vessel is coagulated and severed, providing a flat, basal, tangential approach to the supraclinoid carotid artery and the tumor. Cerebrospinal fluid is removed from the lateral chiasmatic, basal sylvian, and carotid cisterns in order to facilitate brain relaxation and subsequent retraction. An attempt is made to identify the limits of the mass in all directions and identify its relationships to the optic nerve, chiasm, and tracts, the internal carotid artery, and the tentorial edge at the level of the posterior clinoid process. This is often precluded by the bulk of the tumor, and initial internal decompression is required to allow sufficient mobilization of the tumor capsule so that the full extent of the mass and its attachments may be appreciated.

Internal decompression of the tumor is carried out using a high-power (about 60 W), defocused laser beam in a continuous fashion. Continuous suction-irrigation is used to minimize the spread of heat to surrounding tissues. This internal decompression must be carried out with great care because it is possible to encounter large arterial trunks that have been encased by

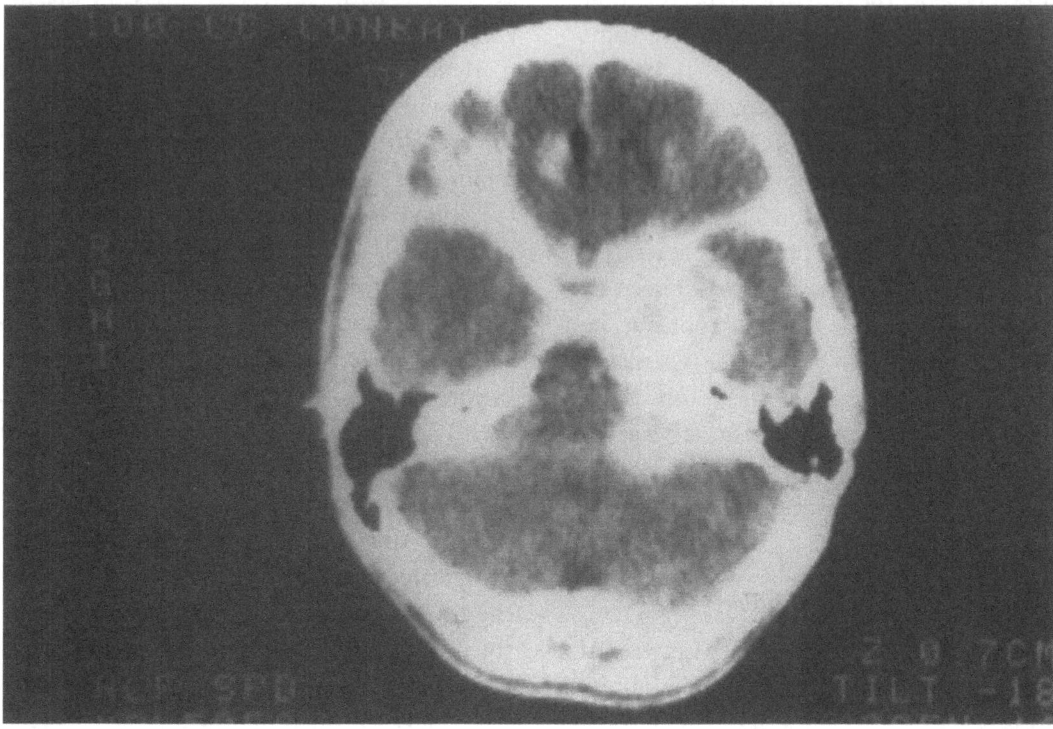

FIGURE 5-6. CT scan of a medial third sphenoid wing meningioma.

the tumor mass. It is occasionally of value to identify the vessel outside the mass and then divide and evaporate the tumor as the plane around the vessel is followed into the mass. When working very close to the vessel, to other structures that must be preserved, or deep in the tumor mass adjacent to the distal tumor capsule, one may use the laser in a pulsed rather than a continuous fashion, which will decrease the spread of heat to adjacent tissue. If available, the superpulse mode will achieve the same effect. Excessive displacement of the tumor should not be attempted until the carotid artery and optic nerve are identified. In most instances the optic nerve will be displaced ventrally and be markedly compressed. Arachnoid strands can be divided and the nerve separated from tumor capsule. The carotid artery is also often markedly displaced, but an adequate plane of dissection is often present and allows the vessel to be freed from the tumor. The careful internal decompression and extracapsular dissection are continued until sufficient tumor mass has been removed such that the remaining mass may be retracted superiorly with the frontal lobe to expose and inspect the free edge of the tentorium. Once these attachments have been severed, attention is returned to the major vascular structures. Further internal decompression is carried out as necessary to allow mobilization of the capsule sufficient to expose the proximal anterior and middle cerebral arteries and any association they have with the tumor.

When the major vascular structures are identified and separated from the tumor, internal decompression and piecemeal capsule removal are continued to minimize traction on the brain. After removal of the tumor is completed, a low-power, defocused laser beam is used to thoroughly coagulate the entire dural surface along the sphenoid, with special attention directed toward the area of previous attachment. Hemo-

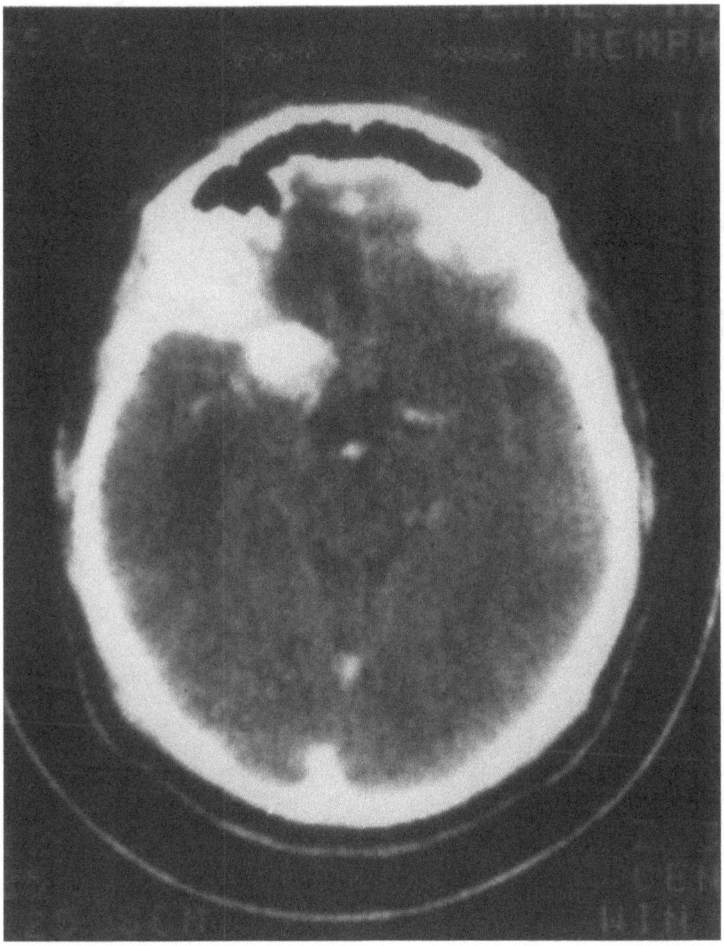

FIGURE 5-7. CT scan of a middle-third sphenoid wing meningioma.

stasis is achieved using the bipolar cautery and Gelfoam soaked in thrombin. The wound is then closed in a customary fashion.

Meningiomas of the middle and lateral thirds of the sphenoid wing generally reach a larger size before making their presence known, either with the hyperostosing changes of bone or with seizures or symptoms of increased intracranial pressure [31] (Figures 5-7 and 5-8). The surgical removal of these lateral tumors is not as hazardous as with those tumors located on the medial sphenoid wing. A standard pterional craniotomy is used to expose the tumor. The boundaries are identified and outlined with Gelfoam strips. Once again, an internal decompression of the mass is performed as previously described. When the capsule becomes empty and can be manipulated, it can either be evaporated with the laser or excised with microsurgical instruments (Figure 5-9).

Once the tumor mass has been eradicated, the dural and bony attachments of the lesion must be removed. This usually requires coagulation or evaporation of the dura in the middle fossa and along the greater and lesser wings of the splenoidal bone. This is accomplished with a "painting" of the area using a low-energy, defocused laser beam in a continuous fashion. In areas where the bone of the base of the skull has been infiltrated by meningioma, the laser may

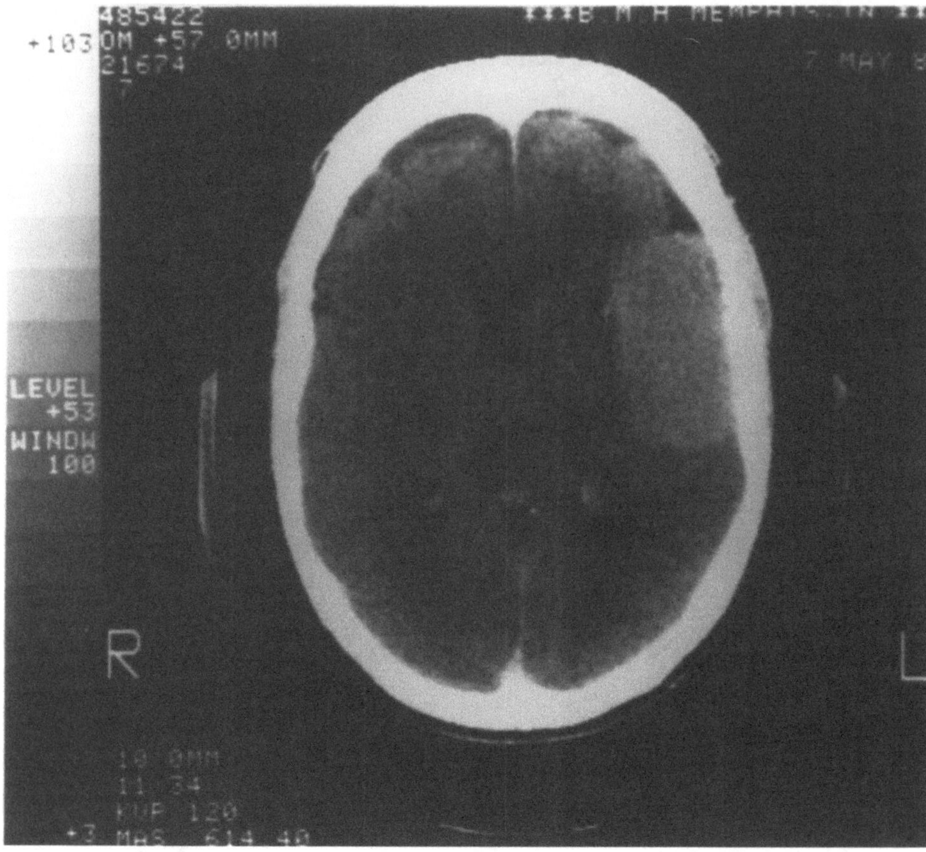

FIGURE 5-8. CT scan of a meningioma attached at the lateral aspect of the sphenoid wing.

again be used to evaporate or devitalize most of this invasion. This represents a substantial advancement in technique, because recurrence of these tumors is often due to this invading portion that previously, either was not recognized or could not be easily or cosmetically removed [5].

Olfactory Groove Meningiomas

These tumors arise over the lamina cribrosa of the ethmoid, indenting the frontal lobes inferiorly, and commonly they are bilateral [2, 31]. Anosmia, the earliest manifestation of the tumor, is nearly always present, although the patient rarely complains of it [31]. In most reported series of intracranial meningiomas, they constitute somewhere between 5% and 13% of these tumors (Figure 5-10).

Although David and Askenasy attempted to organize and classify these tumors into anterior, middle, or posterior groups based on their relation to the floor of the anterior fossa [10], it has been our experience and is the feeling of others [2] that the large size of these tumors at the time of presentation usually precludes any clinically meaningful classification along these lines. It is important to recognize that these tumors are often bilateral [31], and this should be taken into account when planning the operative approach to these tumors.

With high-resolution computed tomography (CT) it is now usually possible to differentiate those tumors with bilateral extension. If the tumor is bilateral, a modified Souttar skin flap and bifrontal free bone flap should be utilized.

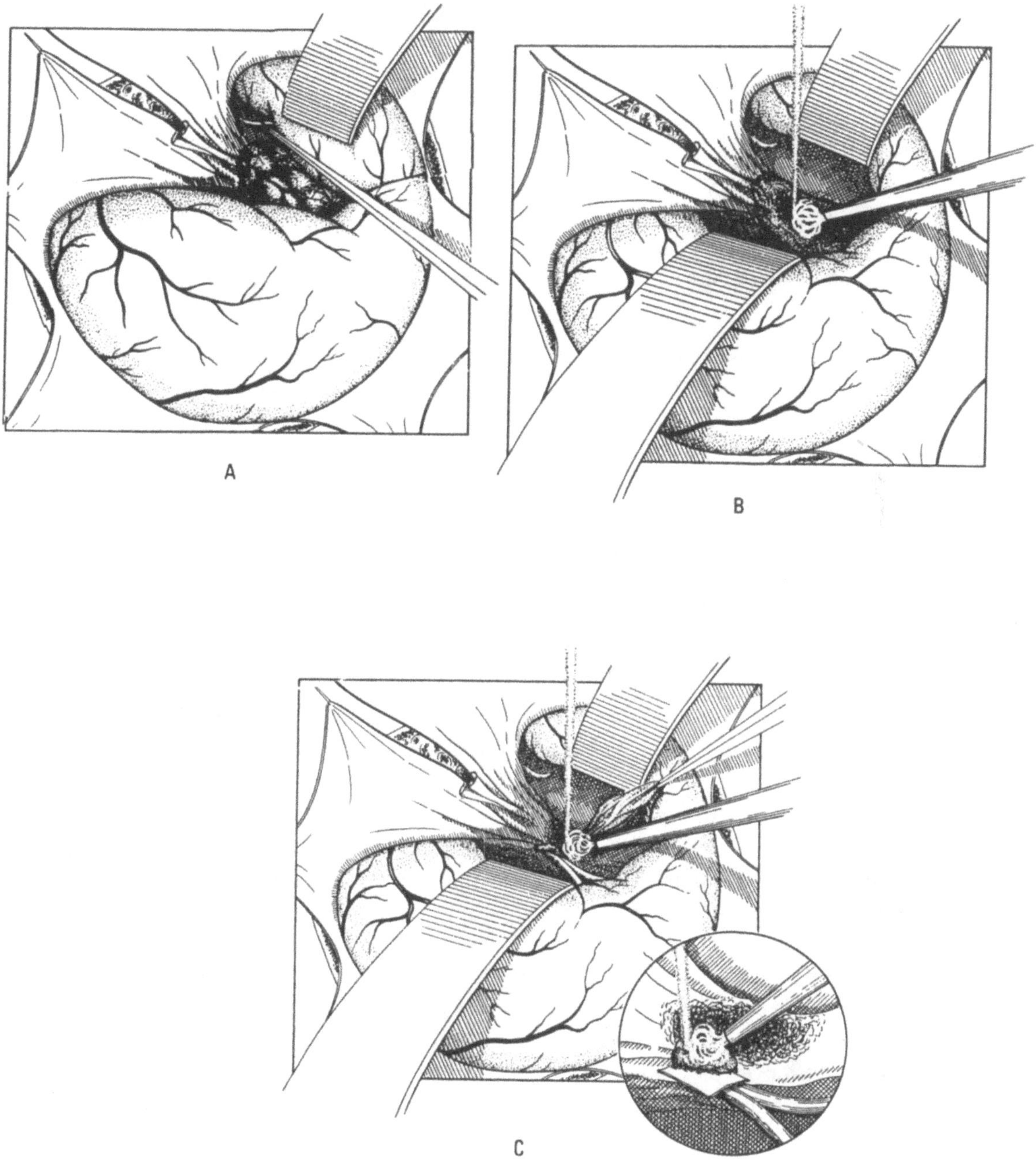

FIGURE 5-9. (A) Sphenoid wing and tumor exposure. (B) Intracapsular decompression of tumor with laser in progress. (C) Tumor capsule emptied and evaporation of capsule in progress.

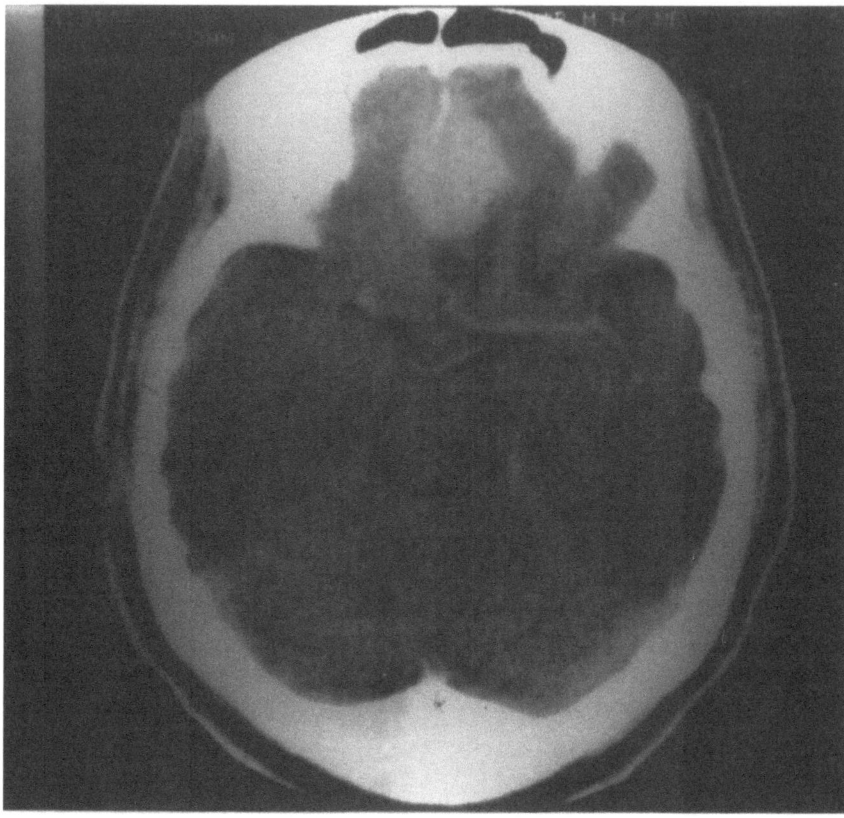

FIGURE 5-10. Olfactory groove meningioma.

Otherwise, the approach is through a standard frontal craniotomy. There is usually remarkable edema associated with these tumors. As a result, an effort should be made to apply only minimal retraction forces in achieving the exposure.

An internal decompression of the tumor is accomplished as described earlier, but extreme care must be taken because of the typical displacement of the anterior cerebral arteries, optic nerves, and hypothalamus that occurs when these tumors are large.

Sellar Tumors

Pituitary adenomas may be classified according to function, anatomy, or histology. We do not routinely use the laser for the removal of these adenomas because they ordinarily may be removed with suction. If a pituitary tumor is too fibrous or dense to prevent its removal with suction, it should probably be approached via a craniotomy [22]. Other indications for craniotomy as the preferred initial approach may include: (1) extension of tumor into the anterior, middle, or posterior fossa; (2) hour-glass-shaped tumors, suggesting a small opening in the diaphragm; or (3) presence of suprasellar tumor with a normal or only slightly enlarged sella turcica [35]. Several excellent reviews have explored the diagnosis and treatment of these lesions and they should be consulted for details [21, 22]. Other lesions occur so infrequently that their discussion is beyond the scope of this work.

Suprasellar Tumors

The major differential diagnosis in tumors of this area is betwen meningiomas and pituitary

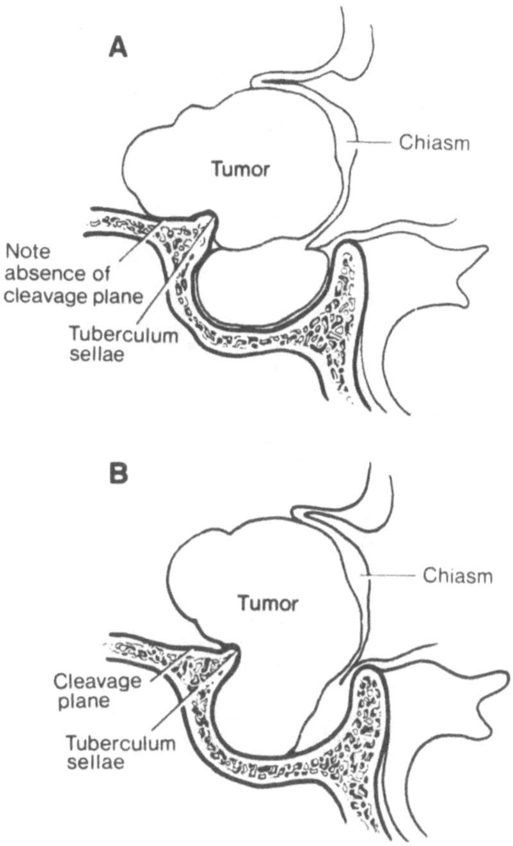

FIGURE 5-11. (A) Sagittal section through the sella turcica shows the intimate relationship between tumor and planum sphenoidale seen with meningiomas. (B) Sagittal section through the sella shows the cleavage plane between tumor and planum sphenoidale seen with pituitary adenoma.

adenomas with suprasellar extension. It is usually possible to make this distinction using CT and angiography, with the remaining few difficult cases aided by the use of high-resolution sagittal reformatted CT images [7] (Figure 5-11). When the tumor is a pituitary adenoma, it is usually decompressed from below via a transsphenoidal approach and followed with radiation therapy. When pituitary tumors are fibrous or dense, they are difficult to remove via the transsphenoidal route (Figure 5-12). A recent study has shown that magnetic resonance imaging (MRI) can help differentiate tumor consistency [35], and this may help the surgeon decide when to approach these tumors transcranially.

We prefer to approach fibrous or dense adenomas with suprasellar extension through either a pterional or frontal craniotomy on the nondominant side. Several surgeons have reported a preference for a bifrontal approach, and this is an alternative. Exposure is achieved in a customary fashion, and the laser and operating microscope are brought into the operating field. Great care must be exercised because of the proximity of the carotid arteries and the optic nerves, but it is possible to use moistened cottonoids to protect these structures from the carbon dioxide beam.

A defocused beam is then used to coagulate the tumor capsule and begin an intracapsular decompression of the mass. The internal decompression is performed as described earlier. In most instances, capsular remnants must be left behind because they adhere to the hypothalamus, but it is usually possible to completely decompress the optic apparatus. It is usually necessary to follow these subtotal removals with radiation therapy. The meningiomas are approached via a craniotomy.

This group of meningiomas consists only of those tumors arising from the tuberculum sellae, planum sphenoidale, diaphragma sellae, and/or the anterior clinoid processes. These tumors usually comprise only about 10% of all intracranial meningiomas [7, 9, 12, 26, 31, 37]. Their size, close proximity to the optic apparatus and major vessels, and their vascularity and usually hard consistency have made them a considerable technical challenge for the neurosurgeon [37] (Figure 5-13).

The most common presenting complaint is usually visual loss, with the characteristic picture often described as a bitemporal hemianopia that occurs as a result of upward pressure on the optic chiasm. This classic presentation is used to attempt to differentiate these tumors from those of the olfactory groove, because they tend to

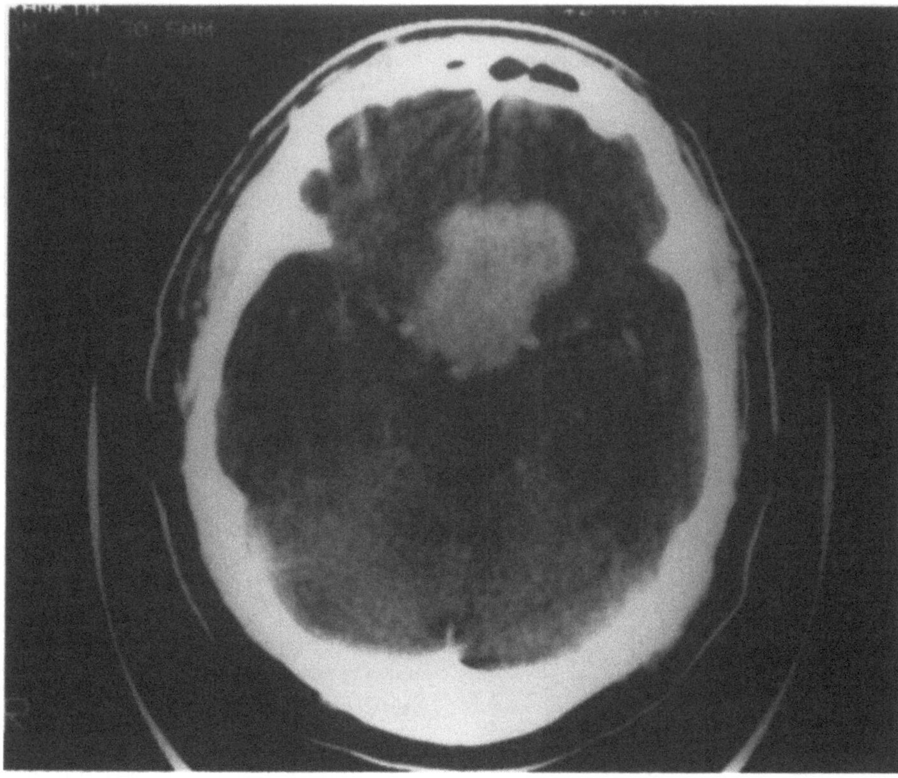

FIGURE 5-12. CT scan of large pituitary tumor with suprasellar extension that was of firm consistency and required laser removal. Note that this usually occurs in only about 2% of these tumors.

press on the optic nerves from above and cause scotomata that are usually easily differentiated from field cuts. Less commonly, one sees headache, mental changes, and seizures as the initial complaint with these tumors [37].

The tumor may be approached frontally, bifrontally, or pterionally. In most cases we prefer the pterional approach from the nondominant side. The craniotomy is performed in the customary fashion, with the sphenoid ridge being removed extradurally down to the level of the orbitomeningeal artery. The dura is then opened close and parallel to the floor of the anterior and middle fossae. A relaxing incision is also made in the dura in the direction of the sylvian fissure to facilitate dural retraction and exposure. The frontal and temporal lobes are gently retracted to allow cerebrospinal fluid to drain from the chiasmatic, carotid, and sylvian cisterns and increase the amount of cerebral relaxation. Self-retaining retractors are placed, and the operating microscope and laser are brought into the operating field. The olfactory tract is then identified; the point where it crosses the sphenoid wing usually serves as a reliable landmark of the entry of the optic nerve into the optic canal.

Once the tumor and the extent of its relations to the surrounding neurovascular structures have been identified, tumor removal is begun. The initial step is an internal decompression performed as described earlier, using continuous suction-irrigation to protect the surrounding structures. Once an adequate debulking is completed, the capsule becomes sufficiently thin and easily mobile. At this point the capsule is either dissected with microsurgical technique or evaporated in order to remove it from the optic

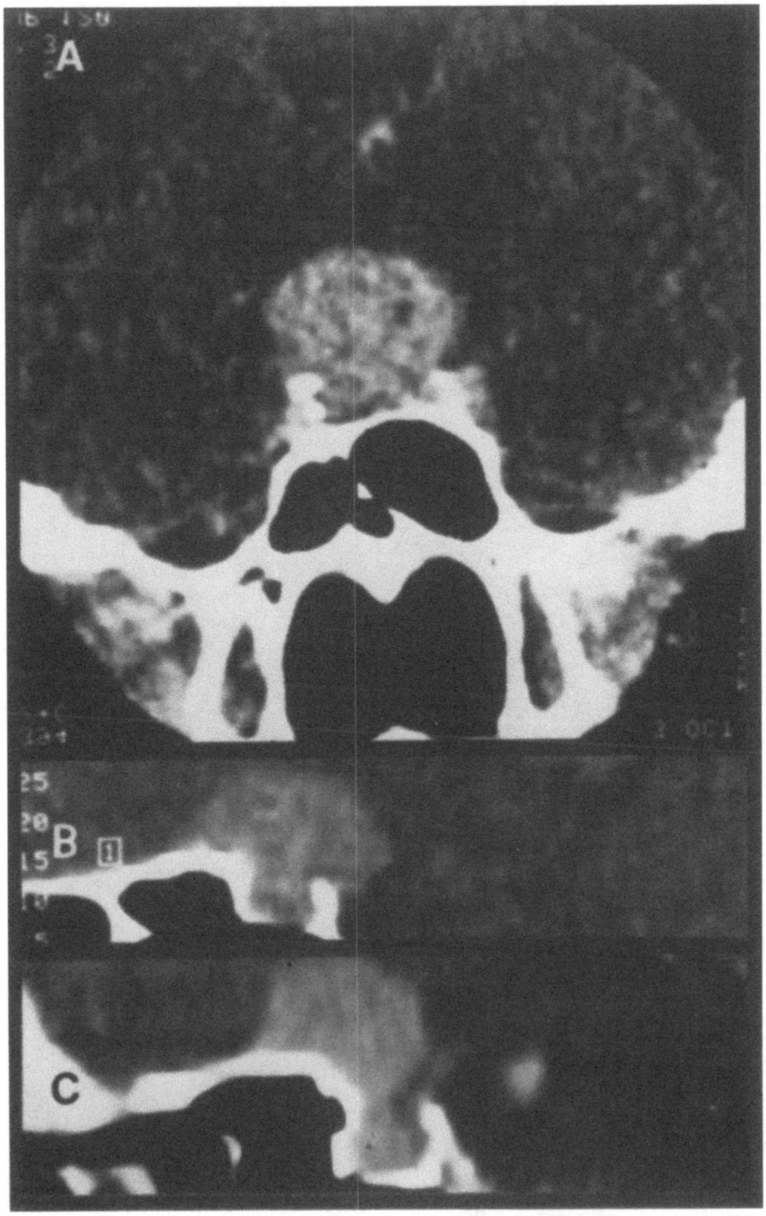

FIGURE 5-13. (A) Coronal CT scan of suprasellar mass. (B) Reformatted sagittal image of a high-resolution CT scan shows the appearance of a meningioma with suprasellar extension. (C) Appearance of an additional meningioma to demonstrate the consistency of the sign.

nerves, chiasm, and blood vessels. The dural attachment is then heavily coagulated or evaporated using a low-power, defocused laser beam in a continuous fashion.

Hemostasis is achieved with bipolar coagulation, the defocused laser beam, and Gelfoam soaked in thrombin; the wound is closed in a customary fashion.

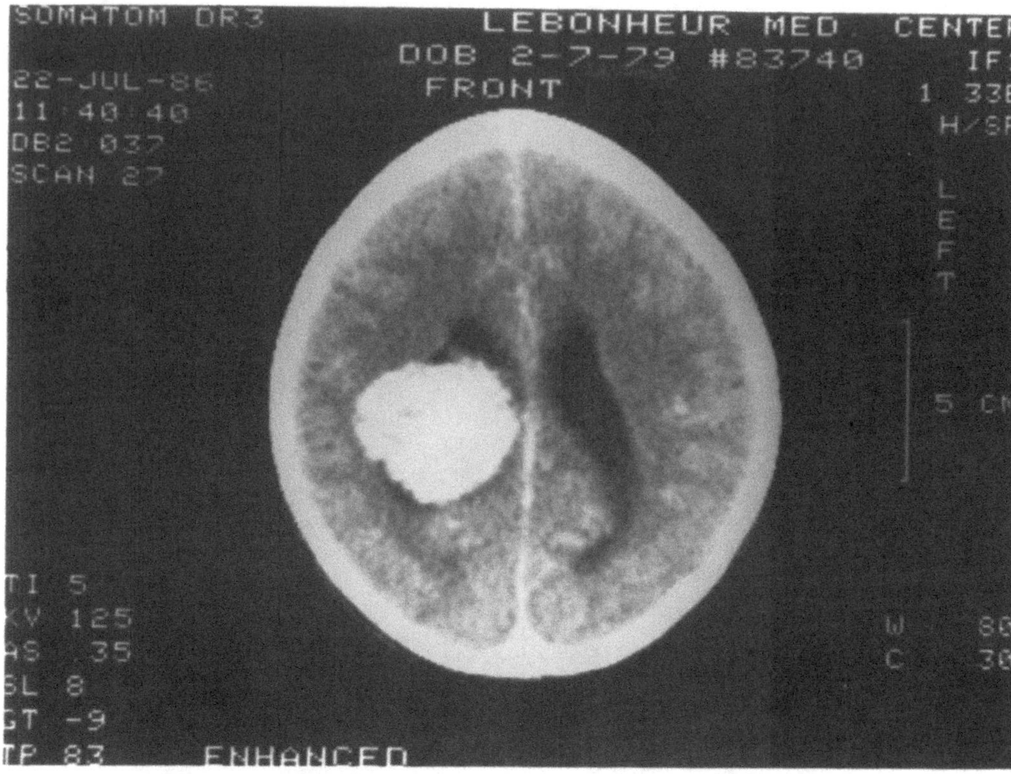

A

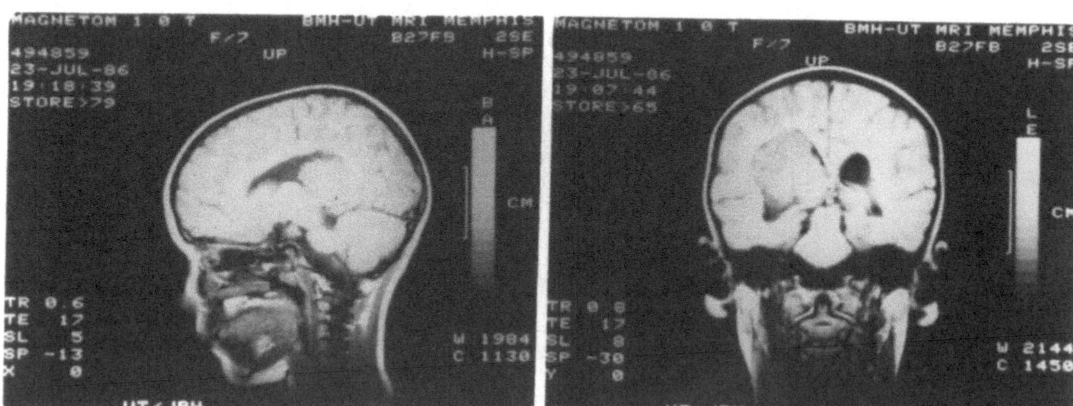

B

FIGURE 5-14. (A) CT scan of choroid plexus papilloma. (B) MRI scan of same patient.

Intraventricular Tumors

The most common benign intraventricular tumors include the meningiomas, choroid plexus papillomas, and subependymomas.

The choroid plexus papillomas are soft, vascular, irregular tumors that resemble a purplish to gray cauliflower. They tend to conform to the contours of the ventricle and may extend to adjacent ventricles or the subarachnoid space. This neoplasm accounts for about 0.5% of all intracranial tumors, but for about 4% of tumors in patients under the age of 12 [8, 32]. Due to this pediatric preponderance, this lesion is discussed in Chapter 8 (Figure 5-14).

Subependymoma is a rare, slow-growing, noninvasive tumor of the central nervous system that may be located in the ventricular system, the septum pellucidum, the aqueduct, or the proximal spinal cord [23, 24]. It has been estimated that only 37% of subependymomas become symptomatic, with the remainder being incidental findings at necropsy [33].

This benign tumor may be completely removed without sacrificing contiguous normal tissue. The laser is an ideal adjunct in the removal of these tumors because of their limited accessibility and the extreme importance of minimizing mechanical forces applied to the ependymal lining that may be contiguous with the tumor mass (Figure 5-15).

Meningiomas of the ventricular system are relatively rare and have been found to comprise from 0.5% to 2.0% of various series of intracranial meningiomas [13, 19, 26, 31]. There would appear to be a tendency for these tumors to occur more often in the lateral ventricles [13, 19], on the left more than the right [3, 13, 19], although they have also been reported in both the third and fourth ventricles [28, 38]. Most of the lateral ventricular meningiomas originate in the posterior portion of the lateral ventricle, especially in the region of the trigone, and receive their blood supply primarily from the choroidal arteries [3, 27]. These tumors arise from the arachnoid of the choroid plexus and may be fibrous, meningotheliomatous, or mixed [20] (Figure 5-16).

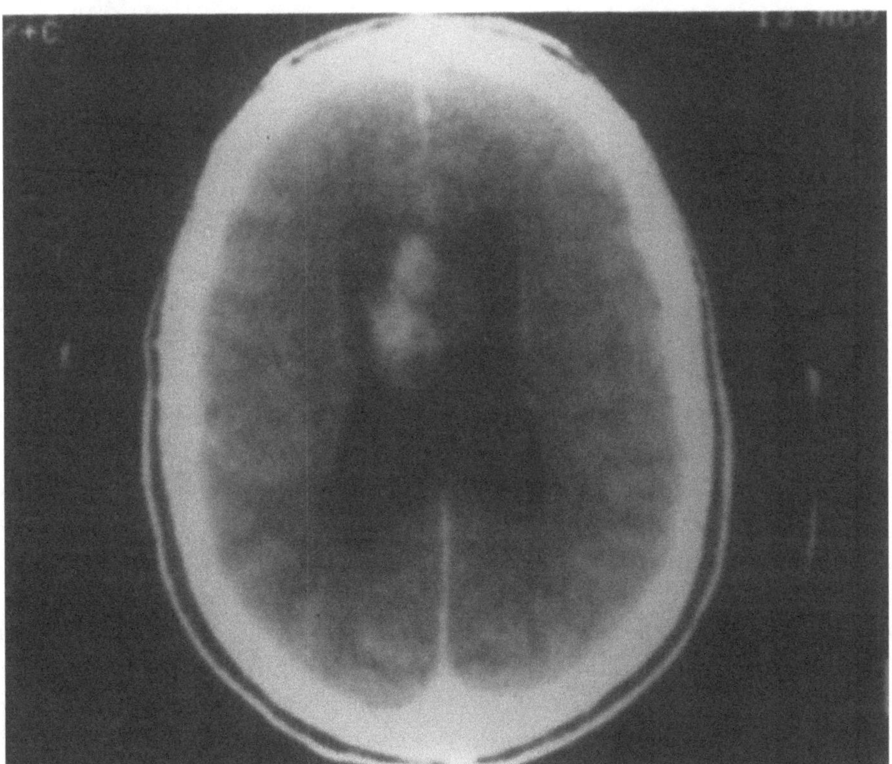

FIGURE 5-15. CT scan of a subependymoma of the lateral ventricle.

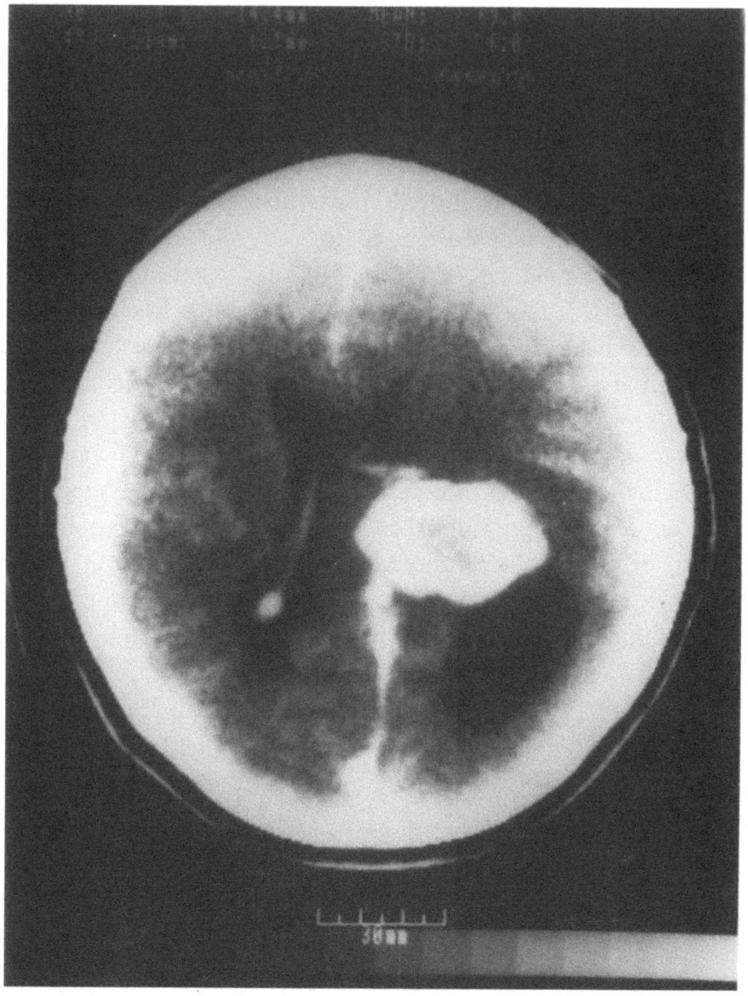

FIGURE 5-16. CT scan of an intraventricular meningioma. Note that this tumor is typical in its left, posterior lateral ventricular location.

As with other intraventricular tumors, the intraventricular meningioma continues to present a significant technical challenge. There are a variety of approaches to these tumors described in the literature [11, 26, 36], but the basic concepts include planning to avoid functional areas, using minimal retraction of the hemisphere, and controlling the main blood supply of the tumor as early as possible [36]. Since the principles of laser removal of these lesions are the same, regardless of their location in the ventricle, the approach and techniques of removal of the trigonal tumors will be described, recognizing that adaptation may be necessary for the removal of tumors in the body. Frontal and temporal horns will require certain changes as a result of the subtle differences in each of these locations.

Most surgeons recognize that one single approach to the trigonal tumor is not the best for all tumors. We prefer the posterior parietal approach just above the lambdoidal suture but also recognize that certain circumstances will arise whan a lateral temporal parietal, middle temporal gyrus, superior parietal occipital, or some combination of these incisions will provide a safer and better exposure of a given tumor. The relative merits of each of these approaches for trigonal tumors have been discussed, and the reader is referred to that discussion for more detailed information [36]. Also, we prefer an incision rather than a cortical resection because of the increased functional loss that may accompany resection in this area.

The cortical incision may be performed in a standard fashion using bipolar coagulation or, alternatively, using a low-wattage, defocused laser beam. It is very important to recognize that one of the keys to the successful removal of these tumors is that one should not attempt to visualize the borders of the tumor by retracting on the white matter. Rather, an intracapsular removal should be accomplished using a defocused laser beam, with the borders of the tumor seen only when sufficient decompression has been carried out to allow the tumor capsule to be folded in on itself. The surgeon must be prepared to deal with blood loss, because the choroidal artery tributaries supplying the tumor cannot be controlled until some of the tumor mass has been removed. The use of the laser provides the capability to remove these masses from within the ventricle through a small exposure, with improved hemostasis, and without applying mechanical forces to the choroid plexus that can result in undetected bleeding at a distance from the operative field.

Other Meningiomas

The remaining 1% to 2% of supratentorial meningiomas are comprised of those found in the middle fossa, the orbit, and miscellaneous rare ectopic sites such as the paranasal sinuses, the neck, and the temporal bone. The principles of the use of the laser for removal of these tumors are consistent with techniques already described.

References

1. Ausman JI, French LA, Baker AB: Intracranial neoplasms. In Baker AB, Baker LH (eds): *Clinical Neurology* Hagerstown, MD, Harper & Row, 1974, p. 1–103.
2. Bakay L, Cares HL: Olfactory meningiomas. *Acta Neurochir* 26:1–12, 1972.
3. Bernasconi, V, Cabrini GP: Radiological features of tumors of the lateral ventricles. *Acta Neurochir* 17:290–310, 1967.
4. Boldrey E: The meningiomas. In Minckler S (ed): *Pathology of the Nervous System.* New York, McGraw-Hill, 1971, pp 2125–2144.
5. Bonnal J, Brotchi J: Surgery of the sagittal sinus in parasagittal meningiomas. *J Neurosurg* 48: 935–945, 1978.
6. Bonnal J, Brotchi J, Stevenaert A, et al: L'ablation de la portion intrasinusale des mengiomes parasagittaux rolandiques, suirie de plastie du sinus longitudinal superieur. *Neurochirurgie* 17:341–354, 1971.
7. Clark WC, Acker JD, Robertson JH, et al: Reformatted sagittal images in the differential diagnosis of meningiomas and pituitary adenomas with suprasellar extension. *Neurosurgery* 18:555–558, 1986.
8. Cobb CA, Youmans JR: Glial and neuronal tumors of the brain in adults. In Youmans JR (ed): *Neurological Surgery.* Philadelphia, Saunders, 1982, pp 2798–2801.
9. Cushing, HW, Eisenhardt L: *The meningiomas: Their classification, regional behavior, life history, and surgical end results.* Springfield, IL, Thomas, 1938.
10. David M, Askenasy H: Les meningiomes olfactifs. *Rev Neurol* 68: 489–531, 1937.
11. De La Torre E, Alexander E, Davis CH, et al: Tumors of the lateral ventricles of the brain: Report of eight cases with suggestions for clinical management. *J Neurosury* 20: 461–470, 1963.
12. Finn JE, Mount LA: Meningiomas of the tuberculum sellae and planum sphenoidale. *Arch Ophthalmol* 92:23–27, 1974.
13. Fornari M, Savoiardo M, Morello G: Meningiomas of the lateral ventricles. *J Neurosurg* 54:64–74, 1981.
14. Giombini S, Solero CL, Morello G: Late outcome of operations for supratentorial convexity meningiomas. *Surg Neurol* 22:588–594, 1984.
15. Grant FC: A clinical experience with meningiomas of the brain, *J Neurosurg* 11:479–487, 1954.
16. Hartmann K, Klug W: Recidivation and possibilities of surgery in meningiomas of the middle and posterior third of the longitudinal sinus. In Klug W, Brock M, Klinger M, et al (eds): *Advances in Neurosurgery, Meningiomas, Multiple Sclerosis, Forensic Problems in Neurosur-*

gery. Berlin, Springer-Verlag, 1975, pp 100–107.

17. Kapp JP, Gielchinsky I, Deardourff SL: Operative techniques for management of lesions involving the dural venous sinuses. *Surg Neurol* 7:339–342, 1977.
18. Kearns TP, Wagener HP: Ophthalmologic diagnosis of meningiomas of the sphenoid ridge. *Am J Med Sci* 226:221–228, 1953.
19. Kobayashi S, Okazaki H, MacCarty CS: Intraventricular meningiomas, *Mayo Clin Proc* 46: 735–741, 1971.
20. Landenheim JC: *Choroid Plexus Meningiomas of the Lateral Ventricles*. Springfield, IL, Thomas, 1963.
21. Landolt AM, Wilson CB: Tumors of the sella and parasellar area in adults. In Youmans JR (ed): *Neurological Surgery*. Philadelphia, Saunders, 1982, pp 3107–3162.
22. Laws ER: Transsphenoidal approach to lesions in and about the sella turcica. In Schmidek HH, Sweet WH (eds): *Operative Neurosurgical Techniques*. New York, Grune & Stratton, 1982, pp 327–350.
23. Lobato RD, Cabello A, Carmena JJ, et al: Subependymoma of the lateral ventricle. *Surg Neurol* 15:144–147, 1980.
24. Lobato RD, Sarabia M, Castro S, et al: Symptomatic subependymoma: Report of four new cases and literature review. *Neurosurgery* 19:594–598, 1986.
25. Logue V: Parasagittal meningiomas. In Krayenbuhl H (ed): *Advances and Technical Standards in Neurosurgery*, Vol 2, New York, Springer-Verlag, 1975, pp 171–198.
26. MacCarty CS, Piepgras DG, Ebersold MJ: Meningeal tumors of the brain. In Yeomans J (ed): *Neurological Surgery*. Philadelphia, Saunders, 1982, pp 2936–2966.
27. Mani RL, Hedgcock MW, Mass SI, et al: Radiographic diagnosis of meningiomas of the lateral ventricle. *J Neurosurg* 49:249–255, 1978.
28. Markwalder TM, Markwalder RV, Markwalder HM: Meningioma of the anterior part of the third ventricle. *J Neurosurg* 50:233–235, 1979.
29. Masuzawa H, Tamura A, Sano K: Recurrence of parasagittal meningioma and sinus-plasty using falx. *Sixth International Congress of Neurological Surgery*, São Paulo, Brazil, June 1977 [Abstract], *Excerpta Medica*, International Congress Series No. 418, p 121, 1977.
30. Northfield DWC: *The Surgery of the Central Nervous System: A Textbook for Postgraduate Students*. Blackwell, Oxford, England, 1973.
31. Quest DO: Meningiomas: An Update. *Neurosurgery* 3:219–225, 1978.
32. Ringertz N, Raymond A: Ependymomas and choroid plexus papillomas. *J Neuropathol Exp Neurol* 8:355–380, 1949.
33. Scheithauer BW: Symptomatic subependymoma: Report of 21 cases with review of the literature. *J Neurosurg* 49:689–696, 1978.
34. Schmidek HH, Kapp JP: Traumatic and neoplastic involvement of the cerebral venous system. In Kapp JP, Schmidek HH (eds.), *The Cerebral Venous System and It's Disorders*, New York, Grune & Stratton, 1984, pp 581–596.
35. Snow RB, Lavyne MH, Lee BCP, et al: Craniotomy versus transsphenoidal excision of large pituitary tumors: The usefulness of MRI in guiding the operative approach. *Neurosurgery* 19:59–64, 1986.
36. Spencer DD, Collins WF: Surgical management of lateral intraventricular tumors. In Schmidek HH, Sweet WH (eds), *Operative Neurosurgical Techniques*. New York, Grune & Stratton, 1982, pp 561–574.
37. Symon L, Rosenstein J: Surgical management of suprasellar meningioma. *J Neurosurg* 61:633–641, 1984.
38. Tsuboi K, Nose T, Maki Y: Meningioma of the fourth ventricle. *Neurosurgery* 13:163–166, 1983.
39. Zulch KJ: *Brain Tumors. Their Biology and Pathology*, 3rd ed. New York, Springer-Verlag, 1986, pp 357–393.

6. LASER SURGERY FOR INTRACRANIAL GLIAL TUMORS

Michael Salcman

Technical advances in neurosurgical instrumentation, anesthesia, and adjunctive medication now permit the removal of benign and malignant brain tumors from virtually all intracranial sites with acceptable morbidity and minimal mortality. The advent of the operating microscope, the carbon dioxide laser, and the ultrasonic aspirator have created a virtual revolution in our ability to perform radical resections in formerly inaccessible locations. Because tumors of glial origin are the most common supratentorial neoplasms, it is of considerable practical importance to determine, if possible, the role of the microscope and the laser in the contemporary management of these lesions. The clinical and theoretical reasons for a primary radical resection of an intrinsic tumor may include any or all of the following: mechanical cytoreduction, adequate sampling of tissue for diagnostic purposes, the "setting up" of other therapies through removal of resistant cells, and the amelioration of acute symptoms and signs that would otherwise prevent a patient from receiving further therapy. The rationale for a subsequent reoperation in a glioma patient can be equally strong if it is carried out with minimal risk and within the context of a true multimodality therapeutic program. The advent of computed tomography (CT)–guided stereotactic surgery has left little justification for the performance of open craniotomy for diagnostic purposes alone. This chapter will briefly review the role of radical resection in the treatment of glial tumors and the experience in our clinic with the use of the carbon dioxide laser for both primary and secondary procedures.

Robertson, J.H. and Clark, W.C. (eds), Lasers in Neurosurgery.

Rationale for Radical Resection

The cellular and structural diversity of glial tumors, and glioblastoma in particular, has been the subject of much recent discussion [3, 20, 27]. Large cell populations within the tumor mass are likely to be inherently resistant to particular forms of therapy due to a variety of intrinsic cellular and extrinsic environmental factors. The cells in each particular tumor vary in their metabolic, kinetic, antigenic, morphological, and genetic characteristics to such a degree that no single therapeutic modality is likely to prove effective at a clinically tolerable dose. The difficulties posed by drug-resistant cells, cells that shed or hide surface antigens, and by noncycling cells that can repair sublethal radiation damage are compounded by limited drug or antibody access due to variable blood supply (including partial blood-brain barrier effects) and the depressed metabolism and oxygen levels found within the tumor center. Of all available therapeutic modalities, surgery is the least affected by cellular heterogeneity, oxygen tension, capillary structure, or cell cycle kinetics. The central portions of the tumor that are inherently the most resistant to radiation and chemotherapy are also the simplest and safest to resect from a technical point of view. The concept of tumor heterogeneity gives new urgency to the need for reduced tumor burden prior to the application of other therapies. If, as we believe, all therapeutic modalities should be given in close physical and temporal coordination, then gentleness of surgical technique and optimization of the neurological status of the patient become absolute priorities of the therapeutic plan.

Support for the utility of radical resection for solid tumors is quite extensive in both the neurological and nonneurological literature. Solid tumors elsewhere in the body are rarely cured unless they can be completely excised at the initial operation [7]. In our own literature, the extent of surgical resection can be clearly related to the length of survival for meningioma, astrocytoma, and medulloblastoma (1, 11–13, 20). Even in the case of glioblastoma, there is a tendency for prolonged survival to be associated with more radical surgery. The evidence is based on a retrospective analysis of 603 cases in which extensive surgical resection, partial surgical resection, or simple biopsy was performed without subsequent irradiation or chemotherapy [21]. In another study of 98 glioblastoma patients, the length of survival correlated inversely with the amount of residual tumor present on the postoperative scan [2]. The positive impact of surgery on the quality of survival has been demonstrated by Shapiro [27], and the beneficial role of reoperation for glial tumors has been extensively discussed by us elsewhere [20, 25]. One can assume that the technical sophistication with which reoperation is carried out may have a great impact on the quality of survival in either a positive or negative sense. In primary procedures, the neurological status of patients tends to improve or stabilize after surgery, but this can be more difficult to accomplish in the face of other concomitant therapies and after repeated mechanical disturbance of the brain. Therefore, the laser and the microscope were introduced into glioma surgery in the hope of increasing the safety of radical resection in the context of combined modality therapy.

Surgical Technique

Successful extirpation of an intrinsic glial tumor without further increase in neurological deficit is a difficult neurosurgical exercise and cannot be achieved on a routine basis without attention to detail and seriousness of purpose. Optimal results are achieved when maximal resection of the tumor has been combined with minimal disturbance of the surrounding brain. The general condition of the patient, the presence or absence of specific neurological deficits, the prospect for useful recovery, and the precise location of the lesion all have considerable bearing on the selection of a specific operative approach. For example, a tumor located close to a cortical surface is generally attacked through that surface if the associated cortical function is already lost, the prospect for recovery is small, or the potential loss of function (e.g., quadrantanopia or weakness restricted to the distal leg) is considered justified by both patient and physician in view of the potential gains of the procedure. For most hemispheric neoplasms, the decision whether to approach to the tumor directly or by a paramedian route is fundamental in determining patient position and the design of an appropriate scalp incision and bone flap. These general considerations have been discussed elsewhere [21], and useful guides have been given to the location of the motor strip and the major language areas.

Although the operations are conducted through relatively large bone flaps, the cortical incisions are usually no more than 2 cm in length. These incision are always made perpendicular to the long axis of functional areas within the hemispheres. For example, when the cortical incision must be made in the vicinity of the motor strip, it should be drawn at an acute angle to a line extending back from the pterion at a 45 degree angle to the skull base, cutting across the motor homunculus at a single point.

The incision should always be drawn toward the motor strip and never along its long axis. This initial incision can be made with the laser, but we prefer to carry out the initial steps in the procedure with a two-point suction cautery and conventional microinstruments. The Scarff modification of the original Greenwood bipolar forceps combines the advantages of restricted bipolar coagulation with suction at the tips of a bayonet forceps that also can be used for grasping; as a consequence, the operator's other hand is free to hold another bayonet forceps, a microdissector, or microscissors. Although the initial subpial incision for lobectomies is made with the unaided eye, I prefer to use the operating microscope in making the small cortical incisions required for deep hemispheric work in critical areas. The suction of the two-point cautery is pinched off and the cautery used to paint the incision on the pial surface; the incision is opened with the no. 11 blade and large microscissors. The incision is deepened by spreading with the two-point forceps; no cortical plug is resected. Copper blades are attached to a Leyla self-retaining retractor, and the lips of the cortical incision are gently spread apart; the blades are always oriented parallel to the long axis of the incision, because a transverse orientation tends to cut into the brain and produce subpial hemorrhage. At this point, use of the operating microscope is absolutely essential, because a 5- to 8-cm tumor cannot be gently and safely removed through a 2-cm incision without it. Some deep lesions are better approached by microsurgical dissection through a sulcus so that no incision at all is made in the cortical crown of a gyrus [15].

The improved illumination provided by the microscope readily permits exploration of a large space through a narrow aperture and facilitates the delineation of edematous white matter from either a low-grade glioma or the peripheral fringe of a glioblastoma. Resection of the tumor must be restricted to those areas of tissue that are clearly abnormal by virtue of their altered consistency, texture, or color. Most soft tumors can be resected with just the large two-point suction cautery, a large microscissors for cutting coagulated blood vessels, and a large microfreer dissector for establishing planes. Firm areas in fresh oligodendrogliomas, calcified astrocytomas, or previously irradiated glioblastomas are best handled with the carbon dioxide laser. With the two-point suction cautery in one hand and the micromanipulator of the laser in the other, it is possible to gently and efficiently remove large tumors with a minimum loss of blood. The resection is always begun in the center of the tumor and carried out circumferentially towards the periphery. The details of the laser technique employed are described in the next section. As soon as edematous white matter is reached, fluid will be seen to glisten under the illumination of the microscope, and, in some areas, actual weeping of the tissue will be observed. Throughout the resection, the size of the cavity should be measured along its major axes and these measurements compared with radiographic determinations made by CT: it goes without saying that both the actual scans and the measurements should be immediately available on the x-ray viewbox of the operating theater.

At the conclusion of the resection, scrupulous hemostasis must be obtained through patient irrigation of the field and liberal use of the two-point cautery. The return from the irrigating fluid should be crystal clear prior to the use of oxidized cellulose or microfibrillary collagen to line the walls of the cavity. The oxidized cellulose should be laid down in thin wisps so as not to decrease the size of the resection cavity; because gelatin sponge swells and because it does not provide as satisfactory a surface for platelet adhesion, I tend to avoid leaving it in tumor resection beds. When the self-retaining retractor blades are removed, the two edges of the cortical incision should just come to rest against each other without any obvious holes or bruises in the cortical surface. At the conclusion of a transsulcal approach there should be no evidence of subpial hemorrhage. The dura is always closed in a watertight fashion, and the bone flap is secured with heavy silk sutures. The scalp is closed in multiple layers, and a closed drainage system is inserted into the subgaleal space.

Laser Technique

Use of the laser is generally reserved for those portions of the tumor that are unusually firm, calcified, or moderately vascular [22]. The longer and narrower the transcortical aperture required to reach the tumor, the more the laser and the microscope are employed. The majority of our cases have been performed with the laser coupled to the microscope; the joystick of the micromanipulator is held in one hand and the two-point suction cautery is held in the other. When the carbon dioxide laser is run at less than 30 W in the continuous mode or in most pulsed-mode sequences and the beam is aimed between the tips of the bipolar, the available suction is sufficient to keep the microsurgical field clear of vapor. Used in this way, the two-point suction cautery is readily available to seal vessels larger than 0.5 mm when these are revealed by laser dissection or inadvertently transsected by the beam. The suction cautery is also useful in gently clearing carbonized tumor and char from the surface of the resection bed and can quickly remove pieces of tumor that have been incised or softened by the beam. The simultaneous use of the laser and the two-point suction cautery enables the operator to maintain absolute control over visibility and blood loss while maximizing the speed of tissue removal at relatively low laser power.

Vaporization of the tumor is produced through the use of a defocused beam and a relatively rapid to-and-fro motion across the face of the tissue; the movement resembles that employed in the use of a high-speed drill when sculpting a cranioplasty or thinning a critical surface of bone. Because the attachment of the microslad to the undersurface of the microscope decreases the working distance available for hand-held instruments, it is necessary to use a 300-mm objective on the microscope and to defocus the beam by turning the lens wheel of the microslad to 400 mm. The effective working diameter of the laser beam is then approximately 1.2 mm, and this decreases the power density to 20 W to a level where the beam can be more safely used near critical structures. A cutting action is provided when the lens wheel is turned to 300 mm, and the beam is refocused to a spot size of 1 mm or less; special dissection techniques (detail below) also can be obtained by placing the laser in pulse mode.

During laser resection, all major vessels and cranial nerves are covered by wet cottonoid strips, and intermittent irrigation is employed to cool the working surface and loosen char. The suction of the two-point suction cautery can be supplemented by a microsucker held in the hand of an assistant or by the suction provided along the deep edge of special nonreflecting retractor blades designed for the self-retaining retractor. Inadvertent reflection of the laser beam may result in small areas of damage on the side of the field opposite to the shiny-surfaced instrument responsible for the "bounce." Beam-bounce can be eliminated through the use of instruments that are both blackened and roughened; a metal surface that is smooth but black may still reflect the laser. Of course, careful aiming, frequent use of the power pedal, and copious irrigation are the best protection against a misdirected beam. When instructing others in the use of the laser, the supervising surgeon must have control of the power pedal.

It is not widely appreciated that the gentleness and safety of laser technique in any tumor operation, but especially in deep hemispheric locations, depend as much on the thermal properties of the tissues as they do on the physical properties of the beam. The bioheat equation is a nonlinear description of the manner in which tissue temperature changes with time in response to heat conduction, heat convection, the injection of external thermal energy (i.e., the laser), and the influence of cellular metabolism. The bioheat equation for the brain can be written as follows:

$$\frac{\partial T}{\partial t} = \frac{K_b}{\sigma_b C_b} \nabla^2 T - \frac{\sigma_c}{C_b} f\, T + \frac{L(r,t)}{\sigma_b C_b} + W_b$$

where C_b, σ_b, and K_b are the specific heat, tissue density, and thermal conductivity of the brain and f is the cerebral blood flow.

Because tissue cooling by conductive means is relatively slow, and the heat produced by the metabolic work of the brain (W_b) is infinitesimal in comparison to the heat injected by the laser (L), the rate of temperature change in tissues at the edge of the laser beam is primarily determined by the rate of convective cooling or blood flow. Thermal cooling curves measured in human brain tumors indicate that these lesions are far less efficient at dissipating heat than are normal tissue [24]. When the laser is used in a pulsed mode or when it is moved rapidly over the surface of the tissue, blood flow in tissue subjacent to the plane of impact has an opportunity to provide tissue cooling; the ability of normal tissues to cool is greater than that of neoplastic tissues and may serve as an extra safety factor at the margin of the lesion. The surgeon must always remember, however, that tissue cooling by convective means can easily be overwhelmed by a stationary lasere beam because the half-time for cooling from a steady state temperature is approximately 1.5 minutes at a blood flow of 60 ml/100gm/minute [23]. Thermal injury is also efficiently prevented within the ventricle by the great heat capacity of the cerebrospinal fluid. Even a thin film of fluid over the thalamus or the head of the caudate nucleus can protect such structures from the action of the laser upon a nearby intraventricular tumor [7].

Clinical Results

Our clinical experience with laser surgery consists of 220 cases performed over a six-year period between October of 1980 and October of 1986 (Table 6-1). Laser-assisted operations for intrinsic brain tumors accounted for more than half of these procedures (56%), the majority being performed for the various grades of astrocytic tumors including glioblastoma multiforme. We recently published a statistical analysis of the first 3 years of this experience [26]. During the 36-month period, 421 operations for tumors of the brain and spinal cord were performed in our clinic. Of these 111 (26%) were carried out with the aid of the laser. To compare some of the salient features of the cases carried out with and without the laser, all of the laser charts were reviewed as well as 287 of the 310 nonlaser charts or 95% of the cases overall. The diagnostic categories in both series are tabulated in Table 6-2. The frequency of cranial tumors in both the laser and nonlaser series is approximately the same with the exception that pituitary tumors and metastatic tumors are much more frequent in the nonlaser series and the converse is true for melignant astrocytomas and posterior fossa tumors. In Table 6-3, a comparison is made between laser and nonlaser craniotomies; transsphenoidal and CT-guided stereotactic procedures have been specifically

TABLE 6-1. Laser Procedures, 1980–1986

Type of Tumor	No. of Cases
Astrocytoma	100
Meningioma	27
Metastatic brain tumor	14
Schwannoma	7
Medulloblastoma	10
Choroid plexus papilloma	4
Other gliomas	16
Pituitary adenoma	2
Chordoma	2
Craniopharyngioma	2
Other tumors	7
Spinal tumors	16
Syringotomy	11
Dorsal root entry zone lesions	2
Total	220

TABLE 6-2. Cranial Operations by Type of Tumor, 1980–1983

Histology	Laser Cases No.	Laser Cases %	Non laser cases No.	Non laser cases %
Astrocytoma, grades 3, 4	51	48.6	86	33.9
Meningioma	12	11.4	36	14.2
Astrocytoma, grades 1, 2	9	8.6	22	8.7
Metastatic brain tumor	7	6.7	31	12.3
Acoustic schwannoma	5	4.8	5	2.0
Medulloblastoma	4	3.8	4	1.6
Choroid plexus papilloma	4	3.8	1	0.4
Oligodendroglioma	2	1.9	5	2.0
Ependymoma	2	1.9	7	2.8
Hemangioblastoma	2	1.9	2	0.8
Pituitary adenoma	2	1.9	29	11.5
Ganglioglioma	2	1.9	0	0
Chordoma	1	1.0	1	0.4
Craniopharyngioma	0	0	4	1.6
Pinealoma	0	0	3	1.2
Dermoid/teratoma	0	0	5	2.0
Colloid cyst	0	0	3	1.2
Neuroblastoma	0	0	4	1.6
Lymphoma/sarcoma	0	0	3	1.2
Myeloma	0	0	1	0.4
Other	2	1.9	1	0.4
Total	105		253	

excluded from this analysis. There was no statistically significant difference in the mean estimated blood loss (637 vs 670 ml), the average length of stay (24.7 vs 23.8 days), the mortality rate (4.5% vs 5.6%), or the neurological morbidity rate (6.3% vs 5.6%) between laser and nonlaser cases, respectively. One significant finding was that the mean operative time was longer for laser cases (299 vs 238 minutes). The number of reoperations was also significantly greater in the laser series (63% vs 31.9%), and this was undoubtedly due to the greater percentage of malignant astrocytoma cases in the laser group.

Since our therapeutic philosophy in regard to the treatment of recurrent glial tumors certainly contributed to the high percentage of malignant astrocytoma cases in the laser group, a comparison was made between laser and nonlaser craniotomies for this tumor alone (Table 6-4). The difference in reoperation rate is even more extreme for this subgroup than for all tumors types. Fully 82% of the laser procedures for malignant astrocytoma were reoperations in comparison to 50% of the nonlaser cases ($\chi^2 = 13.6$; $p = 0.0002$). The mortality and morbidity rates were not significantly different in the two groups, but the length of stay for laser patients tended to be less. Once again, the operating time was significantly increased in laser cases and the estimated blood loss tended to be lower.

Since the period covered by our initial analysis, another three-year experience has been obtained, and, although the total number of laser procedures is about the same in each 36-month interval, the pattern of use appears to be changing (Table 6-5). Operations for astrocytoma, other glial tumors, and other intrinsic tumors represented 67% of the cranial laser procedures in the period from 1980 to 1983 and 62% in the second period from 1983 to 1986; the percentage of astrocytoma cases in each period was 57% and 47%, respectively. Never-

TABLE 6-3. Craniotomy for Tumor, 1980–1983

	Laser	Non Laser	χ^2/Z	p
No. cases	105	216		
No. reoperations	64(60.1%)	70(32.7%)	23.67	0.000001
Mortality	5(4.5%)	16(5.6%)	0.81	0.37
Mean operating time	299.3±123	237.6 ± 85.7	4.62	0.00001
Mean length of stay	24.7±17.1	23.87± 17.3	0.74	0.46
Mean estimated blood loss	637.9±756.5	670.7 ±771.8	0.36	0.72
Morbidity, CNS	7(6.3%)	12(5.6%)	0.21	1.07

TABLE 6-4. Craniotomy for Malignant Astrocytoma, 1980–1983

	Laser	Non Laser	χ^2/Z	p
No. cases	51	83		
No. reoperations	42(82.4%)	42(50.6%)	13.6	0.0002
Mortality	4(7.8%)	2(2.4%)	2.18	0.14
Mean operating time	246 ± 60.9	221 ± 60.2	2.32	0.02
Mean length of stay	21.3± 12.8	27.4± 21.7	2.05	0.04
Mean estimated blood loss	457 ±416.5	522 ±430.4	0.86	0.40
Morbidity, CNS	4(7.8%)	4(4.8%)	0.514	0.47

TABLE 6-5. Laser Operations

	No. Operations	
Type of Tumor	1980–1983	1983–1986
Astrocytoma	60	40
Meningioma	12	15
Metastatic brain tumor	7	7
Schwannoma	5	2
Medulloblastoma	4	6
Choroid Plexus Papilloma	4	0
Other gliomas	8	8
Pituitary adenoma	2	0
Chordoma	1	1
Craniopharyngioma	0	2
Other tumors	2	5
Spinal tumors	6	10
Syringotomy	0	11
Dorsal root entry zone tumors	0	2
Total	111	109

theless, the relative use of the carbon dioxide laser for cranial gliomas did decline in comparison to an increasing number of spinal procedures and meningioma resections. This does not appear to be a result of a change in operative philosophy on our part so much as a change in the surgical case mix.

Discussion

With the possible exception of the operating microscope, it is unlikely that the introduction of any single surgical instrument can ever be shown to affect such gross parameters of outcome as morbidity, mortality, length of stay, and average blood loss. It is not surprising, therefore, that no such differences can be detected for tumor cases carried out with and without the laser. Several authors have claimed to demonstrate a decrease in estimated blood loss [9, 14], but no series has ever employed the laser in a random manner. The highly selective nature of laser use is indicated by the somewhat different tumor histologies in the laser and nonlaser groups (see Table 6-2), the difference in the reoperation rate between the two series overall and for malignant astrocytoma alone (see Tables 6-3 and 6-4), and the fact that the laser was used in only 32% of the craniotomies and 26% of all tumor procedures. It can be argued, however, that since the laser was generally employed for the more difficult cases, any tendency for decreased blood loss, length of stay, and equivalent morbidity is supportive evidence for the effectiveness of the instrument. The tendency for longer operating times in laser cases (see Table 6-3 and 6-4) may reflect the difference in tumor difficulty as well as the painstaking nature of the surgical technique. Recurrent tumors often have a more ligenous feel to them, secondary to increased fibrosis, calcification, and radiation necrosis. Removal of such tumors from eloquent areas of the brain, already partially damaged by prior operations, is certainly facilitated by the microsurgical use of the carbon dioxide laser. Nevertheless, there is no way to quantitatively prove this without a randomized study. It should be emphasized that it is reoperation per se rather than the laser that contributes to longer survivals in some patients with malignant astrocytoma.

The first brain tumor exposed to laser irradiation was a glioblastoma multiforme, and the operation was performed with a ruby laser operating in the pulse mode [18]. Similarly, the initial neurosurgical application of the carbon dioxide laser occurred in a patient with a glioblastoma [16, 28]. By 1982, Heppner and Ascher had operated on 329 brain tumors with the laser, of which fully 107 were glioblastoms, 62 were astrocytomas, and only 89 were meningiomas, schwannomas, or metastatic brain tumors [10]. In their series, vaporization of the brain surface after resection of malignant astrocytomas did not appear to influence the recurrence rate over 5 years [10], and this result is consistent with the failure of either argon or carbon dioxide laser resection to improve the recurrence rate of the experimental 9L gliosarcoma in the rat [4].

On the other hand, numerous investigators have testified to the technical benefits afforded by laser surgery in difficult glioma cases [6, 8]. In the context of complex multimodality therapy for recurrent glioblastomas, a consecutive series of 40 patients subjected to reoperation with the laser and the microscope had a median survival of 37 weeks from the time of the second operation to either the third procedure or death [25]. This series demonstrated very low morbidity and mortality as well as a length of survival after reoperation identical to that obtained after conventional primary procedures and radiation. We feel that maximal surgical cytoreduction, when achieved with a minimum risk to life and neurological morbidity, offers the optimal conditions for the possible success of any adjuvant therapy. Shapiro has also emphasized the potential utility of reoperation as well as the relative lack of serious morbidity from modern glioma surgery [27]. The coupling of the laser to the operating microscope appears to be essential for safe and extensive removal of deep hemispheric tumors through narrow transcortical exposures on a repetitive basis.

Some authors have used nonquantitative means to assess the usefulness of laser techniques in glioma surgery. Perria compared 42 cases performed with the carbon dioxide laser during 1979 and 1980 with 42 conventional operations carried out before 1977 [14]. Of the 42 cases, 13 were meningiomas and only eight were glioblastomas; although the latter cases were performed with the laser coupled to the microscope, the usefulness of this approach was rated similar to that of the nonmicrosurgical use of the laser for meningiomas. In another clinical series, 18 of 80 surgeries using the carbon dioxide laser were carried out for gliomas, and the use of the laser was considered "helpful" in comparison to the "very helpful" rating given for its use in meningioma and acoustic schwannoma surgery [5]. Of course, the utility of an instrument for a particular tumor type can be judged by a wide variety of quantitative criteria including crude survival, morbidity, blood loss, and palliation within the context of other therapies.

Several investigators have claimed that the use of the carbon dioxide laser decreases operating time and blood loss while improving the extent of the resection of glioma patients. Such impressions either have been gleaned from relatively small experiences (i.e., seven glioblastomas and four astrocytomas out of a total tumor group of 25 cases) or have been based on studies with faulty statistical design [9, 14]. In one study the mean blood loss for eight glioblastomas removed with the laser was 544 ml and this was compared to a mean loss of 1150 ml for eight cases performed without the laser in an earlier era [14]. We were unable to statistically confirm these impressions of decreased blood loss and operating time; indeed, operating time with the laser was found to be uniformly increased for all tumor types, including malignant astrocytoma.

In conclusion, it is not possible to statistically demonstrate that the carbon dioxide laser is a necessary surgical adjunct for tumors of a specific histological type in any particular intracranial location. In our clinic, the laser was only employed in one-fourth of the procedures carried out for central nervous system tumors and was "essential" in only a fraction of this number. However, many of these procedures were re-operations carried out for malignant astrocytomas located in deep sites and near eloquent cortex. Sweeping claims in regard to the overall superiority of laser surgery cannot be supported by an analysis of such crude outcome measures as operative mortality, neurological morbidity, average length of stay, mean operating time, or estimated blood loss. As is probably true with any surgical instrument, the applicability of the laser to a particular tumor and the benefits derived from the use of this tool are highly dependent upon the individual vagaries of the clinical situation as well as the skills and judgment of the surgeon involved. Only the individual operator can determine whether the laser has helped him navigate through troubled water. Nevertheless, we firmly believe that the carbon dioxide laser and the microscope are valuable surgical adjuncts in the gentle extirpation of glial tumors from difficult locations and in circumstances (i.e., reoperation) in which tissue conditions have been impaired by prior and concomitant therapies.

References

1. Adegbite AB, Khan MI, Paine KWE, et al: The recurrence of intracranial meningioma after surgical treatment. *J Neurosurg* 58:51–56, 1983.
2. Andreou J, George AE, Wise A, et al: CT prognostic criteria of survival after malignant glioma surgery. *Am J Neuroradiol* 4:488–490, 1983.
3. Bigner DD: Biology of gliomas: Potential clinical implications of glioma cellular heterogeneity. *Neurosurgery* 9:320–326, 1981.
4. Edwards MSB, Boggan JE, Bolgerm CA, Davis RL: Effect of microsurgical and carbon dioxide and argon laser resection on recurrence of the intracerebral 9L rat gliosarcoma. *Neurosurgery* 14:52–56, 1984.
5. Edwards MSB, Boggan JE, Fuller TA: The laser in neurological surgery. *J Neurosurg* 59:555–556, 1983.
6. Fasano VA, Lombard GF, Ponzio RM: Preliminary experiences with the use of three lasers (CO_2, Nd:YAG, argon) in some posterior fossa tumors in childhood. *Childs Brain* 10:26–38, 1983.
7. Gastrointestinal Tumor Study Group: Adjuvant therapy of colon cancer: Results of a prospectively randomized trial. *N Engl J Med* 310:737–743, 1984.
8. Gongbai C, Qiwu X: Carbon dioxide laser vaporization of brain tumors. *Neurosurgery* 12: 123–126, 1983.
9. Hara M, Takeuchi J, Okada J, et al: Evaluation of brain tumor laser surgery. *Acta Neurochir (Wien)* 53:141–149, 1980.
10. Heppner F, Ascher PW: The CO_2 laser in neurosurgery. *Int Adv Surg Oncol* 5:385–396, 1982.
11. Laws ER, Taylor WF, Clifton MB, et al: Neurosurgical management of low-grade astrocytoma of the cerebral hemispheres. *J Neurosurg* 61:665–673, 1984.
12. Mirimanoff RO, Dosoretz DE, Linggood RM, et al: Meningioma: Analysis of recurrence and progression following neurosurgical resection. *J Neurosurg* 62:18–24, 1985.
13. Park TS, Hoffman HJ, Hendrick EB, et al: Medulloblastoma: Clinical presentation and management: Experience at the Hospital for Sick Children, Toronto, 1950–1980. *J Neurosurg* 58:543–552, 1983.
14. Perria C, Francaviglia N, Borzone M, et al: The value and limitations of the CO_2 laser in neurosurgery. *Neurochirurgia* (Stuttg) 26:6–11, 1983.
15. Pia HW: Microsurgery of gliomas. *Acta Neurochir* 80:1–11, 1986.
16. Polanyi TG, Bredemeier HC, Davis TW: A CO_2 laser for surgical research. *Med Biol Eng* 8: 541–548, 1970.
17. Robinson WL, Salcman M: Intraventricular tumors: Treatment with CO_2 laser. Presented at the Congress of Laser Neurosurgery III, Chicago, Il, May 1984.
18. Rosomoff HL, Carroll F: Reaction of neoplasm and brain to laser. *Arch Neurol* 14:143–148, 1966.
19. Salcman M: Biophysical rationale of hyperthermia for brain tumors—an update. Continuing Medical Education Program, 1985 Japan Neurosurgical Society (in press), 1986.
20. Salcman M: Resection and reoperation in neuro-oncology: Rationale and approach. *Neurol Clin* 3:831–842, 1985.
21. Salcman M: Supratentorial gliomas: Clinical

features and surgical therapy. In Wilkins RH, Rengachary SS (eds): *Neurosurgery*. New York McGraw-Hill, 1985, pp 579–590.

22. Salcman M: The use of the laser in neurological surgery. *Neurology and Neurosurgery, Updata Series* 5:2–8, 1985.
23. Salcman M, et al: Measurement of CBF by microwave-induced thermal clearance. (in preparation), 1986.
24. Salcman M, Samaras GM: Interstitial microwave hyperthermia for brain tumors: Results of a phase-1 clinical trial. *J Neuro-Oncol* 1:225–236, 1983.
25. Salcman M, Kaplan RS, Ducker TB, et al: Effect of age and reoperation on survival in the combined modality treatment of malignant astrocytoma. *Neurosurgery* 10:453–463, 1982.
26. Salcman M, Robinson W, Montgomery E: Laser microsurgery: A review of 105 intracranial tumors. *J Neuro-Oncol* 3:363–371, 1986.
27. Shapiro WR: The treatment of neuroectodermal brain tumors. *Ann Neurol* 12:231–237, 1982.
28. Stellar S, Polanyi TG, Bredemier HC: Experimental studies with the carbon dioxide laser as a neurosurgical instrument. *Med Biol Engng.* 8: 549–558, 1970.

7. TUMORS OF THE POSTERIOR FOSSA AND SKULL BASE IN ADULTS

Jon H. Robertson
W. Craig Clark

Posterior fossa tumors

Posterior fossa tumors in adults may be subdivided into those related to the cerebellum and those in the cerebellopontine angle (CPA). The most common cerebellar tumors are astrocytomas and hemangioblastomas, followed by meningiomas. Because both astrocytomas and hemangioblastoma are best resected using techniques other than the laser, this portion of the discussion will necessarily concentrate on meningiomas. Medulloblastomas are primarily a pediatric tumor and are discussed in Chapter 8.

The acoustic neuroma is the most common of all CPA lesions; in most series of CPA tumors acoustic tumors comprise about two-thirds [16]. Meningiomas comprise 3% to 13% of all CPA tumors and are second only to acoustic neuromas in this location [2, 19, 26]. Other more rare lesions include epidermoid tumors (2%–6%) [2, 32], schwannomas of other cranial nerves (2%) [17], and arachnoid cysts (1%) [2, 28].

CEREBELLAR CONVEXITY MENINGIOMAS

These tumors usually constitute about 8% of the posterior fossa meningiomas. They are usually found in close proximity to the transverse sinus and may be attached to the torcular Herophili [23]. If tumor involvement occurs on the non-dominant side or if the sinus is occluded by tumor, the sinus usually can be resected if necessary. The full extent of any venous sinus involvement is routinely ascertained with pre-operative arteriography.

The tumors are approached through a routine suboccipital craniectomy whose superior border is the transverse sinus. The dura is opened and reflected upward on the sinus. Great care should be taken in this maneuver in case the tumor is adherent to the dura of the sinus. If the tumor is merely adherent to the sinus, it is removed as described earlier for parasagittal tumors (Chapter 5). If it is adherent only to the dura, the dura is removed along with the tumor mass, and a free graft of pericranium or fascia lata femoris is placed. In cases where the tumor is extremely adherent to both the dura and the tumor bed in the cerebellar hemisphere, an internal decompression is carried out as described previously to allow the tumor and its dural attachment to be evaporated and folded inward on itself. This facilitates both exposure and microdissection of the capsule from the cerebellum. A careful, watertight closure of the dura, combined with meticulous hemostasis and closure of the wound, completes the procedure.

CPA TUMORS

There are a variety of approaches to CPA tumors that may be utilized under certain circumstances. These include translabyrinthine, subtemporal-

Robertson, J.H. and Clark, W.C. (eds), Lasers in Neurosurgery.

transtentorial, translabyrinthine-transtentorial, suboccipital-transmeatal, and translabryinthine-suboccipital [6–10, 12–14, 24, 31, 33]. The pros and cons of these various approaches remain an item of controversy, and a discussion of this can be found elsewhere [5, 29]. Generally speaking, we prefer a translabyrinthine approach for all but the largest tumors when audition is not functional. The suboccipital-transmeatal approach is utilized when an attempt will be made to conserve hearing (i.e., tumor <2.5 cm, speech discrimination score $\geqslant 50\%$, and no more than 50 dB hearing loss) or when the tumor is larger. A combined approach may be used in the largest of tumors. Acoustic tumor removal will be described using all three approaches. CPA meningiomas are usually removed through a standard suboccipital approach.

ACOUSTIC NEUROMAS

The acoustic neuroma is a benign tumor primarily formed of Schwann cells investing the vestibular nerve. In spite of its name, it is this origin on the vestibular nerve and not the auditory nerve that allows the preservation of hearing in some cases. Although an acoustic neuroma arises from the vestibular nerve, more than 70% of patients with an acoustic neuroma note hearing loss as the initial symptom. Further, by the time medical attention is sought, hearing loss is present in over 95% of patients [1, 11, 21].

Within the past decade, computed tomography (CT) has advanced to the point where a plain and contrast-enhanced CT scan confirm the diagnosis in a majority of cases. When the tumor is small, CO_2-CT cisternography may

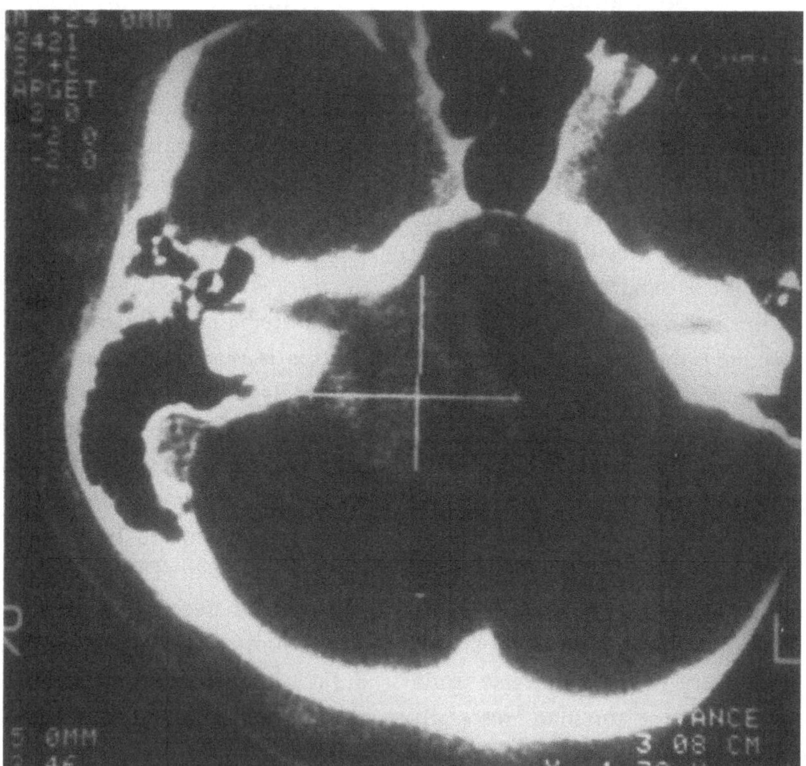

A

FIGURE 7-1. (A) Contrast enhanced, high-resolution CT scan showing the typical appearance of an acoustic neuroma. (B) CT appearance of a partially cystic acoustic neuroma. (C) CO_2CT cisternogram showing how gas enhancement caps the intracanalicular acoustic tumor at the level of the porus acousticus.

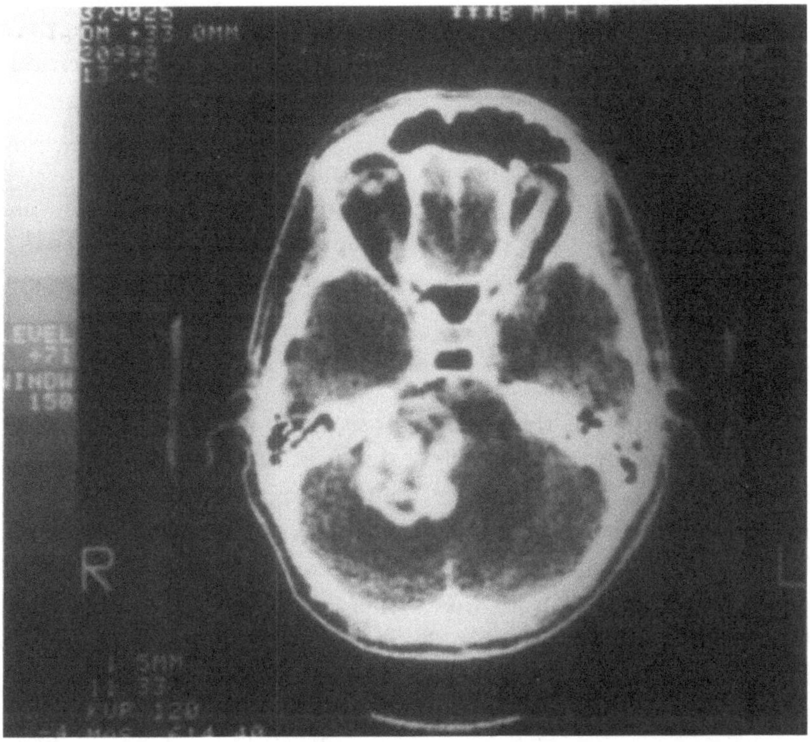

B

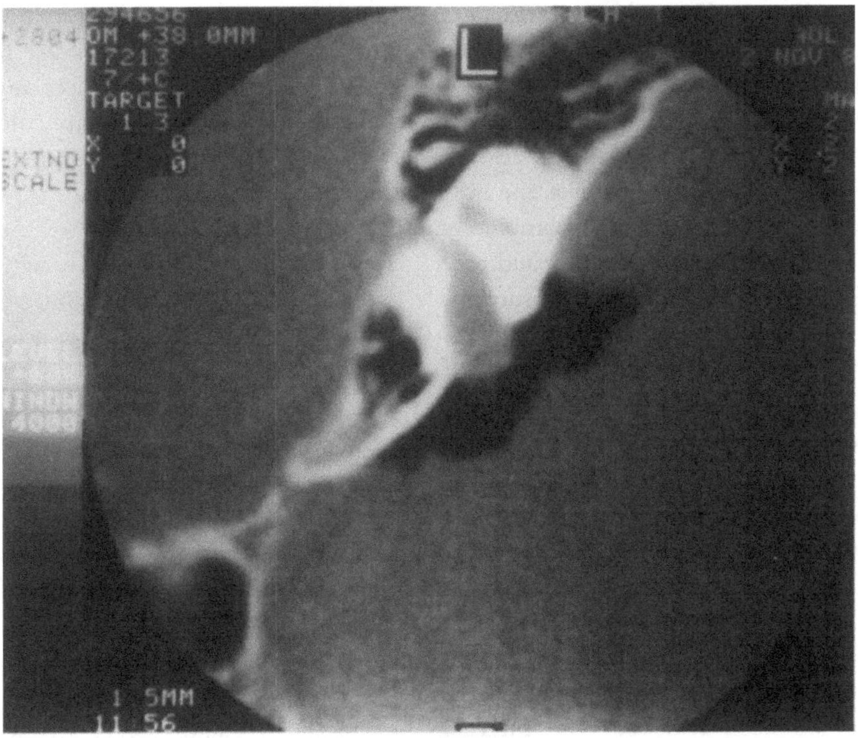

C

greatly aid the diagnosis [4], since magnetic reasonance imaging (MRI) is still not universally available. When it is available, MRI may replace both the CT scan and CO_2-CT cisternography because of its increased sensitivity and lack of bone artifact in the posterior fossa (Figure 7-1A, B, C).

Translabyrinthine Approach. An incision is made 3 cm posterior to the auricular fold, extending from above the auricle to just short of the mastoid process. Soft tissue is retracted and elevated. A simple mastoidectomy is then performed. If exposure is limited by a constricted mastoid space, the sigmoid sinus is skeletonized, the adjacent dura elevated medially from the overlying bone anterior and posterior to the sinus, and the sinus then depressed from the operative field with bone wax. A labyrinthectomy is done with removal of otic capsule from over the three semicircular canals and the vestibule. The tympanic segment of the facial nerve is skeletonized.

The superior vestibular nerve canal is skeletonized, using the ampullae and cribriform areas of the horizontal and superior semicircular canals as landmarks. The dura of the canal is skeletonized by removal of the adjacent bone superior, posterior, and inferior to the internal auditory canal. Bone is also removed from over the posterior fossa dura. Care is taken to completely remove the bone overlying the internal auditory canal and CPA, so as to provide exposure for tumor removal. Particular care is taken in removing bone from above the most lateral end of the internal auditory canal [10].

The dura surrounding the internal auditory canal is opened with a defocused carbon dioxide laser beam. The subarachnoid cistern next to the inferior pole of the tumor is incised, and cerebrospinal fluid is released in order to further decompress the posterior fossa structures.

A continuous, defocused laser beam is used to cavitate the tumor mass. When most of the tumor mass has been removed, the internal auditory canal dura is incised. The most lateral fibers of the superior vestibular nerve are identified first. These fibers are elevated from the underlying bone of the vertical crest of the internal auditory canal. Immediately beneath this bony structure, the facial nerve is seen. The incision is now completed in the dura overlying the internal auditory canal, and the tumor occupying the canal is exposed. This residual tumor and the attached vestibular nerve are carefully elevated from the underlying facial nerve.

Suboccipital Approach. A variety of incisions and skin flaps have been described for this approach, but we prefer a paramedian, lazy S-shaped incision centered over the mastoid groove. The craniectomy is extended to the transverse sinus superiorly, the lateral sinus laterally, and the foramen magnum inferiorly. Sufficient bone is removed medially to allow good visualization of the tumor. The dura is then opened with a Y-shaped incision and the cerebellar cisterns are entered to obtain release of cerebrospinal fluid and cerebellar relaxation. The cerebellum is gently retracted with a self-retaining retractor in order to expose the tumor. We have generally found it unnecessary to resect any of the cerebellum in achieving adequate tumor exposure.

The lower cranial nerves are first identified and dissected from the tumor capsule. They are protected with Gelfoam or wet cottonoids. The tumor capsule is evaporated with a defocused laser beam, and an intracapsular decompression is carried out. Because of the unique protective function of water to absorb and prevent dissipation of the heat generated by absorption of the carbon dioxide laser, it is important to isolate cranial nerves or vital blood vessels in the operative field with Gelfoam or wet cottonoids. Surface vessels on the tumor capsule may be coagulated with the biploar cautery or a defocused laser beam. Vessels larger than a millimeter in diameter are best managed with bipolar cautery.

The need to cavitate a tumor is dependent upon the size and ease of separation of tumor from the surrounding structures of the CPA. If

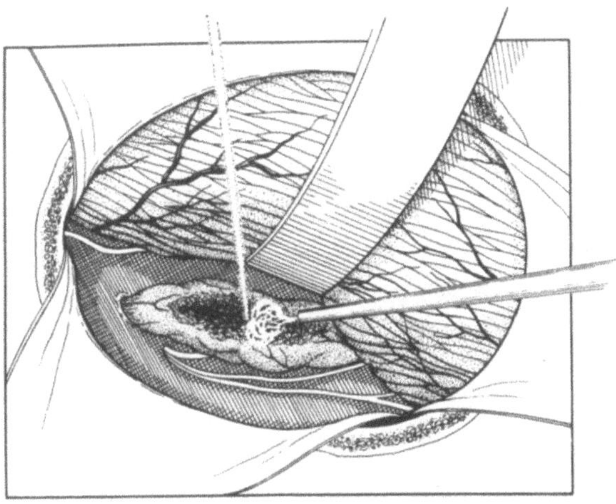

FIGURE 7-2. Carbon dioxide laser cavitation of tumor body. This debulking facilitates mobilization of the tumor capsule.

the inferior, medial, and superior surfaces of tumor are not well visualized, the tumor should be internally decompressed. The ease of resecting the internal mass of an acoustic tumor will vary with the tissue consistency and vascularity. The carbon dioxide laser allows rapid vaporization of the interior of the tumor with continuous coagulation (Figure 7-2). The smoke of vaporized tissue and the charred surface debris are easily removed with continuous suction-irrigation.

The amount of laser energy used in cavitating an acoustic tumor will vary depending upon the size of the tumor and the preference of the surgeon. We have preferred a high-energy (50–80 W), defocused laser beam, which quickly guts the tumor, whether it is solid or cystic. Obviously, less energy (20–40 W) would be used in a small tumor and as the capsule of the tumor is approached during the internal decompression.

The method of applying the carbon dioxide laser beam is critical in obtaining the desired effect. In cavitating the tumor, the laser beam is used in a continuous fashion, controlled by stepping on a foot pedal to activate the laser. Depending on the level of energy, the laser beam is moved slowly or rapidly in a sweeping motion to "paint" the exposed surface of tumor. As vaporization of the tumor proceeds, coagulation of the majority of the tumor vessels is evident. If larger vessels in the substance of the tumor are encountered, bipolar cautery is used. Continuous suction-irrigation is used to prevent unwanted spreading of thermal effects.

The effect of the carbon dioxide laser occurs at the tissue surface. The problem with controlling the depth of laser energy penetration at higher wattage levels, as seen with other lasers, is not encountered. Whether a focused, low-energy or a defocused, high-energy laser beam is used, rapid movement of the beam in a continuous fashion will prevent deep vaporization and unwanted tissue penetration [26].

Cavitation of the tumor allows room to begin separation of the tumor capsule from the adjacent structures of the CPA. If an arachnoidal plane provides easy dissection, the capsular vessels of the tumor are coagulated with the bipolar cautery as the capsule is freed. Microdissection proceeds with blunt dissection of the capsule away from the major blood vessels, the brainstem, and the cranial nerves. In small and moderate size tumors that are gutted with the carbon dioxide laser, the tumor capsule may shrink away from the surrounding structures. This may be due to the thermal effect of laser energy and assists in capsule dissection and preservation of anatomical planes.

However, if the tumor capsule is densely adherent to the elements of CPA, the carbon dioxide laser allows vaporization of the tumor capsule with minimal trauma. To remove tumor or capsule precisely without injury to the structure to which it is attached, a focused, low-energy laser beam (4–8 W) is applied in pulsed bursts at a duration of a fraction of a second (Figure 7-3). The precise thermal effect attained with the carbon dioxide laser can be limited to a 1-mm surface area and may be diminished further by the application of water.

A thin, fragile facial nerve with that last bit

of tumor capsule attached can often become a lost nerve because of trauma exerted in blunt microdissection. The ability to remove fragments of tumor or capsule without pulling or picking bluntly offers hope for preserving the anatomical continuity of the vital structures found in the CPA. The unique effect observed with removal of tumor by the carbon dioxide laser is not possible with other techniques currently used.

In removing the portion of the tumor that extends into the internal auditory canal, the dura mater over the posterior rim of the canal is coagulated and curetted before bone drilling. The exposure of the tumor within the canal and the neural elements may be performed before or after the tumor mass in the CPA has been internally decompressed, depending upon the size of the tumor.

The use of the carbon dioxide laser for this stage of acoustic tumor surgery is not recommended because of the difficulty in controlling the thermal effect while removing bone. The dura mater of the petrous bone covering the posterior rim of the canal can be coagulated with the laser. However, a higher level of carbon dioxide laser energy is required in bone removal, with spread of thermal energy. Visualization and protection of the contents of the internal auditory canal with wet cottonoids is not possible until the posterior rim of the canal has been removed. For these reasons, we have continued to expose the involved portion of the canal by using a high-speed surgical drill with continuous irrigation, exercising great care at the lateral extent of the canal.

Combined Approach. If additional exposure is necessary at any point, the inferior end of the skin incision can be extended posteriorly, making it possible to elevate more completely the soft tissue from over the suboccipital. The previously applied bone wax is removed from the sigmoid sinus. The dura of the suboccipital is exposed with the use of bone-biting rongeurs. A cruciate incision is made in the dura, the dural edges raised, and traction sutures placed.

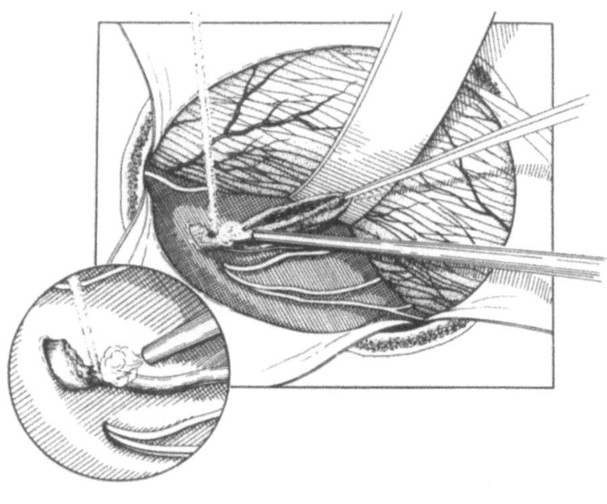

FIGURE 7-3. Precise removal of tumor fragments from the facial nerve.

Using the carbon dioxide laser as described above, the posterior tumor mass is removed. The surgeon may remove tumor from an angle anterior to the sigmoid sinus or from an angle posterior to the sinus by rotation of the operating table. Moist sponges are used throughout the procedure to protect the sigmoid sinus. When most of the posterior tumor mass is removed, final tumor resection is completed along with the tumor that is in the internal auditory canal [10].

MENINGIOMAS (CPA)

Meningiomas arising along the posterior surface of the petrous bone adjacent to the porus acusticus in the CPA comprise 40% of the posterior fossa meningiomas. They cause symptoms similar to those associated with acoustic neuromas and cannot be distinguished with assurance on clinical findings alone [18]. The more recent use of high resolution CT and MRI have greatly aided this differential, with meningiomas tending to show less erosion of the porus and being closely applied and contiguous with the dura overlying the petrous ridge (Figure 7-4). Other signs that aid in this differential are the ten-

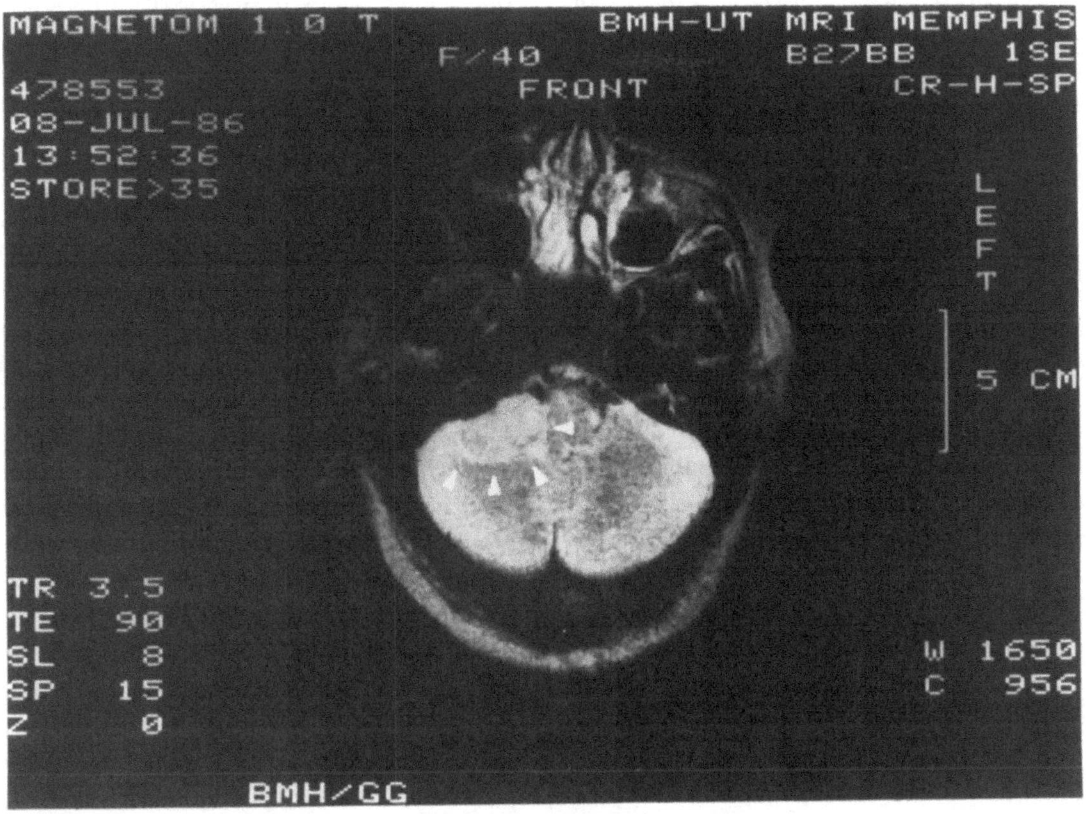

FIGURE 7-4. Magnetic resonance scan showing a small CPA meningioma at the anterior lip of the porus acusticus.

dencies for meningiomas to show less marked elevations of the cerebrospinal fluid protein [23] and more common involvement of the fifth and lower four cranial nerves [18].

The surgical approach most often used for these tumors is the standard suboccipital craniectomy as described earlier for use in the removal of acoustic tumors. Basically, the craniectomy is extended to the transverse sinus superiorly, the lateral sinus laterally, and the foramen magnum inferiorly. The dura is then opened with a Y-shaped incision, and the cerebellar cisterns are entered to obtain release of cerebrospinal fluid and cerebellar relaxation. The cerebellum is gently retracted with a self-retaining retractor to expose the tumor. We have generally found it unnecessary to resect any of the cerebellum in achieving adequate tumor exposure.

The lower cranial nerves are first identified and dissected from the tumor capsule. They are protected with Gelfoam or wet cottonoids. The tumor capsule is evaporated with a defocused laser beam, and an intracapsular decompression is carried out as previously described. The amount of power used is based on the texture of the tumor and the surgeon's personal preferences. However, we have found that tough, fibrous tumors and those with calcification generally require from 40 to 80 W of defocused carbon dioxide laser power to aggressively proceed with the debulking of the tumor mass. A word of caution is in order since the amount of power and duration of application of the beam must be decreased as the opposite capsular wall is approached. Further, important structures such as the anterior inferior cerebellar artery (AICA) and the facial nerve may be displaced in almost any direction, or completely concealed by the tumor. This displacement is usually far more variable than that seen with acoustic neuromas [17], even though these structures are usually extracapsular. Routine electromyographic monitoring and direct facial nerve stimulation are used in an effort to preserve facial function.

Once the internal decompression is completed, a thin capsule is all that remains. The capsular wall is carefully involuted and contiguous structures are dissected off the capsule. The tumor capsule is coagulated with bipolar cautery as mobilization proceeds. If the laser is used to vaporize the capsule, the operator should protect the structures that have been dissected free with Gelfoam or wet cottonoids.

TENTORIUM CEREBELLI MENINGIOMAS

Meningiomas of the tentorium comprise 30% of posterior fossa meningiomas. These tumors commonly invade the venous sinuses and may extend above as well as below the tentorium [22] (Figure 7-5A, B). Castellano and Riggiero analyzed Olivercrona's series of meningiomas and concluded that tentorial meningiomas are best removed from above whether they present on the superior or inferior surface of the tentorium It is now probably more reasonable to conclude that the approach to these tumors should be individualized, based on the location of the main mass of the tumor. Small tumors growing downward into the posterior fossa are best reached by a subtemporol-occipital approach with tentorial splitting. Tentorial meningiomas with a large element in the posterior fossa or those involving the posterior petrous ridge are better reached by a combined supratentorial and infratentorial approach [17].

The skin incision is begun about 6 cm above the ear and again is extended in an S-shaped fashion centered over the mastoid groove. The inferior portion of the incision in the neck is outlined, prepared, and draped so the incision can be extended as far inferiorly as needed to achieve adequate exposure. Initially a temporo-occipital free bone flap is elevated, with additional bone removed as necessary to allow flat, direct access over the petrous bone to the tentorium. The dural flap is based on the lateral sinus to avoid interrupting bridging veins before they are well exposed. Occipital bridging veins are coagulated with bipolar forceps and cut well away from the dura and lateral sinus. The occipital lobe is gently retracted a little further to expose the tentorium and the incisura. If no tumor is visible, gentle palpation with microinstruments will often reveal the location of the tumor arising from the underside of the tentorium. The tentorium is then incised well away from the tumor attachment and the lateral sinus, with hemostasis usually possible with bipolar coagulation. It is occasionally necessary to use metallic clips, but they are not routinely required. The tentorium is then further opened using a low-power, defocused laser beam and bipolar coagulation. Extension of the opening is carried forward to the incisura and posteriorly to the transverse sinus. Care must be taken not to injure the trochlear nerve at the incisura or the transverse sinus at the posterior aspect of the incision. This then results in an opening into the CPA from above and may suffice for tumor removal, provided the tumor is not large. If there is a large extension into the CPA or if the tumor arises from the posterior surface of the petrous ridge, the incision should be extended and a suboccipital craniectomy performed as described earlier in the discussion of CPA meningiomas.

Once the tumor is exposed, an internal decompression is performed with the defocused laser beam, with great care exercised not to place the brainstem or the cranial nerves under compression or traction by manipulating the tumor. Even though there is a higher incidence of meningiomas of the angioblastic variety in this region, we have not yet encountered one where hemostasis could not be achieved by alternately using the carbon dioxide laser and bipolar coagulation. Because of this increased incidence of angioblastic meningiomas, the neodymium:yttrium-aluminium-garnet (Nd:YAG)

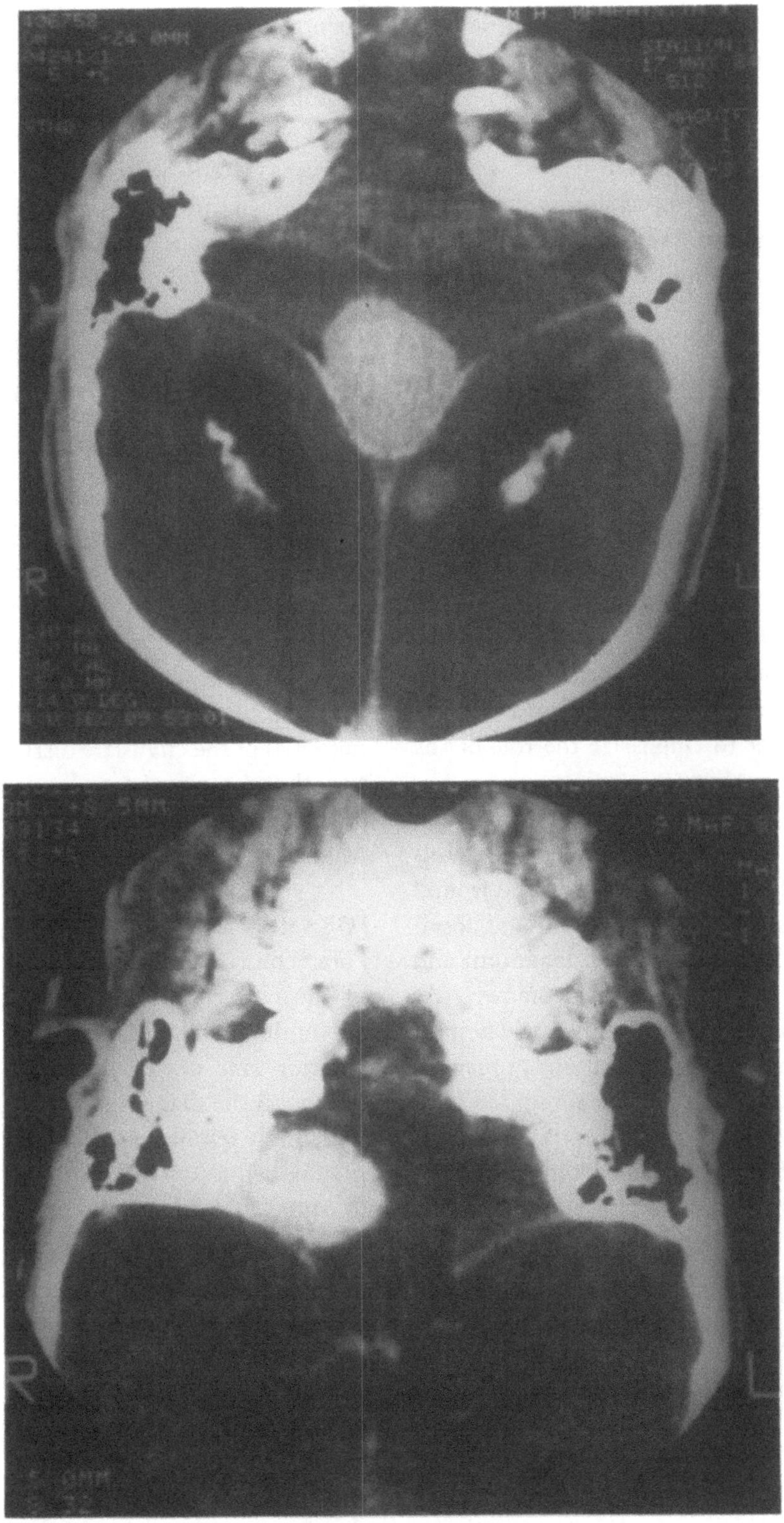

FIGURE 7-5. (Top) CT appearance of a tentorial meningioma in axial section. (Bottom) A coronal CT demonstrating the tentorial orgin of a meningioma.

laser would at least have theoretical advantages due to its superior hemostatic abilities (see Chapter 4). However, great caution would be in order as a result of its decreased precision and widespread heating effects in the proximity of the brainstem and cranial nerves.

Once the internal decompression is complete, the capsule should be sufficiently pliable to allow it to be folded inward on itself, allowing the operator to avoid retracting on the brainstem or cranial nerves. The residual pieces of capsule may be removed piecemeal by microdissection or laser evaporation.

Skull Base Tumors

Tumors of the skull base may constitute one of the more difficult and challenging areas facing the neurosurgeon. A complete exposition regarding these lesions is beyond the scope of this text. However, a few selected lesions will be presented in order to emphasize the role of the laser in their management.

Some of the tumors usually classified as tumors of the skull base include sellar, juxtasellar, and parasellar lesions; lesions of the frontal fossa, temporal bone, and infratemporal fossa; lesions of the clivus and foramen magnum; and lesions of the jugular fossa and foramen. As mentioned earlier, the laser is only rarely helpful in pituitary tumors, and applications in planum sphenoidale and tuberculum meningiomas have already been described (see Chapter 5). The laser is used in the management of glomus jugulare tumors only when these lesions are large. This discussion will concentrate on tumors of the clivus and foramen magnum.

CLIVUS LESIONS

The primary diagnostic considerations in lesions of the clivus are meningiomas and chordomas. This is usually a fairly straightforward differentiation based on the tendency of chordoma to infiltrate bone. Clivus meningiomas are theoretically susceptible to surgical removal and cure.

Clivus meningiomas account for 10% of all posterior fossa meningiomas [23]. In a series reported before the use of microsurgical techniques, 16 of 29 patients with clivus meningioma died within 2 weeks of operation, and the 1-year survival after diagnois was 25% [3]. A more recent series has been reported that utilized an inventive transection of the nondominant venous sinus at the junction of the lateral and sigmoid sinuses and the tentorium to expose the clivus and achieve complete removal in many [16]. The clivus meningiomas may be approached in a variety of ways. These include the transclival approach through either a transseptal or sublabial incision, a transtentorial approach through the middle fossa, or approaches through the posterior fossa.

Regardless of the approach selected, removal is carried out as with other meningiomas, by first performing a careful internal decompression with the defocused laser beam. The removal is then completed as previously described. Meningiomas of the clivus are distinctly uncommon, and the clinician must be ever aware of the possibility of this lesion in order to make the diagnosis [10].

FORAMEN MAGNUM MENINGIOMAS

Foramen magnum meningiomas account for 8% of the posterior fossa meningiomas [23]. The site of dural attachment is most often along the anterior rim of the foramen magnum [15]. Although the diagnosis is most often confirmed with high resolution CT, preoperative arteriography delineates the relationship of the tumor to the vertebral artery, and MRI shows the direction and degree of brainstem and spinal cord displacement.

A midline incision extends from the level of the inion to about C_3. A wide craniectomy is performed to completely expose the inferior portion of the cerebellar tonsils; the incision is extended to expose the spinal cord down to about C_2-C_3. The dura is opened with a Y-shaped incision and retracted with sutures. Cerebellar relaxation is obtained by removal of cerebrospinal fluid from the cistern. The entrance of the vertebral artery into the intrathecal space is identified by finding the uppermost dentate ligament. The upper cervical and spinal accessory nerves are identified and protected. The tumor is cavitated using a defocused laser beam as described previously. The capsule is collapsed and mobilized with bipolar cautery. Microdissection defines the anatomical limits for tumor removal. Intraoperative monitoring with somatosensory evoked potentials has been helpful.

GLOMUS JUGULARE TUMORS

Glomus tumors are the most common neoplasms of the middle ear and second only to acoustic tumors as the most common tumors in the temporal bone. They may initially occur from the second to the eighth decade and are six times more common in women than men, with the duration of symptoms prior to diagnosis ranging from 1 month to 28 years. Characteristically, they occur predominately in middle-aged women [25].

High-resolution CT is now considered the primary radiological modality for evaluation of glomus jugulare tumors. If the jugular plate is eroded or if a lesion presents with neurological signs, the limits of the lesion are defined by axial and coronal CT, and arteriography is performed to confirm the diagnosis, determine the arterial feeders, assess the patency of the jugular vein and sigmoid sinus, and assess for possible embolization (Figure 7-6A, B). Because the evaluation of the bony anatomy plays such a key role in the neuroradiological assessment of glomus jugulare tumors, it is presently unclear what role MRI may play. For the present, high-resolution CT remains the methodology of choice.

Surgical Resection. Our surgical technique has been reported previously [25]. Although this technique is unchanged in principle, certain modifications have been incorporated and will be outlined here.

The surgical procedure consists of three phases: (1) exposure of the base of the skull through the neck; (2) exposure of the tumor within the temporal bone and jugular fossa; and (3) removal of the tumor and closure of the wound. It should be emphasized that we continue to feel that tumors of the glomus jugulare should be managed by a surgical team consisting of neurosurgeon, otologist, and otolaryngologist [25].

SKULL BASE EXPOSURE. A postauricular incision is extended into the neck (Figure 7-7), skin flaps are elevated, and the ear canal transected at the bony-cartilaginous junction. Cartilage is resected from the membranous ear canal and the meatus closed permanently. The facial nerve is identified at the stylomastoid foramen and followed distally to its second bifurcation. A large musculoperiosteal flap consisting of the temporal muscle, mastoid periosteum and subcutaneous tissue, and the sternocleidomastoid muscle is outlined so that it is based inferiorly and maintained for later use in closure. The tip of the mastoid is resected, with special care taken not to injure the facial nerve.

The neurovascular structures of the upper neck are identified. The soft tissue along the base of the skull between the posterior end of the digastric groove to the lateral lip of the jugular foramen is resected along with the styloid process and attached tendons. The posterior three-fourths of the bony circumference of the jugular foramen is freed of soft tissue attachments. The tip of the lateral process of the first cervical vertebra is resected if necessary for exposure. If the tumor is large, the soft tissue is elevated from the glenoid fossa, and the condyle of the mandible is retracted anteriorly.

TEMPORAL BONE EXPOSURE. A simple, well-beveled mastoidectomy is performed with a high-speed drill and suction-irrigation. The mastoid and tympanic segments of the facial nerve are skeletonized. The posterior bony canal wall is removed. All bone is removed from the facial nerve, which is elevated from the facial canal, extending from the geniculate ganglion to the stylomastoid foramen. At the stylomastoid foramen, continuity is established with

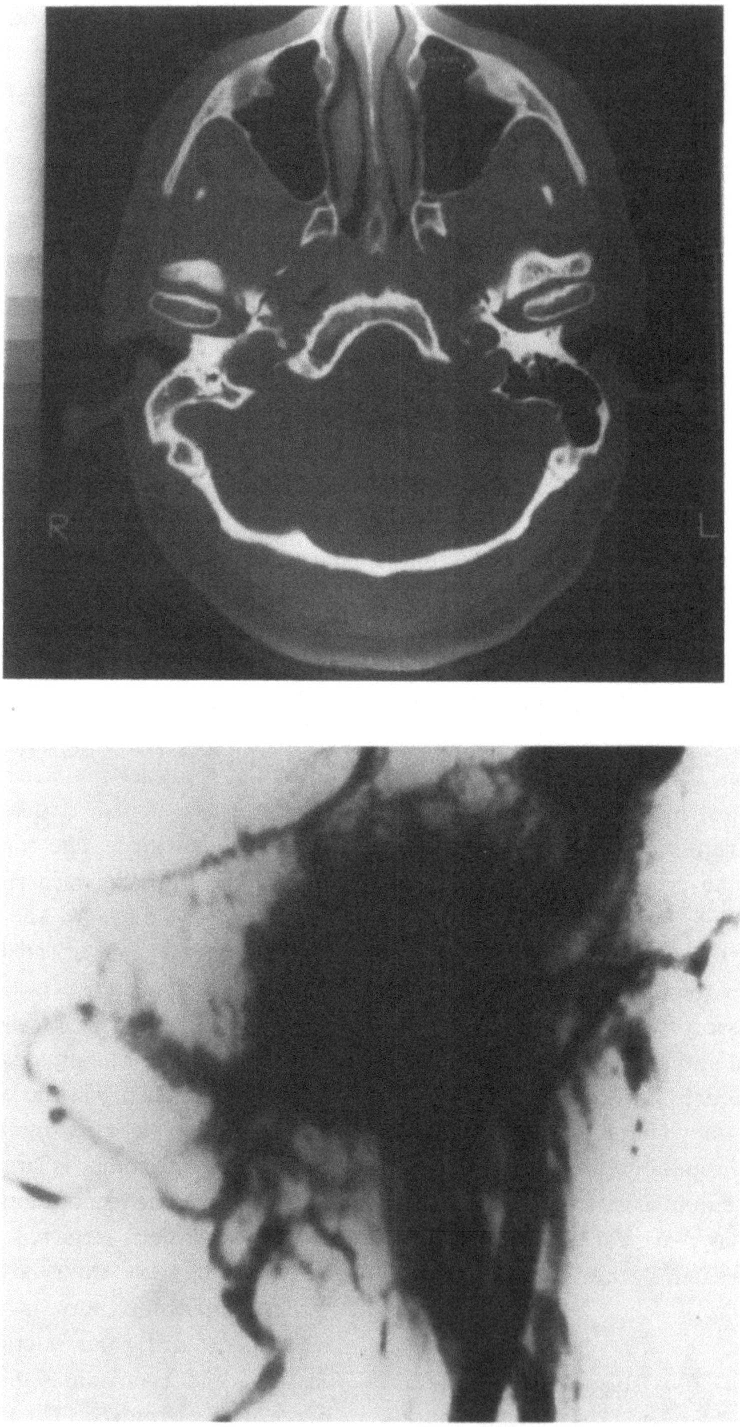

FIGURE 7-6. (Top) High-resolution CT scan showing a normal, intact jugular plate (on *left*) and an eroded jugular plate (*right*) in a case of glomus jugulare tumor. (Bottom) Typical angiographic appearance of glomus jugulare tumor seen with selective external carotid artery catheterization.

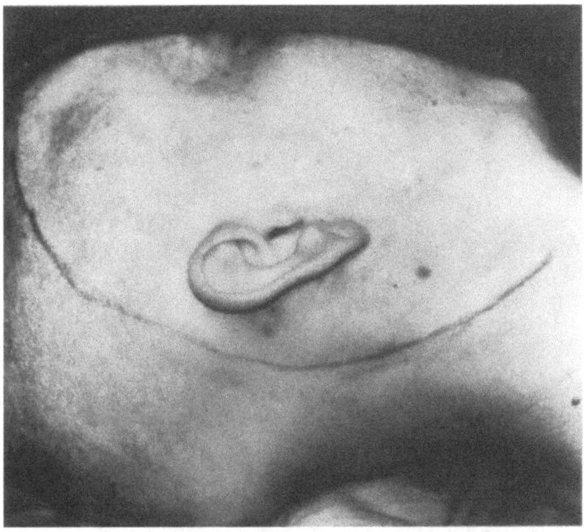

FIGURE 7-7. Surgical incision. Note the extension of the incision into the neck.

the earlier nerve dissection. A tangential groove is drilled through the bone of the anterior epitympanum to soft tissue depth as described by Fisch [8]. The facial nerve is then transposed anteriorly into this groove and distally along the substance of the parotid gland, and sutured permanently in this position.

The sigmoid sinus is skeletonized, with the adjacent posterior fossa dura exposed anteriorly and posteriorly to the sigmoid. Using the skull-base exposure already achieved, the bone of the base of the skull is removed between the posterior end of the digastric groove and the jugular foramen until soft tissue is reached, thereby skeletonizing the tumor mass or the jugular bulb. Care is taken to avoid entering the cochlea or semicircular canals unless sensorineural function has been lost.

Anteriorly, the bony anterior wall of the tympanum and hypotympanum is removed. In large tumors the bone of the glenoid fossa may also be removed to more fully expose the internal carotid artery. The internal carotid artery is skeletonized from the level of the carotid foramen inferiorly to the genu of the artery adjacent to the cochlea and eustachian tube. The horizontal segment of the carotid may be skeletonized if necessary for exposure. The tumor mass in the middle ear is mobilized inferiorly in continuity with the primary mass in the hypotympanum. The tympanic membrane and bony meatal skin are included in the resection. The stapes is carefully protected.

A variety of methods for ligation of the sigmoid sinus have been described. We currently pass a silk ligature through the dura adjacent to and around the sigmoid sinus. The sinus is doubly ligated and divided. The internal jugular vein is ligated and divided in the neck. Care must be taken during ligation that the ligatures are placed beyond any tumor extension that is present within the sinus or venous lumen.

TUMOR REMOVAL. The lateral wall of the sigmoid sinus is resected from the point of sinus ligation to the junction with the tumor or bulb. Working alternately from below and above, the tumor is mobilized. Very careful dissection is required in elevating the tumor from the medial wall of the jugular fossa and away from cranial nerves. Either the carbon dioxide or the Nd:YAG laser may occasionally be useful in the removal of large tumor masses (Figure 7-8). Bleeding from the inferior petrosal sinus is controlled by direct packing with oxidized regenerated cellulose (Surgicel) and bone wax.

Larger tumors often are attached to the internal carotid artery and may extend into the posterior fossa. Frequently, dura may have been pushed medially by the tumor and may be preserved as the intracranial portion of the tumor is removed, thereby minimizing the risk of postoperative cerebrospinal fluid leakage. Less frequently there is no layer of dura between the tumor and the contents of the posterior fossa.

The eustachian tube is then closed, and the facial nerve is maintained in its new anterior location. Fat from the abdominal wall is placed into the surgical defect. The previously prepared musculoperiosteal flap is placed over the fat, and the wound edges are closed in layers.

Conclusion

The laser in combination with microsurgical technique provides a distinct advantage in the management of benign extraaxial lesions found

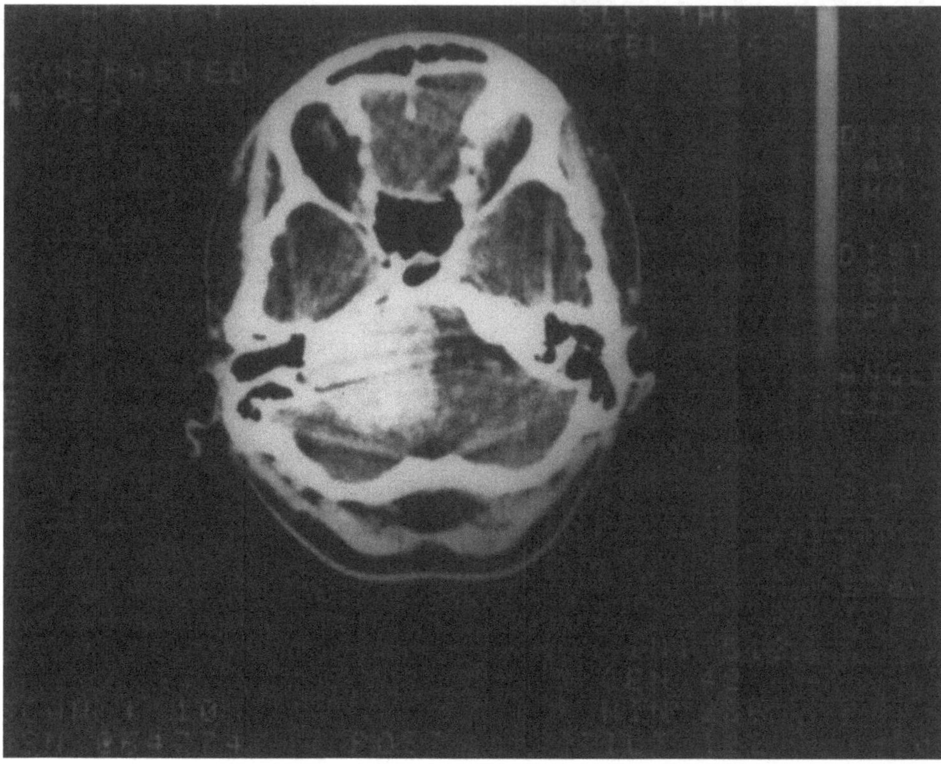

FIGURE 7-8. A glomus jugulare tumor with a large posterior fossa extension.

in difficult locations. The advantage of the laser over conventional techniques is mostly due to its ability to remove tissue without applying traction or pressure [19, 28]. Other advantages may include improved hemostasis and less interference with electrophysiological monitoring. Further advances will be forthcoming as the interaction between laser light and tissue is better understood.

References

1. Brackmann DE: Acoustic neuroma surgery: Otologic Medical Group result. In Silverstein H, Nouell H (eds): *Neurological Surgery of the Ear*. Aesculapius, Birmingham, AL, 1979, pp 248–259.
2. Brackmann DE, Bartels LJ: Rare tumors of the cerebellopontine angle. *Otolaryngol Head Neck Surg* 88:555–559, 1980.
3. Cherington M, Schneck SA: Clivus meningiomas. *Neurology* 16:86–92, 1966.
4. Clark WC, Acker JD, Robertson JH, et al: Neuroradiological detection of small and intracanalicular acoustic tumors. An emphasis on CO_2–CT cisternography. *Neurosurgery* 11:733–738, 1982.
5. Cohen NL, Berg H, Hammerschlag P, Ransohoff J: Acoustic neuroma surgery: An eclectic approach with emphasis on preservation of hearing. *Ann Otol Rhinol Laryngol* 95:21–25, 1986.
6. DiTullio MV, Malkasian D, Rand RW: A critical comparison of neurosurgical and otolaryngological approaches to acoustic neuromas. *J Neurosurg* 48:1–12, 1978.
7. Drake CG: Surgical treatment of acoustic neuroma with preservation or reconstitution of the facial nerve. *J Neurosurg* 26:459–464, 1967.
8. Fisch U: Infratemporal fossa approach for extensive tumors of the temporal bone and base of the skull. In Silverstein H, Norrell H (eds): *Neurological Surgery of the Ear*. Aesculapius, Birmingham, AL, 1977, pp 45–53.
9. Fisch U: Otoneurosurgical approach to acoustic neurinomas. *Prog Neurol Surg* 9:318–336, 1978.
10. Gardner G, Robertson JH, Clark WC: 105 patients operated upon for cerebellopontine

angle tumors: Experience using combined approach and CO_2 laser. *Laryngoscope* 93:1049–1055, 1983.

11. Hart RG, Davenport J: Diagnosis of acoustic neuroma. *Neurosurgery* 9:450–463, 1981.
12. House WF: Final thoughts. *Arch Otolaryngol* 80:756, 1964.
13. King TT: Combined translabyrinthine-transtentorial approach to acoustic nerve tumors. *Proc R Soc Med* 63:780–782, 1970.
14. Kurge TL, Doyle JB: Extradural intracranial (middle fossa) approach to the internal auditory canal. *J Neurosurg* 19:1033–1037, 1962.
15. MacCarty CS, Piepgras DG, Ebersold MJ: Meningeal tumors of the brain. In Yeomans J (ed): *Neurological Surgery*. Philadelphia, Saunders, 1982, pp 2936–2966.
16. Malis LI: Tumors of the skull base. Presented at the American Association of Neurological Surgeons, Denver, CO, April 1985.
17. Martuza RL, Parker SW, Nadol JB, et al: Diagnosis of cerebellopontine angle tumors. *Clin Neurosurg* 32:177–213, 1984.
18. Maxwell RE, Chou SN: Posterior fossa meningiomas. In Schmidek HH, Sweet WH (eds): *Operative Neurosurgical Techniques*. New York, Grune & Stratton, 1982, pp 517–533.
19. Moller A, Hatam A, Olivercrona H: The differential diagnosis of pontine angle meningioma and acoustic neuroma with computed tomography. *Neuroradiology* 17:21–23, 1978.
20. Nehls DG, Spetzler RF, Shetter AG, Sonntag VKH: Application of new technology in the treatment of cerebellopontine angle tumors. *Clin Neurosurg* 32:223–241, 1984.
21. Ojemann RG, Montgomery WW, Weiss AD: Evaluation and surgical treatment of acoustic neuroma. *N Engl J Med* 287:895–899, 1972.
22. Pool FL, Pava AA, Greenfield EC: *Acoustic Nerve Tumors: Early Diagnosis and Treatment*, 2nd ed. 2 Springfield, IL, Thomas, 1970.
23. Quest DO: Meningiomas: An update. *Neurosurgery* 3:219–225, 1978.
24. Rand RW: Suboccipital transmeatal microneurosurgical resection of acoustic tumors. *Ann Surg* 174:663–671, 1971.
25. Robertson JT, Clark WC, Robertson JH, Gardner G: Glomus jugulare tumors. In Youmans J (ed): *Neurological Surgery*, 3rd ed. Philadelphia, Saunders, 1988, (in press).
26. Robertson JH, Clark WC, Robertson JT, et al: Use of the carbon dioxide laser for acoustic tumor surgery. *Neurosurgery* 12:286–290, 1983.
27. Robinson K, Rudge P: The differential diagnosis of cerebellopontine angle lesions. *J Neurol Sci* 60:1–21, 1983.
28. Rousseaux M, Lesion F, Petit H, Tomim M: Les Kystes arachnoidiens de l'angle ponto cerebelleux. *Neurochirurgie* 30:119–124, 1984.
29. Shea MC, Robertson JT: Acoustic neuroma removal: A comparative study of translabyrinthine and suboccipital approaches. *Am J Otol* 1:94–99, 1979.
30. Strait TA, Robertson JH, Clark WC: Use of the carbon dioxide laser in the operative management of intracranial meningiomas. *Neurosurgery* 10:464–467, 1982.
31. Tator CH, Nedzelski JM: Facial nerve presentation in patients with large acoustic neuromas treated by a combined middle fossa transtentorial translabyrinthine approach. *J Neurosurg* 57:1–7, 1982.
32. Turner RG, Shepard NT, Frazer GJ: Clinical performance of audiological and related diagnostic tests. *Ear Hear* 5:187–194, 1984.
33. Yasargil MG, Fox JL: The microsurgical approach to acoustic neurinomas. *Surg Neurol* 2:393–398, 1974.

8. USING LASERS IN PEDIATRIC NEUROSURGERY

Marion L. Walker

As pediatric neurosurgery has evolved into a subspecialty, more and more experience has proved that the immature and developing central nervous system is especially vulnerable. This vulnerability includes the diseases that affect the central nervous system in children, as well as the traumatic effects of surgery, radiation therapy, and chemotherapy treatment modalities. Minimization of trauma is a goal while treating any child with a disease of the central nervous system, and this is especially important when treating surgical diseases. For this reason, surgical lasers have rapidly evolved as an important part of the surgical armamentarium for those neurosurgeons treating children. Even though, when compared to other surgical specialties, neurosurgery was late in implementing the use of surgical lasers for clinical treatment of patients, lasers have become increasingly important in all of neurosurgical practice. In pediatric neurosurgery, surgical lasers have special importance. This chapter will review the use of surgical lasers in pediatric neurosurgery and also note how some of these applications are different in the child as compared to the adult. The discussion will include lesions affecting the brain and the spinal cord.

The benefits of laser surgery are threefold: first, decreased blood loss; second, decreased surgical trauma to the immature and developing central nervous system; and, third, increased precision of tumor removal. Although these benefits of laser usage are no different than the benefits afforded to adult patients, they may be more important in the child. Minimization of blood loss is especially significant in an infant. A blood loss of 100 ml in an infant weighting 10 kg can be highly serious. Any surgical modality that will help minimize this loss should be employed.

Likewise, the decreased trauma associated with the use of surgical lasers is important. A child's brain is less firm, poorly myelinated, and has a high water content. The laser allows for less retraction and manipulation of the brain during tumor surgery, and this decreased trauma is very important [1, 6, 26].

The precision of surgical lasers is especially prominent during removal of tumors from vital brain regions. Control of penetrating power, minimal diffusion of heat, and exact placement of the laser beam allow for precision unmatched in any other surgical instrumentation. Because of this, the popularity of tumor excision with laser surgery continues to increase. Lasers are now recognized as the most gentle surgical instruments for tissue dissection and removal. The increased use of lasers in neurosurgery over the past 8 years is directly related to the precision and atraumatic tissue dissection they provide. As experience with lasers in pedatric neurosurgery has increased, indications and contraindica-

Robertson, J.H. and Clark, W.C. (eds), Lasers in Neurosurgery.

tions have been found [5–9, 14, 17, 25–28]. A large body of laser experience is now available for review.

It should also be noted that the laser is most often used as a microsurgical tool in children. Exceptions to this occur in the removal of some spinal cord lesions and will be noted later. For the removal of brain tumors, however, the laser is best used as an extension of the operating microscope using microsurgical techniques.

Different Laser Modalities

Although various laser modalities have been tried in pediatric neurosurgery, no one has yet reported on a significant number of cases using the neodymium:yttrium-aluminum-garnet (Nd:YAG) laser. The Food and Drug Administration (FDA) still has not released the Nd:YAG laser for general neurosurgical use and has been particularly reluctant to approve this laser for pediatric neurosurgery. There are, however, some institutions using the Nd:YAG in pediatric neurosurgery, and more information regarding its value will undoubtedly be available in the future. At this time, however, it is still considered an experimental tool for neurosurgical procedures in children.

The argon laser has been used in a large number of neurosurgical applications [2, 5, 6]. It is, however, not as common in general use, nor as versatile as the carbon dioxide laser. References to laser use in this chapter will refer to the carbon dioxide laser unless otherwise noted.

Use of the Carbon Dioxide Laser on Brain Lesions

The most prominent and useful laser applications on the brain have been related to removal of neoplasms [6–9, 15, 25–28]. The next portion of this chapter will discuss the pros and cons of laser use for pediatric brain tumors. Before that discussion is begun, however, it should be noted that there are other areas of potential laser use in pediatric neurosurgery.

Congenital lesions, e.g., hydrocephalus, developmental cysts, encephaloceles, affecting the brain have not been found to respond well to laser surgical treatment [26]. At this time, standard surgical approaches seem to be more appropriate for these lesions. However, it is likely that different laser wavelengths will become available to allow more appropriate treatment of some of these developmental problems. Laser fenestration of cysts and intraventricular loculations through endoscopes is already beginning. The technique involved in this type of laser surgery will undoubtedly be improved upon and become more widespread in general neurosurgical use over the next few years.

Growing research and early clinical experience suggest that vascular lesions can be treated with both the carbon dioxide and the Nd:YAG lasers [3, 13]. Because these applications have not yet been tried in the pediatric neurosurgical patient, they will not be discussed here.

Use of the Carbon Dioxide Laser on Brain Tumors

The most intense use of the laser in pediatric neurosurgery has been on neoplasms of the brain. A large experience with this application has been gained [5–9, 25–28]. This portion of the chapter will discuss the benefits of carbon dioxide laser surgery on pediatric brain tumors.

A discussion of laser treatment of brain tumors should include an understanding of the advantages and disadvantages of laser therapy. As previously noted in this chapter and elsewhere in this book, use of the carbon dioxide laser will often result in decreased blood loss during the surgical procedure. The neovascularity of most pediatric neoplasms affecting the central nervous system is such that the laser seals the vessels as the tissue is vaporized, thus minimizing blood loss. This can be observed even in lesions where one might not expect it to occur. Choroid plexus papillomas, for example, have often been successfully vaporized using carbon dioxide laser therapy without significant bleeding. This facilitates the debulking of the tumor centrally to allow easier and less traumatic access to the vascular pedicle.

The laser is but one of many surgical tools available to the modern neurosurgeon for tumor removal. Throughout this chapter, I will compare the laser, the Cavitron Ultrasonic Surgical Aspirator (CUSA), and standard surgical suction techniques for removal of various types of tumors. The comparison is based upon my experience using all of these modalities over the past 7 years. The object of tumor removal in the child is to accomplish the removal with the least amount of trauma, the least amount of bleeding, the most complete tumor tissue removal possible, as rapidly as possible, and doing no harm to the surrounding brain. Often standard surgical suction techniques are appropriate. Many tumors in children are soft and can be easily removed by suction. Tumors that are more firm are often best removed using the CUSA or the carbon dioxide laser. In general, I have preferred to remove tumors of the hemispheres with the CUSA because it is faster and because the surrounding brain is not as vital as in some other areas. The laser is used for tumor removal of those lesions adjacent to or within vital brain areas. Even though the CUSA may be used for the major debulking of the tumor, the laser is important for removing tumor that is adjacent to a vital brain area.

This discussion of laser surgery will look at removal of tumors from various brain regions rather than at individual tumors, except when the individual tumors are of special importance.

SUPRATENTORIAL TUMORS

Tumors of the Suprasellar Region. In childhood, tumors of the suprasellar region are most commonly gliomas affecting the hypothalamus and/or optic pathways and craniopharyngiomas. Although other tumor types may occur in this area, these two types are the most important for the purposes of this discussion. Gliomas affecting the optic pathway, especially those involving the chiasm and hypothalamus, are the most common tumors seen in this location in childhood.

Gliomas of the chiasm and hypothalamus are not often treated successfully with laser surgical techniques [26]. These tumors are invasive into the surrounding hypothalamus, and attempts at total removal are often devastating to the patient. Actual removal of all tumor tissue is rarely possible. For this reason, these tumors are generally debulked from their central portions using the carbon dioxide laser, but rarely is the majority of the tumor removed. The biopsy is accomplished, and the patient is then either observed clinically or given radiation therapy. A surprising number of these low-grade neoplasms are very sensitive to radiation therapy, and the prognosis may be quite good despite the location of the tumor [16].

Craniopharyngiomas are generally treated effectively with laser techniques. The central cyst can be evacuated and the tumor attachments to the surrounding brain easily vaporized using microsurgical techniques with the carbon dioxide laser. It has been my experience that these patients can undergo gross total removal of the craniopharyngioma tissue with minimum surrounding trauma (Figure 8-1). I believe that microsurgical techniques and, in particular laser surgical techniques, have allowed more complete and less traumatic removal of these neoplasms than was previously possible. Patients treated in this manner have had better neurosurgical and neuropsychological outcomes than were previously described in the literature. Attempting total removal when feasible and avoiding radiation therapy provide the child the best potential for normal neurological development.

Tumors of the Cerebral Hemispheres. It has been my experience that the majority of the tumors affecting the cerebral hemispheres in children are most efficiently removed using the CUSA. The CUSA allows for a more rapid debulking of the tumor, and, because many of these tumors

A

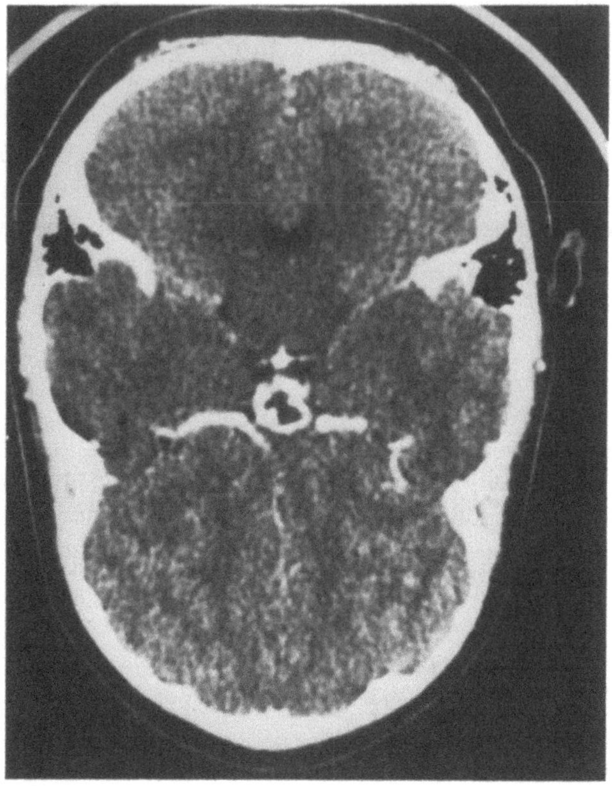

B

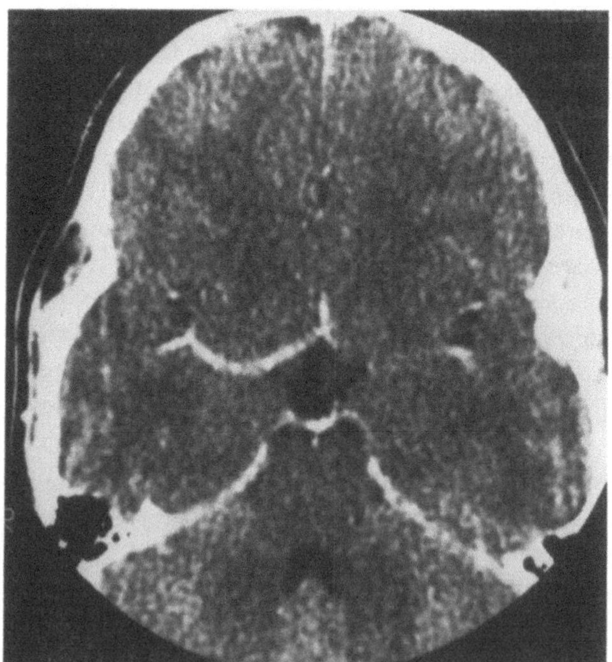

FIGURE 8-1. (A) Contrast-enhanced CT scan showing a suprasellar cystic craniopharyngioma. (B) Contrast-enhanced CT scan taken 2 years following surgical excision of the craniopharyngioma. No evidence of recurrence of the tumor is seen. The attachments of the tumor were easily removed with the carbon dioxide laser.

are not adjacent to vital brain areas, the tumor can be completely excised. Occasionally, however, these tumors are adjacent to vital structures, and the area of the tumor-brain interface is best removed using the precision of the carbon dioxide laser. The choice of instruments is left to the surgeon's judgment at the time of tumor surgery. The carbon dioxide laser does help, however, in making a cortical incision with minimal surrounding trauma. When this is coupled with stereotactic guided craniotomy for small lesions placed near the cortical surface, a minimum of trauma to the developing brain will occur.

Ventricular Tumors. Tumors in the ventricle are usually best treated with laser techniques [26]. Because these tumors are deep within the brain, the laser is an excellent tool for tumor removal. It is often difficult to get the CUSA deep into the ventricle while trying to minimize the exposure. Ventricular tumors are among those that often exhibit the most dramatic response to laser vaporization.

The choroid plexus papilloma is a good example. Although this tumor is vascular and appears vascular on enhanced computed tomography (CT) and angiography, it has been my experience that the majority of these tumors can be vaporized with a minimum of bleeding. This allows for debulking of the tumor centrally and a more atraumatic approach to the vascular pedicle at the base of the neoplasm (Figure 8-2).

Astrocytomas of the ventricle can frequently be vaporized down to their attachment to the ventricular wall. Many of these tumors have a distinct tumor-brain interface and a gross total excision is occasionally possible.

Ependymomas may or may not be easily vaporized using carbon dioxide laser techniques. The difficulty with removing these intraventricular lesions is directly related to their vascularity. Some of these lesions are too vascular for the laser to be used efficiently. When this is the case, the CUSA or other surgical techniques are more appropriate.

Pineal Tumors. Tumors of the pineal region may or may not require an open surgical procedure. One approach to these tumors has been to stereotactically biopsy the tumor to obtain a histological diagnosis. If the diagnosis indicates that an aggressive attempt at tumor removal is necessary, the laser becomes an ideal tool because it allows vaporization of the tumor tissue in these deeply seated neoplasms. Care, however, must always be taken to avoid injuring important surrounding vascular structures.

POSTERIOR FOSSA TUMORS

Tumors of the cerebellum. Tumors of the cerebellum may or may not be appropriate for laser use [26]. Cystic cerebellar astrocytomas with a small mural nodule are usually best treated by standard neurosurgical techniques. The tumor nodule can be removed easily and simply, and the laser does not provide any added benefit to the surgical procedure, unless the nodule is attached adjacent to important brain structures. Solid tumors of the cerebellum, however, are easily vaporized using the laser, and the atraumatic nature of this vaporization is especially important and valuable in removing tumors of the posterior fossa. The laser has been especially valuable in excising those cerebellar astrocytomas that enter the cerebral peduncles. The point of interface between tumor and surrounding normal brain tissue can usually be identified so that a gross total removal is often possible even though the tumor is extending into the cerebral peduncle. The first surgical procedure on a cerebellar tumor extending into the cerebral peduncle is usually the most opportune time to achieve gross total removal. Patience, magnified vision through the operating microscope, a knowledge of the anatomy, and a knowledge of the areas of tumor invasion will often allow the surgeon to achieve the gross total removal desired. The laser is essential for this type of tumor surgery.

Tumors of the Fourth Ventricle. Tumors of the fourth ventricle include medulloblastomas, epen-

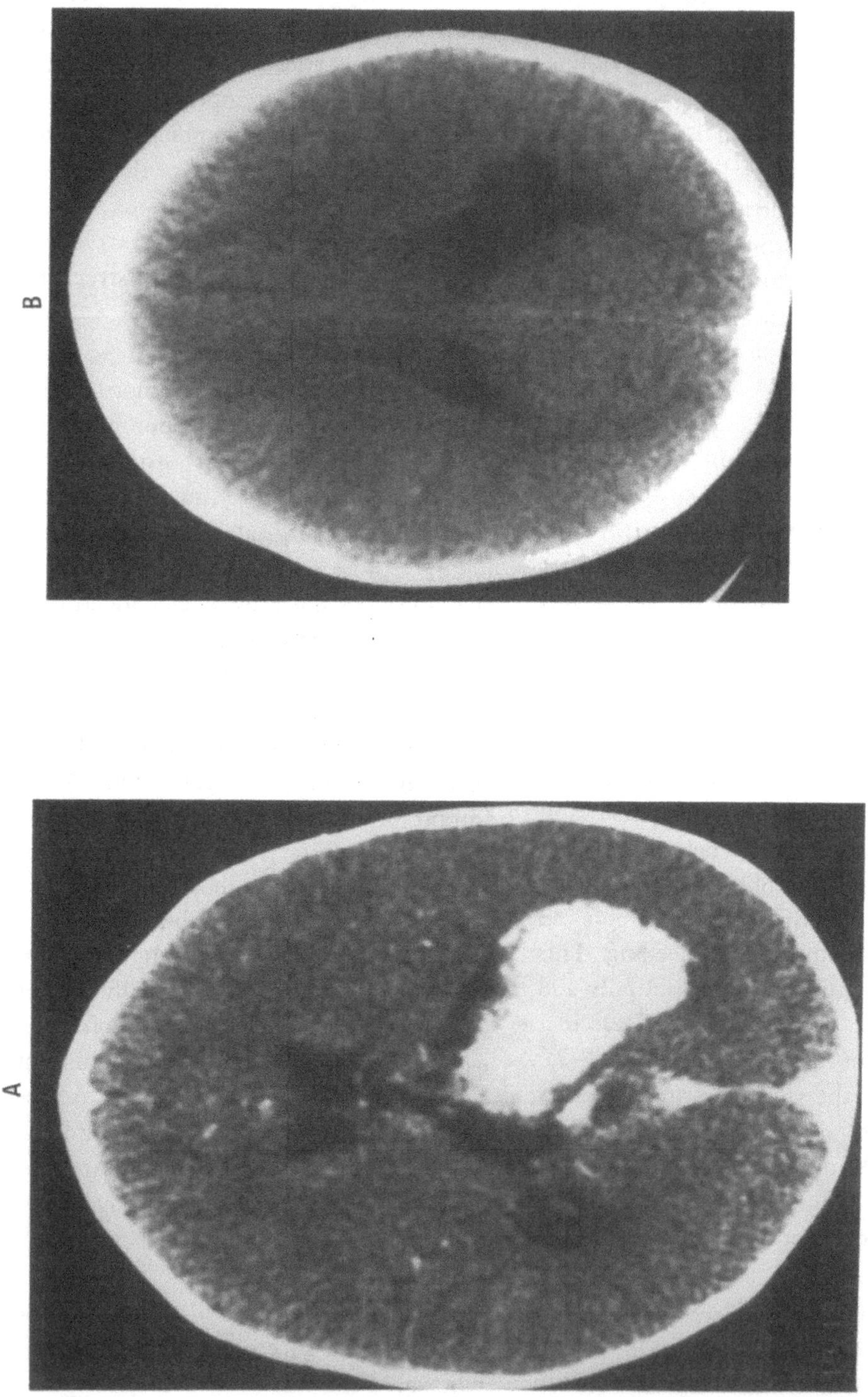

FIGURE 8-2. (A) Contrast-enhanced CT scan showing a large enhancing choroid plexus papilloma with attachment at the atrium of the left lateral ventricle. (B) CT scan taken 1 year following laser surgical excision of the choroid plexus papilloma. No evidence of recurrence or of residual tumor.

dymomas, and choroid plexus papillomas. Although medulloblastomas may technically arise within the cerebellum, they are considered here as fourth ventricular tumors because of their location.

Medulloblastomas are often easily excised using either the CUSA or standard surgical suction. The margins of the tumor, however, are best treated by removing the tumor with the precision available from the carbon dioxide laser. Attachment of the tumor to the cerebral peduncles, the floor of the fourth ventricle, and the cerebral aqueduct are best removed using the carbon dioxide laser. Complete removal may allow the patient to enter a "good risk" protocol for treatment. In the infant this may allow the patient to receive less radiation therapy to the whole brain or to enter a chemotherapy protocol first.

Posterior fossa ependymomas have also been treated using the carbon dioxide laser. This tumor is usually very vascular and often attaches to the floor of the fourth ventricle. The attachment to the floor of the fourth ventricle can be identified and the tumor tissue removed using the carbon dioxide laser. This requires experience in identifying the tumor attachment and skill in selecting and using the appropriate low wattage to avoid injury to structures deep to the tumor that are lying deep to the floor of the fourth ventricle within the pons.

Ependymomas that extend through the foramen of Luschka and into the cerebellopontine angle (CPA), anterior to the brainstem, have been successfully removed by surgical laser. Attachments to vascular structures and cranial nerves can be vaporized. This is an area, however, where it is important to have surgical laser experience and knowledge of appropriate power settings and anatomy before attempting this type of tumor removal. Recent experience suggests that a gross total removal of these malignant neoplasms can be accomplished by using the carbon dioxide laser. This early experience also suggests that the outcome of these patients may be markedly improved when gross total removal can be achieved [2].

Choroid plexus papillomas may occur in any portion of the ventricular system and are occasionally seen in the fourth ventricle in children [12]. These tumors are vascular, but they are treated suprisingly well with the carbon dioxide laser. The laser vaporizes and seals all but the larger vessels. The tumor can be vaporized centrally allowing easier access to the vascular pedicle before complete removal is achieved.

Tumors of the CPA. Tumors of the CPA in childhood include choroid plexus papillomas and ependymomas. The applicability of laser surgery to these lesions has been noted previously.

Other tumors found in the CPA include exophytic neoplasms of the pons and the rare lesions effecting the fifth or eighth cranial nerves in patients with neurofibromatosis. Although the laser is valuable in the treatment of neuromas and schwannomas in this area, these are extremely rare lesions in children. Previous chapters have described the technique of removal of these lesions, and those techniques apply equally well in the pediatric neurosurgical patient.

Exophytic tumors of the pons extending into the CPA are, almost without exception, anaplastic astrocytomas or glioblastomas. Surgical removal does not change the rapidly downward clinical course of these patients.

Brainstem Tumors. One of the most important applications of laser surgical techniques to pediatric brain tumors is to those tumors that are found in the brainstem. Over the past few years, it has become apparent that the "brainstem glioma" is not a uniform brain tumor, but indeed is a collection of different tumors with different histological appearances and biological activities [9, 11, 25, 27].

It has been noted that gliomas of the pons can occur in several locations and have different clinical prognoses [9, 11, 27]. These intrinsic tumors that infiltrate the pons are typically

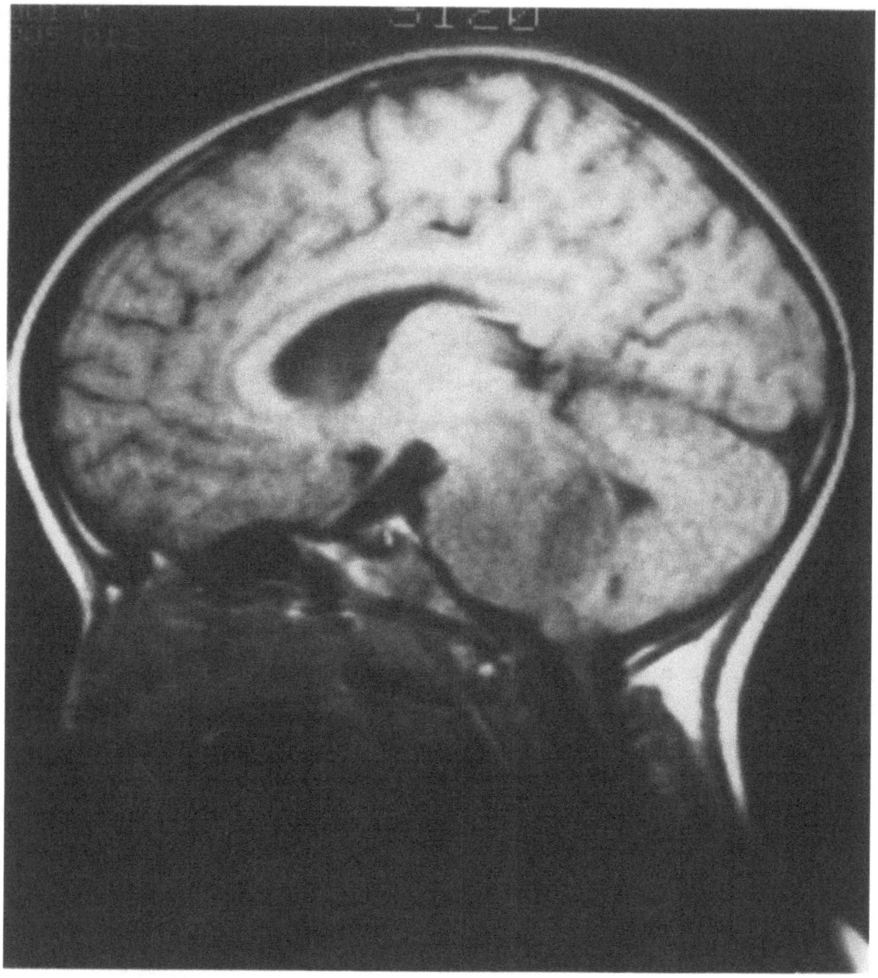

FIGURE 8-3. MRI showing the typical appearance of a pontine glioma. The tumor extends from the pontomedullary junction up to the midbrain.

anaplastic astrocytomas or glioblastomas (Figure 8-3). These tumors have not been successfully treated with laser surgery, and the patients have a rapidly deteriorating clinical course and rarely survive more than a year, even with radiation therapy and/or chemotherapy. Other forms of treatment must be found for these patients. Hyperfractionation radiation therapy is currently being evaluated, and at this early date offers some promise for extended survival.

Tumors of the pons that are exophytic into the fourth ventricle have a much different clinical prognosis. These tumors are often attached to the surface of the fourth ventricle and do not deeply invade the brainstem. They are low-grade astrocytomas and can be successfully removed down to their point of attachment into the pons. It now seems apparent that with gross total removal, these exophytic tumors do not require follow-up radiation therapy, and many of these patients go on to have long-term survivals without evidence of tumor recurrence [10, 11].

Tumors of the pons that are exophytic into the CPA or anterior to the brainstem are generally malignant tumors and have a rapidly deteriorating clinical course [11]. Lasers have not been successful in their treatment.

Intrinsic tumors of the pons that have occasionally been successfully treated with laser surgical techniques are those that are discrete, localized, and small. These tumors are often different from the usual anaplastic astrocytomas that occur in this region. These tumors may be juvenile pilocytic astrocytomas or ganglioneuromas. Removal of these tumors, should be attempted, if possible, and laser techniques are essential for such removal. As previously noted, however, the intrinsic tumor that is diffusely infiltrating the pons is not amenable to surgical therapy.

The area of the brainstem where tumors have been successfully treated has been somewhat of a surprise. Tumors occurring in the medulla oblongata and at the cervicomedullary junction have been treated very successfully with carbon dioxide laser surgical techniques (Figure 8-4) [9, 11, 25–27]. These tumors are almost always low-grade microcystic astrocytomas. They are very similar to the neoplasms found in the spinal cord. Indeed, there are some who believe that these tumors may be extensions of upper cervical spinal cord tumors. The biology of the tumors in this location appears to be different in several ways. First, these tumors are almost universally benign and are of a different type than the tumors that occur higher in the brainstem. As opposed to anaplastic astrocytomas, these juvenile pilocytic astrocytomas behave in much more benign fashion. Secondly, even the tumors that occur in the lower portion of the brainstem that are malignant appear to have a more benign clinical course when compared to the lesions of the pons. Although malignant astrocytomas of the lower brainstem cannot be considered to be cured by surgical therapy, the clinical course is not nearly as rapidly downward and devastating as is often seen with pontine tumors.

SURGICAL TECHNIQUE FOR REMOVAL OF BRAINSTEM GLIOMAS. Because laser removal of brainstem gliomas is so critical, a discussion of the techniques involved will follow.

Surgical treatment of intrinsic astrocytomas of the medulla oblongata requires microsurgical and carbon dioxide laser surgical techniques.

A posterior fossa craniotomy is done in the prone position to minimize the chance of air embolization. A midline opening provides adequate exposure. The posterior arch of C1 is always removed, and occasionally a laminectomy of C2 or lower is necessary when the tumor extends into the upper cervical spinal cord. A standard suboccipital craniectomy is sufficient. Occasionally it is necessary to split the lowermost portion of the inferior vermis to obtain adequate exposure of the lower brainstem. The surgeon must be able to see up beyond the level of the obex, but an exposure of the entire fourth ventricle is usually not necessary. Tumors of the medulla that are surgically accessible will be below the obex and will be visible on the dorsal surface of the lower brainstem; here the opening is made into the medulla to begin tumor removal.

The laser facilitates an atraumatic opening of the dorsum of the medulla. The tumor is immediately beneath the surface, and there is almost always a distinct border between tumor and normal brain. Using the carbon dioxide laser at low-power settings, the tumor-brain interface can be easily identified.

Use of the carbon dioxide laser also allows for continuous electrophysiological monitoring throughout the procedure. Spinal evoked responses and brainstem auditory evoked responses are an important part of this type of surgical therapy. Although it is difficult to maintain spinal evoked responses when opening the dorsal surface of the lower brainstem, the brainstem auditory evoked responses have proven to be extremely valuable. Even though the entry of cranial nerve VIII is above the level of the medulla, the surgery still has a direct effect on the brainstem auditory evoked response. An increase in latency of waves I to V can be seen with retraction and also with heating of the surrounding normal brain tissue when the carbon dioxide laser is used. Removing the offending retractors or stopping the laser and irrigating the wound will return the evoked responses to their baseline. In almost all cases,

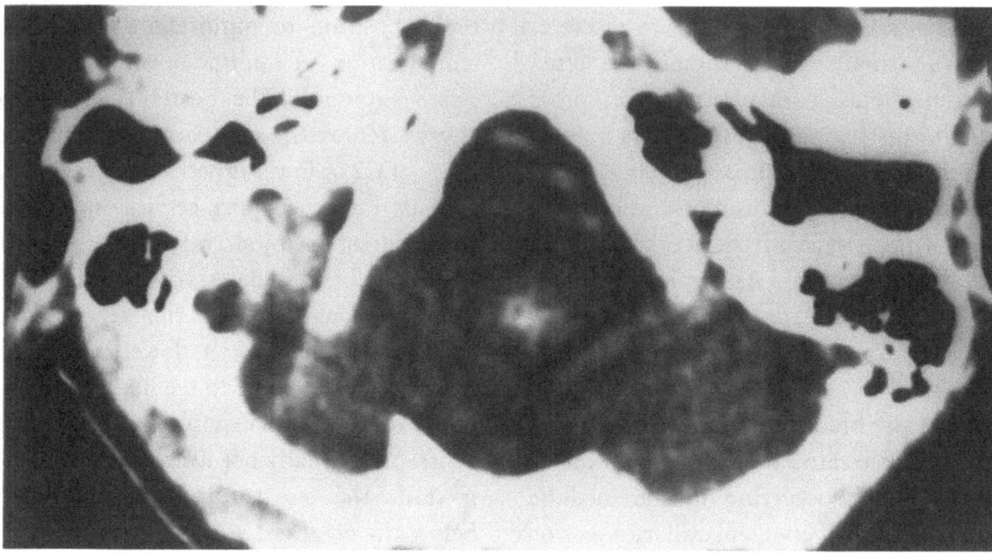

A

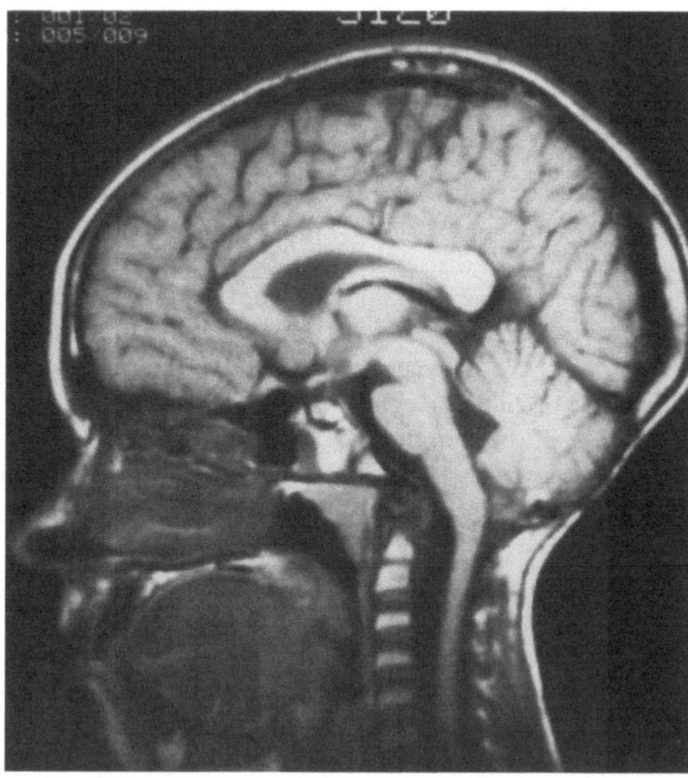

B

FIGURE 8-4. (A) CT scan showing an enhancing lesion within the medulla oblongata. (B) MRI taken 5 years following surgical excision of a lower brainstem astrocytoma. No evidence of residual tumor or recurrence is seen.

the evoked response is improved at the end of the surgical procedure [25].

The carbon dioxide laser appears to allow for greater tissue removal than that which can be safely accomplished using the CUSA. As noted previously, the surgeon can usually visualize the tumor-brain interface quite distinctly, so it is not difficult for the surgeon to know the appropriate time for ending tumor removal. We have found that the CUSA is an effective instrument for debulking large brainstem gliomas. The laser, however, is used to remove the tumor from the surrounding edges at the brain-tumor interface.

Use of the Carbon Dioxide Laser on Spinal Cord Lesions

There are three areas in which the laser has found a role in the treatment of lesions affecting the spinal cord in the pediatric patient: neoplasms, congenital malformations, and the treatment of syringomyelia.

SPINAL CORD TUMORS

Many spinal cord tumors that occur in childhood are fortunately benign. However, because of the location of many of these tumors within the substance of the spinal cord, many of these tumors have been considered inoperable. Recent surgical experience, however, has shown that intrinsic tumors of the spinal cord can be successfully removed using microsurgical and laser surgical techniques. The dorsal surface of the cord is opened in the midline overlying the area of the tumor. Retraction sutures are placed in the pial layer of the cord and exposure of the tumor is easily accomplished. Using laser surgical techniques, the tumor can be vaporized without further mechanical manipulation of the spinal cord. The laser has particular value in this type of surgical procedure. The junction between the tumor and normal spinal tissue is often distinct, and a gross total removal of the tumor can frequently be accomplished [7, 8].

When the laser allows a gross total removal of the tumor, the patients are often improved neurologically. Many of the patients do not require radiation therapy and can be watched clinically for evidence of recurrence before proceeding with any further therapy. This use of laser surgical technique has allowed for a dramatic improvement in the treatment of patients with intrinsic spinal cord tumors. The details of the neurodiagnostic evaluation, the surgical approach, and the use of laser surgical technique have been outlined by Epstein [7, 8]. His vast surgical experience with these lesions has proven the value of laser surgery for intrinsic spinal cord tumors.

LIPOMYELOMENINGOCELE

This congenital malformation is one of the more common lesions of the spine treated surgically by the pediatric neurosurgeon. A better understanding of the surgical anatomy and the embryogenesis of this lesion has lead to a more appropriate surgical approach [4, 17, 19, 20, 22, 23]. McLone has shown that these lesions can be excised without increasing the neurological deficit [17, 20]. Indeed, many of the patients show improvement following laser vaporization of the lipomyelomeningocele (see Chapter 12). McLone's work has led to a better understanding of the embryogenesis and the surgical anatomy. This, in turn, has allowed surgeons to more completely remove the lipomatous tissue. Because this can be accomplished with relatively minor trauma using laser surgical techniques, the outlook for these patients has improved dramatically over the past 10 years. Others have confirmed the surgical anatomy and the usefulness of the carbon dioxide laser in treating these lesions [4, 14, 26].

Knowledge of the embryogenesis is critical to an understanding of the surgical anatomy of lipomyelomeningoceles [18, 22]. Failure of complete closure results in mesenchyme entering a portion of the neural tube, usually at its caudal end. This mesenchyme subsequently develops into lipomatous tissue. This tissue is connected from the region of the central canal and the open neural tube up to the lipomatous tissue extending into the subcutaneous region. The dorsal roots, however, are always anterior and lateral to the lipomatous mass. When the plan of entry of the dorsal roots can be identified, the area of attachment of the lipomatous tissue can easily be seen and the lipomatous tissue can be vaporized with safety. Surgeons who undertake this procedure should be familiar with this abnormal anatomy.

Although it is not necessary to remove all of the lipomatous tissue, a near total removal can usually be achieved using laser surgical techniques. However, when the lipomatous tissue begins to blend with the spinal cord, the procedure should be terminated.

The laser allows vaporization of the lipomatous tissue in an atraumatic manner. However, the lipoma often melts instead of completely vaporizing. This generates additional heat. Care should be taken to irrigate the area of vaporization frequently with saline. As the surgeon approaches the interface between lipomatous tissue and spinal cord, this irrigation should increase in frequency. Damage can be done to the spinal cord through the conduction of heat caused by laser vaporization and melting of the lipomatous tissue.

The complete removal of lipomyelomeningoceles is possible because of the technology now available in neurosurgery, which has ended the deterioration of the patients' neurological status. Many of the patients improve following surgery, especially if the surgery is performed early [17, 20]. It has been my experience that many newborns who have urodynamic testing prior to surgery already show neurogenic impairment of the bladder. If the surgery is performed at an early age, improvement of bladder function can be achieved. If the surgery is delayed, the neurological loss is sometimes not reversible. I recommend that lipomyelomeningoceles be excised as soon as they are found, even in infancy [17, 20]. The child is often operated on as early as 4 to 6 weeks of age. As previously noted, however, the surgeon must have a thorough understanding of the developmental anatomy, the surgical anatomy, and the surgical technique. Because the goal of intervention early in infancy is to preserve normal neurological function, the surgeon must have experience in dealing with this type of malformation. The anatomy is complex and experience is required to achieve the best results.

MYELOMENINGOCELES

The laser can be used very effectively in the closure of myelomeningoceles. One of the critical points of closure of these lesions is to free the edges of the neural placode from the surrounding dermal and epidermal attachments. If pieces of dermis or epidermis are left attached to the neural placode, then subsequent formation of dermoids and epidermoids is likely.

The carbon dioxide laser used in sharp focus at low wattage can vaporize the attachments of the dermal and epidermal layers to the neural placode. Using magnified vision, the surgeon can vaporize the attachments at the lateral portions of the placode and circumferentially around the placode. The neural placode will then be able to be placed back into the spinal canal. Removal of the attachment to the dermis and epidermis can be accomplished bloodlessly and very easily. This is often done instead of the normal sharp dissection. It speeds the surgical procedure and allows for less blood loss.

SYRINGOMYELIA

The treatment of syringomyelia has been a difficult and perplexing problem in neurosurgery. The laser has allowed a different approach to the management of this problem, but has by no means solved the difficulty that these patients present.

Exposure of the spinal cord is accomplished over the area of the syrinx. In children with spina bifida, the opening into the syrinx of the hydromyelic cavity is best accomplished in the midline through a dorsal myelotomy. In patients without spina bifida, the entrance to the syrinx is usually best accomplished at the dorsal root entry zone. This is because the thinnest portion of the syrinx will usually be in that area.

The opening into the syrinx is made using the carbon dioxide laser. A small area of vaporization of tissue allows a communication between the cavity of the syrinx and the spinal subarachnoid space. The surgeon then has the option of placing a small plastic stint between the cavity and the spinal subarachnoid space or placing a shunt. Both have been effective in treating a syrinx. If the stint is chosen, care should be taken to close the arachnoid membrane and reconstruct the spinal subarachnoid space, if possible.

Conclusion

The carbon dioxide laser has found an important place in pediatric neurosurgery. The majority of the lesions treated with this laser technology are neoplasms. Neoplasms of the brain and spinal cord have been successfully treated with the carbon dioxide laser, and many of them are best removed using laser technology. Congenital lesions affecting the spine have also been successfully treated, most prominently, lipomyelomeningoceles and myelomeningoceles. The laser is also useful in treating syringomyelia.

As newer wavelengths become available, a larger number of applications in pediatric neurosurgery will be found. It is anticipated that the use of laser with endoscopic techniques will have an important application for the treatment of congenital anomalies as well as deep-seated lesions in the brain in children.

References

1. Asher PW: The use of CO_2 laser in neurosurgery. In Kaplan I (ed): *Laser Surgery II*. Jerusalem Academic Press, Jerusalem, 1987, pp 76–78.
2. Boggan JE, Edwards MSB, Davis RL, et al: Comparison of the brain tissue response in rats to injury by argon and carbon dioxide lasers. *Neurosurgery* 11:609–616, 1982.
3. Burke LP, Rovin RA, Cerullo LJ, et al: YAG laser in neurosurgery. In Joffe (ed): *Nd:YAG Lasers in Medicine and Surgery*. Elsevier Science Publishing Co, Inc, New York NX, 1983.
4. Chapman PH, Davis KR: Surgical treatment of spinal lipomas in childhood. *Concepts Ped Neurosurg* 3:178–190, 1983.
5. Edwards MSB, Boggan JE: Argon laser surgery of pediatric neural neoplasms. *Childs Brain* 11: 171–175, 1984.
6. Edwards MSB, Boggan JE, Fuller TA: The laser in neurological surgery. *J Neurosurg* 59:555–566, 1986.
7. Epstein F: Surgical treatment of extensive spinal cord astrocytomas of childhood. *Concepts Ped Neurosurg* 3:157–169, 1983.
8. Epstein F, Epstein N: Surgical treatment of spinal cord astrocytoma in children. *J Neurosurg* 57:685–689, 1982.
9. Epstein F, McCleary EL: Intrinsic brainstem tumors of childhood: surgical indications. *J Neurosurg* 64:11–15, 1986.
10. Hoffman HJ, Becker L, Craven MA: A clinically and pathologically Distinct group of benign brainstem gliomas. *Neurosurgery* 7:243–248, 1980.
11. Hoffman HJ, Stroink AR, Davidson G. et al: Pediatric brainstem gliomas: Evaluation of biopsy. *Concepts Ped Neurosurg* 7:105–116, 1987.
12. Humphreys RP, Nemoto S, Hendrick EB, Hoffman HJ: Childhood choroid plexus tumors. *Concepts Ped Neurosurg* 7:1–18, 1987.
13. Jain KK: Complications of use of the neodymium: Yttrium-aluminum-garnet laser in neurosurgery. *Neurosurgery* 16:759–762, 1985.
14. James HE, Williams J, Brock W, et al: Radical removal of lipomas of the conus and cauda equina with laser microsurgery. *Neurosurgery* 15: 340–343, 1984.
15. Kelly PJ, Alker GJ, Jr: A method for stereotaxic laser microsurgery in deep-seated CNS neoplasms. *Appl Neurophysiol* 43:210, 1980.
16. McLaurin R: Hypothalamic gliomas in childhood. *Concepts Ped Neurosurg* 7:19–28, 1986.
17. McLone DG, Naidich TP: Laser resection of fifty spinal lipomas. *Neurosurgery* 18:611–615, 1986.
18. McLone DG, Naidich TP: Spinal dysraphism: Experimental and clinical. In Holtzman RNN, Stein BM (eds): *The Tethered Spinal Cord*. New York, Thieme-Stratton, Inc, 1985, pp 14–28.
19. McLone DG, Dias L, Kaplan WE, Somers MW: Concepts in the management of spina bifida. *Concepts Ped Neurosurg* 5:97–106, 1985.
20. McLone DG, Hayashida SF, Caldarelli M: Surgical resection of lipomyelomeningoceles in

18 asymptomatic infants. *J Ped Neurosci* 12: 239–242, 1985.

21. McLone DG, Mutler S, Naidich TP: Lipomeningoceles of the conus medullaris. *Concepts Ped Neurosurg* 3:171–177, 1983.
22. McLone DG, Suwa J, Collins JA, et al: Neurulation: Biochemical and morphological studies on primary and secondary neural tube defects. *Concepts Ped Neurosurg* 4:15–29, 1983.
23. Naidich TP, McLone DG, *Mutleur S*: A new understanding of dorsal dysraphism with lipoma (lipomyeloschisis): Radiological evaluation and surgical corrections. *AJNR* 4:103–116, 1983.
24. Tomita T, McLone DG: Posterior fossa ependymomas in childhood. Presented at the Annual Meeting of the International Society for Pediatric Neurosurgery, Madrid, Spain, Sept 30–Oct 3, 1986.
25. Walker ML: The use of the CO_2 laser for surgical treatment of intrinsic brainstem gliomas. In Hoffman HH (ed): *Advances in Pediatric Neurosurgery*. State of the Art Reviews in Neurosurgery. Philadelphia, Hanley and Belfus, 1986, pp 133–143.
26. Walker ML, Storrs BB: Lasers in pediatric neurosurgery. *Ped Neurosci* 12:23–30, 1985.
27. Walker ML, Storrs BB: Surgical therapy for intrinsic brainstem gliomas. *Concepts Ped Neurosurg* 5:178–186, 1985.
28. Walker ML, Storrs BB, Goodman SG: Use of the CO_2 Laser for surgical excision of primary brain tumors in children. *Concepts Ped Neurosurg* 3:297–315, 1983.

9. STEREOTACTIC LASER RESECTION OF DEEP-SEATED TUMORS

Patrick J. Kelly
B. A. Kall
S. J. Goerss

The carbon dioxide laser is a precise cutting and vaporizing tool. Its beam can be mechanically directed and computer-monitored in three-dimensional space. Thus, it is applicable to the stereotactic method, especially for the precision resection of intracranial intraaxial neoplasms from neurologically important areas.

In January 1980, we began a program of stereotactic carbon dioxide laser extirpation of deep-seated intracranial lesions. Our first procedures were based on coronal and sagittal reconstructions of computed tomographic (CT) data superimposed on stereotactic x-ray pictures [5, 6]. Later, we incorporated an operating room computer system for the transposition of volumetric information derived from axial stereotactic CT scans into three-dimensional space [1, 4, 7, 9]. The position of a stereotactically directed carbon dioxide laser was displayed on an operating room computer graphics terminal in relation to planar reconstructions of the tumor sliced by computer orthogonal to the surgical approach. In addition, we developed a custom frame to allow rapid stereotactic access to multiple points within the tumor for computer-monitored laser vaporization. Thus, it was theoretically possible to remove all of any intracranial neoplasm detected by CT scanning.

The following chapter will describe our current methodology for computer-assisted stereotactic laser microsurgical extirpation of deep-seated lesions. In addition, we will report on the clinical results in the first 146 patients treated by this method.

Material and Methods

DATA BASE ACQUISITION

Patients undergo stereotactic CT scanning and magnetic resonance imaging (MRI) with their heads fixed in CT- and MRI-compatible stereotactic head-holders. CT and MRI localizing devices attach to the head-holders and create a series of nine reference artifacts on each CT and MRI slice (Figure 9-1). The archived CT data tapes are input to the operating room computer system (Independent Physicians Display Console for General Electric 8800 CT Scanner-Data General Eclipse S140 with a 192-megabyte disc and Ramtek raster display terminal). The surgeon digitizes each CT/MRI slice that demonstrates the tumor as follows. First, the localizing artifacts on each CT and MRI slice are digitized automatically by the computer utilizing cursor and the trackball subsystem of the Ramtek display terminal (Figure 9-2). A tumor volume is created in stereotactic space by an interpolation program that may be sliced orthogonal to

Robertson, J.H. and Clark, W.C. (eds), Lasers in Neurosurgery.

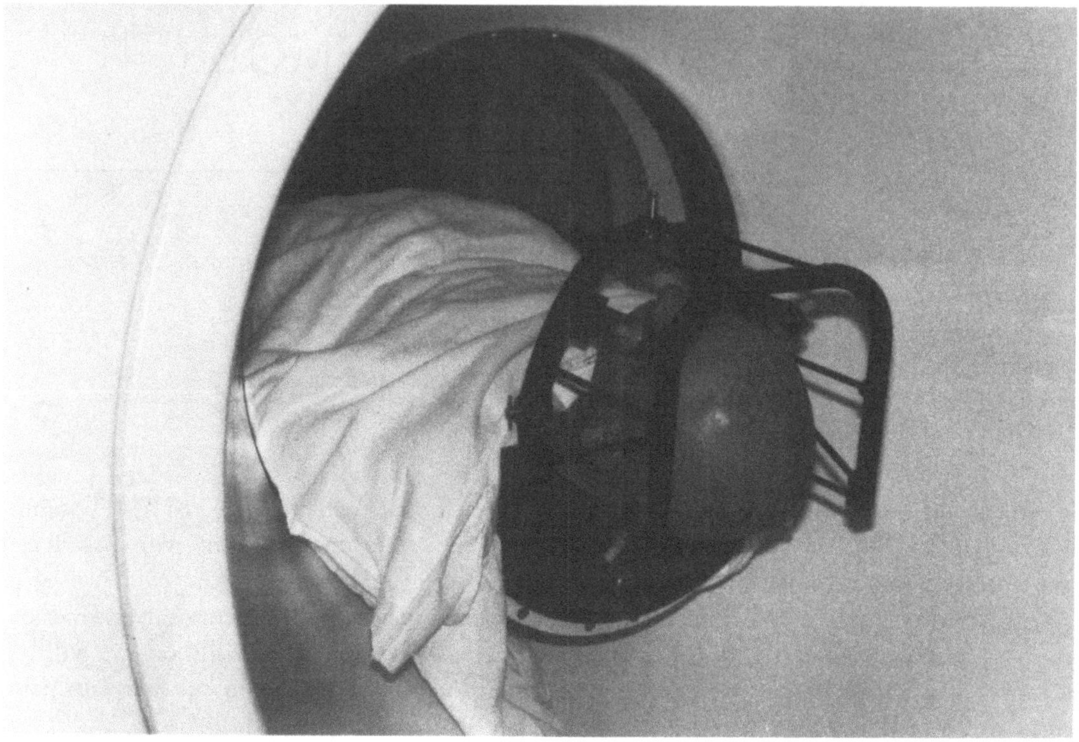

FIGURE 9-1. CT-compatible stereotactic head-holder mounted in a CT table adaptation plate on a GE 8800 CT scanner.

any specified surgical approach angle. Furthermore, the computer calculates the volume of the lesion and the X, Y, and Z mechanical adjustments of the stereotactic frame, which bring a selected point within the tumor volume into the focal point of an arc-quadrant stereotactic frame.

The stereotactic surgical instrument consists of an arc-quadrant frame in which the patient's head is moved within three degrees of freedom to place an intracranial target point into the center of the sphere described by arc and quadrant. Movements of the head in three dimensions are controlled by servomotors and displayed by a digital calibration system (Acu-Rite, Bausch and Lomb). The surgical laser is directed from a carriage that runs perpendicular to the tangent of a 400-mm arc. The center of the arc is at the focal point of the stereotactic frame. An operating microscope is also fixed to the carriage (Acu-Rite, Bausch and Lomb). The laser beam is controlled by X and Y galvanometers operated by a remote joystick. The position of the laser beam is relayed to the computer system by optical encoders activated by the joystick (Figure 9-3).

The surgical procedure is performed under general anesthesia through a linear scalp incision. Prior to the actual craniotomy, the tumor is first traversed by a stereotactic biopsy cannula directed through a twist-drill hole and a series of tiny stainless steel balls at 5-mm intervals along the surgical viewline and deposited (Figure 9-4). Anteroposterior (AP) and lateral radiographs are obtained and used as references for movements of the tumor within the intracranial space following removal of a circular trephine plug and opening of the dura. An incision in the brain is made with the carbon dioxide laser and deepened as the microscope and laser directed toward toward the focal point of the frame are advanced by the carriage. At the outer border of

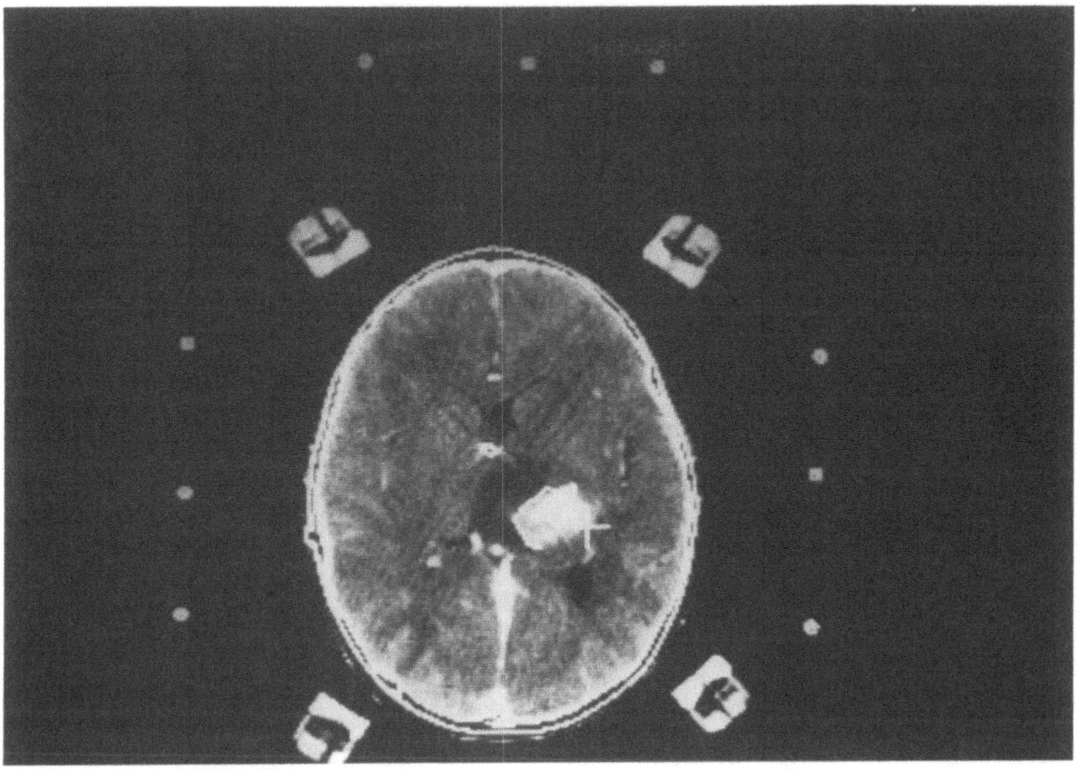

FIGURE 9-2. Each CT slice demonstrates nine reference marks. The height of the slice is related to the distance of the middle reference marks from the others on each localizing set. Reference marks are digitized by an intensity detection program. The surgeon outlines the boundaries of the tumor on each CT slice utilizing cursor and trackball.

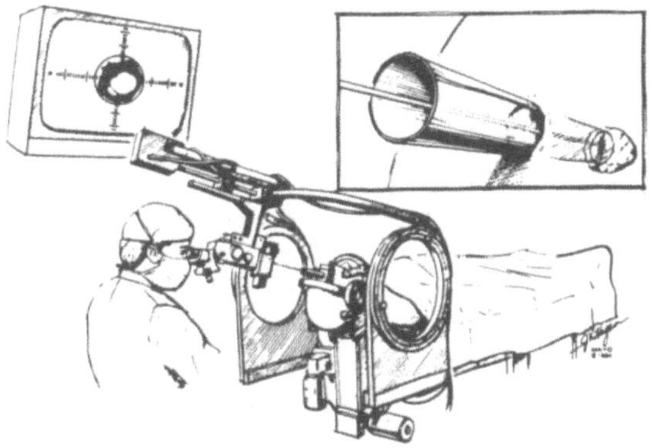

FIGURE 9-3. Custom arc-quadrant stereotactic frame mounted on operating table. A three-dimensional mechanical slide moves the head to place an intracranial target point in the focal point of a 135-mm and a 400-mm arc-quadrant. The microscope and laser manipulator mechanism run on a carriage that travels perpendicular to a tangent of the 400-mm arc. Tumors are vaporized by a stereotactically directed laser aimed through a stereotactically held retractor. The computer display monitor shows the position of the laser (cursor), retractor (circle), and slice from CT- (and/or MRI-) defined tumor volume. Tumor volume is sliced perpendicular to the surgical viewline at the level of depth to which the retractor has been inserted.

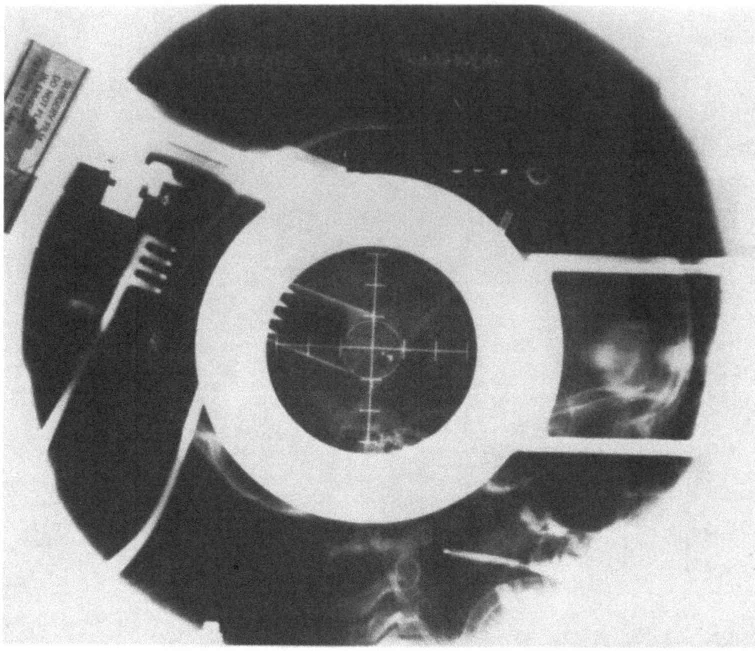

FIGURE 9-4. Lateral stereotactic teleradiograph showing the stereotactic retractor. Also demonstrating the position of steel reference balls, which were inserted along the surgical viewline.

the tumor, a stereotactic retractor is placed, which creates a shaft through the brain to the tumor. The tumor is vaporized slice by slice, progressing from the most superficial layer to the deepest. The surgeon monitors the position of the laser (represented by the cursors) in relationship to reformatted planar tumor boundaries on an operating room graphics monitor (Figure 9-5). Ultimately, a cavity is produced, which is documented by AP and lateral teleradiographs. These may be compared to coronal and sagittal reconstructions of CT data through the tumor.

Results

One hundred and forty-six computer-assisted stereotactic craniotomies have been performed on 140 patients since 1980. Five patients underwent repeat procedures for residual (three patients) and recurrent (two patients) tumors, and one of these patients underwent a third procedure for recurrent tumor. Patients ranged in age from 2 to 78 years, with an average age of 46.8 years. Lesion locations are illustrated in Figure 9-6, and histologies are listed in Table 9-1. Neurological examinations performed one week following the 146 procedures revealed that 67 patients (48%) were improved neurologically and 59 patients (42%) were neurologically unchanged (39 had been normal preoperatively, and remained normal postoperatively, 20 patients

TABLE 9-1. Tumor Histology in 140 Patients Undergoing Computer-Assisted Stereotactic Resections

Astrocytoma, grade IV	32
Astrocytoma, grade III	12
Astrocytoma, grade II	23
Metastatic	38
Oligodendroglioma	9
Vascular	14
Miscellaneous	12
Abscess	1
Choroid plexis papilloma	1
Colloid cyst	1
Ganglioneuroma	2
Lymphoma	2
Meningioma	3
Tub, sclerosis	2
Total	140

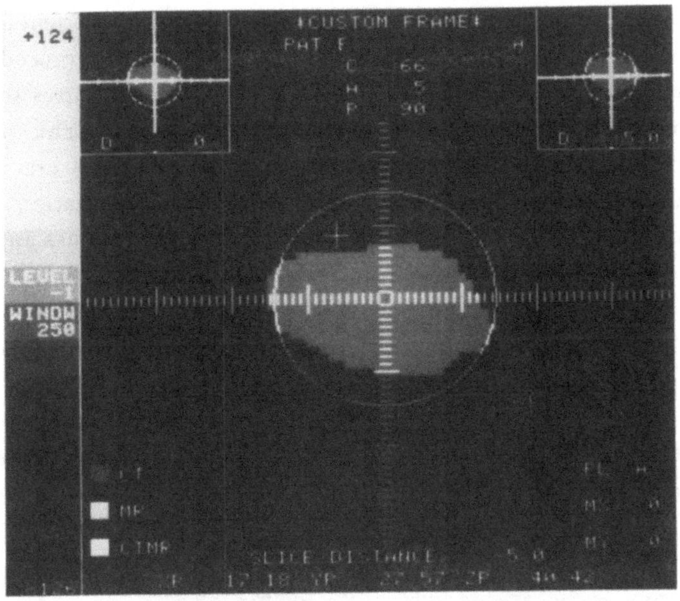

FIGURE 9-5. Computer generated display showing a section of tumor sliced along the surgical viewline, the outline of the stereotactic retractor, and the position of the surgical laser in reference to the tumor represented by a cursor. The "lookahead" sequence shows deeper slices of tumor.

had preoperative neurological deficits that did not improve postoperatively).

Seventeen patients were neurologically worse: seven patients developed superior quadrant visual field deficits following posterior temporal approaches to medial temporal or thalamic lesions, one patient had a complete homonymous hemianopia following an occipital approach to a posterior thalamic lesion, and nine patients experienced worsening of the neurological deficits noted preoperatively. Three

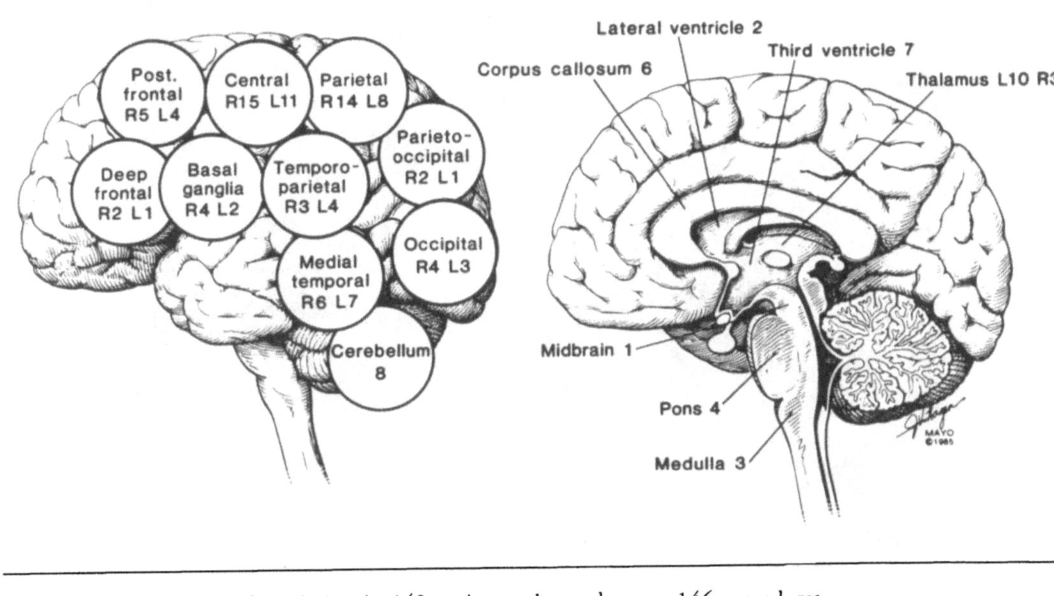

FIGURE 9-6. Location of the lesion in 140 patients who underwent 146 procedures.

deaths occurred within 1 month following surgery: one from massive brainstem edema following removal of a ventral thalamic astrocytoma with brainstem infiltration apparent on MRI, one from a ventricular infection after resection of a previously irradiated teratoma from the third ventricle, and one from a massive pulmonary embolism 2 weeks following resection of a thalamic cavernous hemangioma.

Discussion

Stereotactic laser microsurgical resection of deep-seated intracranial lesions allows a three-dimensional surgical orientation to be maintained in subcortical procedures. Tumors in important subcortical areas may be approached through nonessential brain tissue, and the resection of the lesion is precise and monitored not only by the visualization of the surgeon but also by computer graphics and teleradiography. Thus, aggressive and safe resection of deep-seated neoplasms is possible (Figure 9-7) [8].

With the stereotactic method described, it is possible to resect all tumor detected by CT scanning. Nevertheless, correlation studies of histology from stereotactic serial biopsies and CT-defined tumor boundaries indicated that the

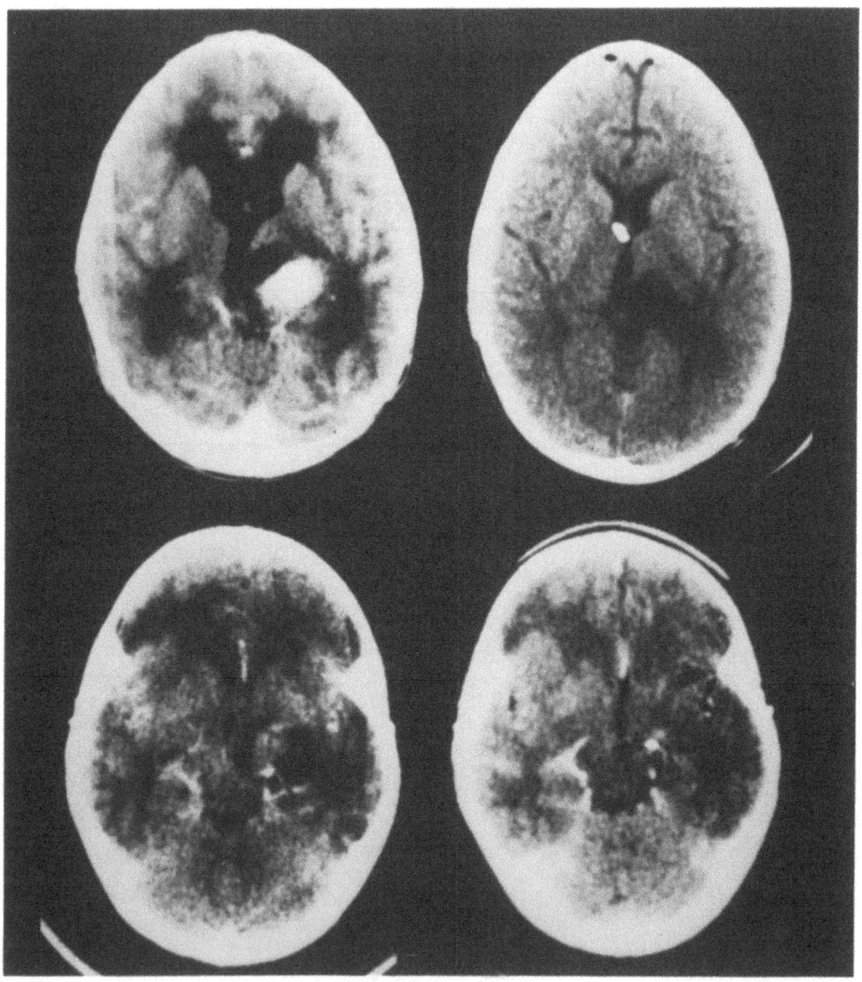

FIGURE 9-7. Representative preoperative and post-operative CT scan in two patients with thalamic pilocytic astrocytomas.

CT scan may not accurately represent the histological limits of primary intracranial neoplasms [2]. Our experience indicates that the histological boundaries of primary glial neoplasms extend beyond the boundaries indicated by CT scanning. Thus, some form of adjuvant therapy must be directed at the cells of the neoplasm remaining in the hypodense zone surrounding the area of contrast enhancement that is resected by the stereotactic procedure. Nevertheless, a significant reduction of tumor cell burden may favorably influence survival and response to external radiation and chemotherapy. In addition, photoradiation therapy is considered to supplement standard radiation therapy and chemotherapy [3]. We believe that this will further reduce the tumor cell population that remains following CT-based stereotactic laser resection of the lesion.

Conclusion

The carbon dioxide laser has been incorporated into a computer-assisted stereotactic system for precision resection of deep-seated intraaxial neoplasms. Stereotactic CT scanning provides a precise three-dimensional, tumor-volumetric data base in relationship to a custom arcquadrant stereotactic frame. A carbon dioxide laser beam is directed by the stereotactic instrument. It is monitored by an interactive computer graphics system in relation to boundaries of the tumor volume, which has been sliced orthogonal to the surgical viewline. Theoretically, the procedure allows removal of all tumor identified by CT scanning. One hundred and forty-six of these procedures have been performed on 140 patients who had a variety of neoplasms in various deep-seated locations, with satisfactory postoperative results.

References

1. Alker GJ, Kelly PJ, Kall BA, Goerss SJ: Stereotactic laser ablation of intracranial lesions. *Am J Neuroradiol* 4:727–730, 1983.
2. Daumas-Duport C, Monsaingeon V, Szenthe L, Szikla G: A double histological code of gliomas according to malignancy and 3-D configuration, as an aid to therapeutic decision and assessment of results. *Appl Neurophysiol* 45:431–437, 1982.
3. Dougherty TJ, Kaufman JE, Goldfarb A, et al: Photoradiation therapy for the treatment of malignant tumors. *Cancer Res* 38:2628–2635, 1978.
4. Goerss S, Kelly PJ, Kall B, Alker GJ Jr: A computed tomographic stereotactic adaptation system. *Neurosurgery* 10:375–379, 1982.
5. Kelly PJ, Alker GJ Jr: A microstereotactic approach to deep-seated arteriovenous malformation: Case report and technical note. *Surg Neurol* 17:260–262, 1982.
6. Kelly PJ, Alker GJ Jr.: A stereotactic approach to deep-seated CNS neoplasms using the carbon dioxide laser. *Surg Neurol* 15:331–334, 1981.
7. Kelly PJ, Alker GJ Jr., Goerss SJ: Computer assisted stereotactic laser microsurgery for the treatment of intracranial neoplasms. *Neurosurgery* 10:324–331, 1982.
8. Kelly PJ, Alker GJ Jr, Kall B, Goerss S: Precision resection of intra-axial CNS lesions by CT-based stereotactic craniotomy and computer monitored CO_2 laser. *Acta Neurochir* 68:1–9, 1983.
9. Kelly PJ, Kall B, Goerss S, Earnest F: Computer-assisted stereotaxic resection of intra-axial brain neoplasms. *J Neurosurg* 64:427–439, 1986.

III. SPINAL APPLICATIONS

10. THE USE OF THE LASER IN THE OPERATIVE MANAGEMENT OF INTRASPINAL TUMORS

W. Craig Clark
Jon H. Robertson

In adults, the ratio between intraspinal and intracranial tumors is roughly one to four [37]. For purposes of discussion, we have divided these tumors into three major categories: (1) those extradural in location; (2) those inside the dura, but outside the spinal cord (intradural-extramedullary); and (3) those inside the spinal cord (intramedullary).

There are several excellent reviews concerning the epidemiology, pathology, and diagnosis of these lesions, and this work will not be reiterated here [22, 23, 30, 31, 37, 38]. Instead, the purpose of this chapter is to discuss specific applications of laser technology in the operative management of various intraspinal lesions and present selected case material to illustrate these applications. We have almost exclusively relied on the carbon dioxide laser unless otherwise noted.

Extradural Tumors

About 30% of all intraspinal tumors are found in the epidural space [37]. Most epidural tumors in the spinal canal will be metastatic in origin, arising from a vertebral body and invading the anterior epidural space [35]. The most common sites of origin of these lesions are from carcinoma of the lung in males and carcinoma of the breast in females. Prostatic carcinoma and tumors of the gastrointestinal tract, as well as thyroid carcinomas, are commonly seen [37].

Most texts and earlier reports recommend immediate decompressive laminectomy, even though this procedure has produced clinical improvement in only 30% to 40% of patients [2, 13, 16, 29, 43, 45]. Recent studies have suggested that the treatment of choice for most patients with metastatic cord compression should be radiotherapy rather than surgery [5, 14, 18], but these studies have compared radiotherapy with a posterior decompressive laminectomy. We are unaware of any study comparing the use of radiotherapy versus anterior surgical intervention and believe surgical intervention is warranted when (1) the known tumor is resistant to radiation, e.g., renal carcinoma, melanoma, and soft tissue sarcoma; (2) the nature of the primary tumor is not known or the diagnosis is in doubt; (3) relapse occurs after radiotherapy, and no further radiation can be administered; or (4) symptoms progress despite ongoing radiotherapy [42].

The major problems associated with a posterior decompressive laminectomy are that only a small amount of the total tumor volume can be

Robertson, J.H. and Clark, W.C. (eds), Lasers in Neurosurgery.

exposed for decompression, and, if the vertebral body is already destroyed by tumor, removal of the posterior elements can result in segmental instability and further damage to an already compromised spinal cord [44].

When performing a posterior decompressive laminectomy, we have not used the laser for attempted decompression of the neural elements for two reasons. First, the tumor that is visible posteriorly can usually be stripped from the dura fairly easily, and the use of the laser only increases the anesthetic time in patients who are often poor surgical risks. Second, the anterior origins of these masses make this procedure strictly palliative and diagnostic, since the majority of the compressive epidural metastatic tumor will not be visualized via a posterior decompressive laminectomy [8].

Other authors have used criteria similar to those outlined above for anterior surgical intervention, because they feel that the majority of epidural metastatic tumors involve the vertebral body and lie anterior to the spinal cord [35, 36] (Figure 10-1). If this approach is selected, there may be a role for the carbon dioxide laser because this represents at least an attempt at a gross total removal of the epidural mass. This strategy involves a fairly extensive surgical dissection, with the operative approach being anterior, transthoracic, retroperitoneal, or via a costotransversectomy, and requiring resection of the involved vertebral body. Several reviews have examined the merits of these approaches [1, 6, 26, 35, 36, 40], and a complete exposition of these various operative strategies is beyond the scope of this chapter. Once the desired anterior or anterolateral exposure is achieved, the operating microscope and carbon dioxide laser are brought into position. A corpectomy is performed using either a high-speed drill or curette in order to expose the tumor mass. The carbon dioxide laser is then used at a power setting of 60 to 80 W and defocused in order to evaporate tumor from the anterior and lateral epidural space. As the bulk of the tumor is evaporated, the power is decreased and the beam changed from continuous to pulsed bursts of radiation to decrease the spread of heat to the dura and the adjacent spinal cord. The continuity of the dura is preserved, if at all possible, to maintain the natural insulating properties of the cerebrospinal fluid around the spinal cord. The dura provides the limit of tumor dissection or evaporation (Figure 10-2).

Once the neural tissues are decompressed, stabilization of the spine may be required. Stabilization is usually performed if more than 50% of the width of the vertebral body was removed or if the spine has been rendered unstable by a previous laminectomy or tumorous involvement of the posterior elements [35] and may be performed using instrumentation, bone grafting, cement, or some combination of these [25, 35, 36].

We have been unable to document any statistically significant difference in outcomes of patients operated on with the laser versus those operated on with conventional microsurgical technique. The prognosis and result of any treatment strategy is more a function of the neurological status and ability to ambulate at the time of presentation rather than any particular mode of treatment.

Intradural Tumors

EXTRAMEDULLARY

The vast majority of tumors in this location are either meningiomas or neurinomas [17, 21, 23, 28, 37]. Both of these tumor types are encapsulated, benign, and usually separate easily from the spinal cord. They are small, rounded tumors and only become symptomatic late in their course as a result of very slow growth. Meningiomas are most often found in the thoracic region (81%), with far fewer located in the cervical (16%) or lumbar (3%) areas [37]. Neurinomas are fairly evenly distributed throughout the spine, with thoracic neurinomas comprising 39% of the total, lumbar, 32%, and cervical, 23% [21]. Neurinomas occasionally present as

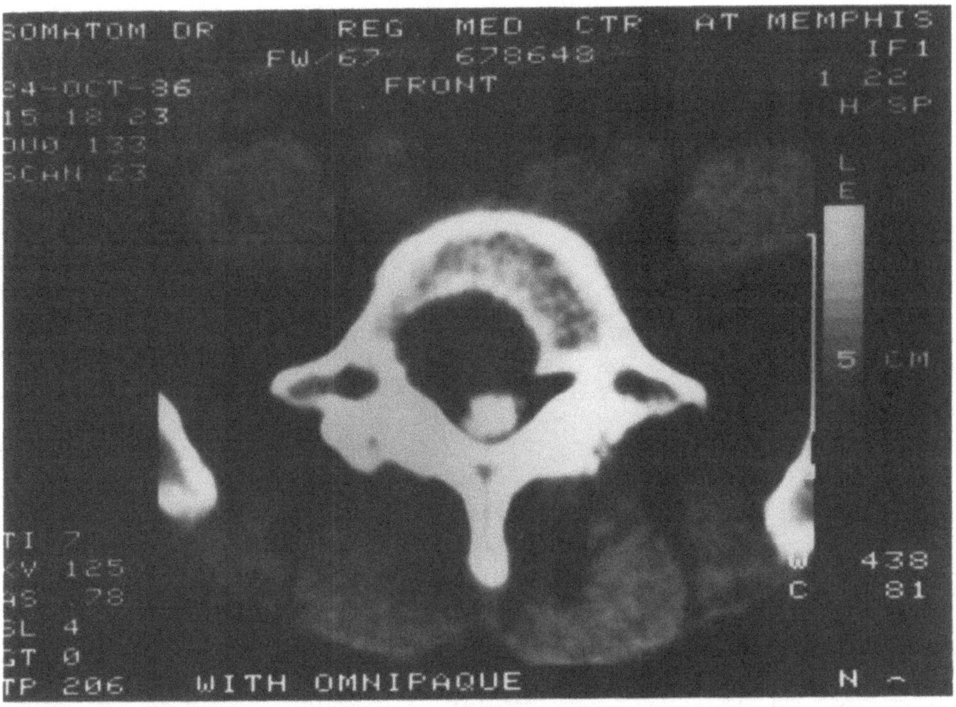

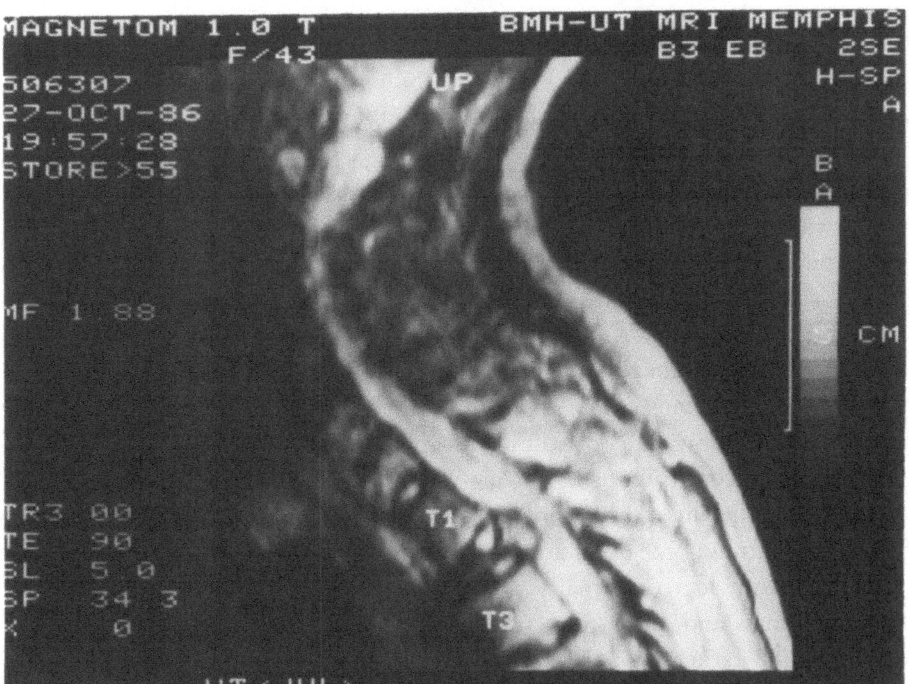

FIGURE 10-1. (Top) CT scan of lumbar spine demonstrating vertebral body and tumor involvement of the anterior epidural space. (Bottom) Sagittal MRI scan demonstrating loss of vertebral body height with concomitant anterior thoracic spinal cord compression with metastatic breast carcinoma.

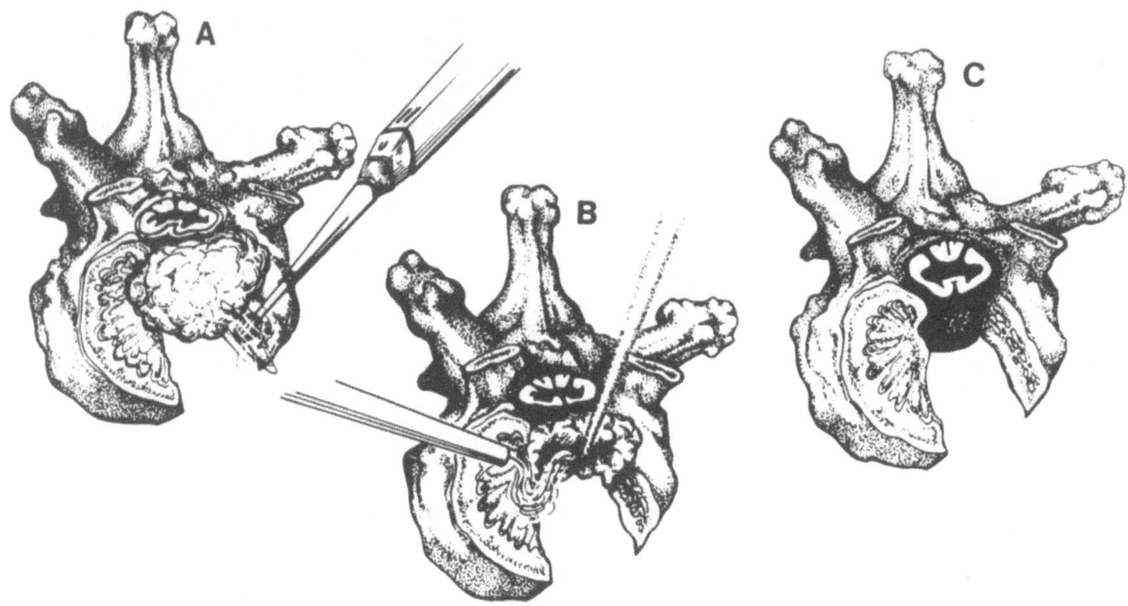

FIGURE 10-2. (A) corpectomy is performed using a high-speed drill or curette. (B) The microscopically-controlled carbon dioxide laser is then used to evaporate tumor from the vertebral body and the anterior eqidural space. (C) The dura provides the limit of dissection and tumor vaporization. If more than 50% of the vertebral body was removed, stabilization may be required. See text.

tumors both within and outside the spinal canal, e.g., the dumbbell tumors [23].

Most subdural meningiomas are attached to the anterolateral wall of the dura, with only a few attached to the posterior wall [23]. When a meningioma is attached to the posterior or posterolateral wall of the dura, it is often possible to incise the dura around the tumor's attachment, achieve dural hemostasis with bipolar coagulation, and simply lift the tumor from its bed in the spinal cord (Figure 10-3). If the tumor capsule is adherent to the cord or there is difficulty in identifying the dural attachment, the laser may be used to internally decompress the tumor mass and allow retraction only on the tumor itself rather than the spinal cord. This decompression is performed in a fairly standard fashion using about 40 watts of defocused laser power in a continuous fashion. After the majority of the tumor is decompressed, the power is decreased and the laser is used in pulsed bursts to prevent the spread of heat through the remaining tumor tissue and capsule to the cord below. Evoked potential monitoring can be used as a guide of when to stop the dissection, when to add irrigation to help dissipate heat, etc. We also advocate the use of continuous suction-irrigation to aid the control of heat generated during the laser dissection.

In anterolateral meningiomas, the spinal cord appears displaced backwards and to the opposite side with the nerve roots and dentate ligaments stretched (Figure 10-4). The dentate ligaments are secured with a small suture for retraction and then sectioned. An effort should be made to preserve any nerve roots, but this is often very difficult to do. The spinal cord is then rotated delicately by retracting slightly on the dentate ligaments and the tumor is exposed. When the tumor is large and the space available insufficient, the operator may remove one or more articular facets on the side of the tumor to

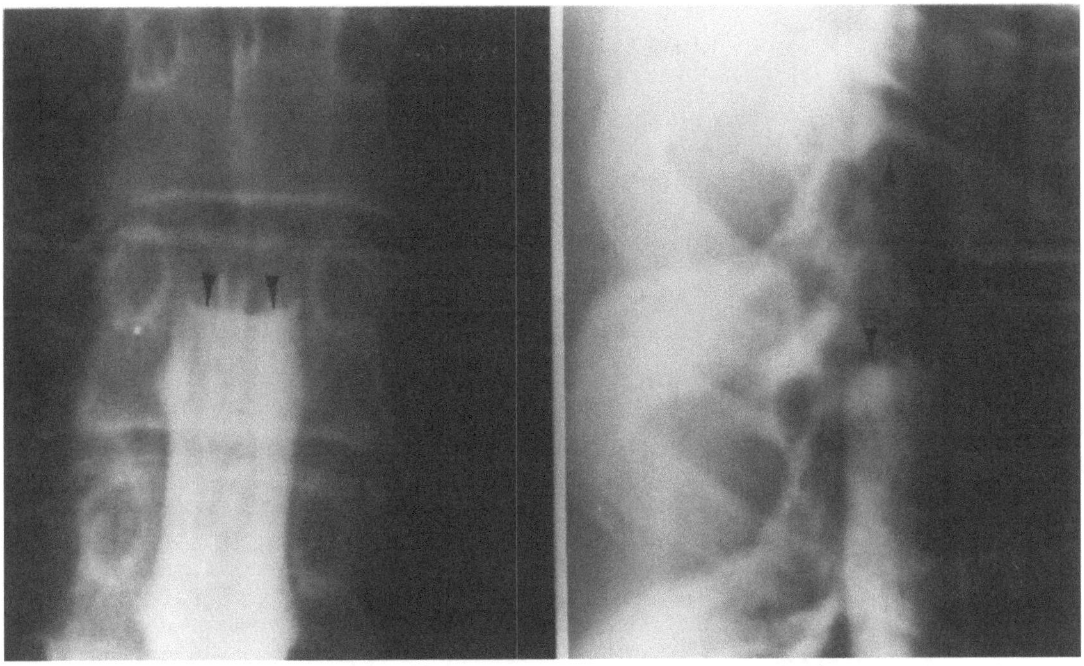

A

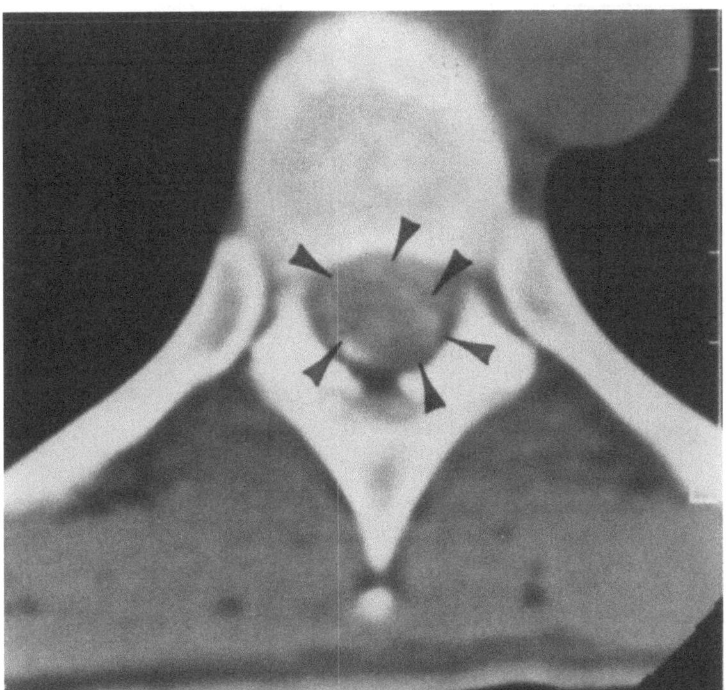

B

FIGURE 10-3. (A) Water-soluble contrast myelogram demonstrating a thoracic intradural, extra-medullary tumor. (B) Axial CT scan demonstrating the well-defined intradural tumor mass (*arrowheads*). Note that the spinal cord is severely compressed by this mass.

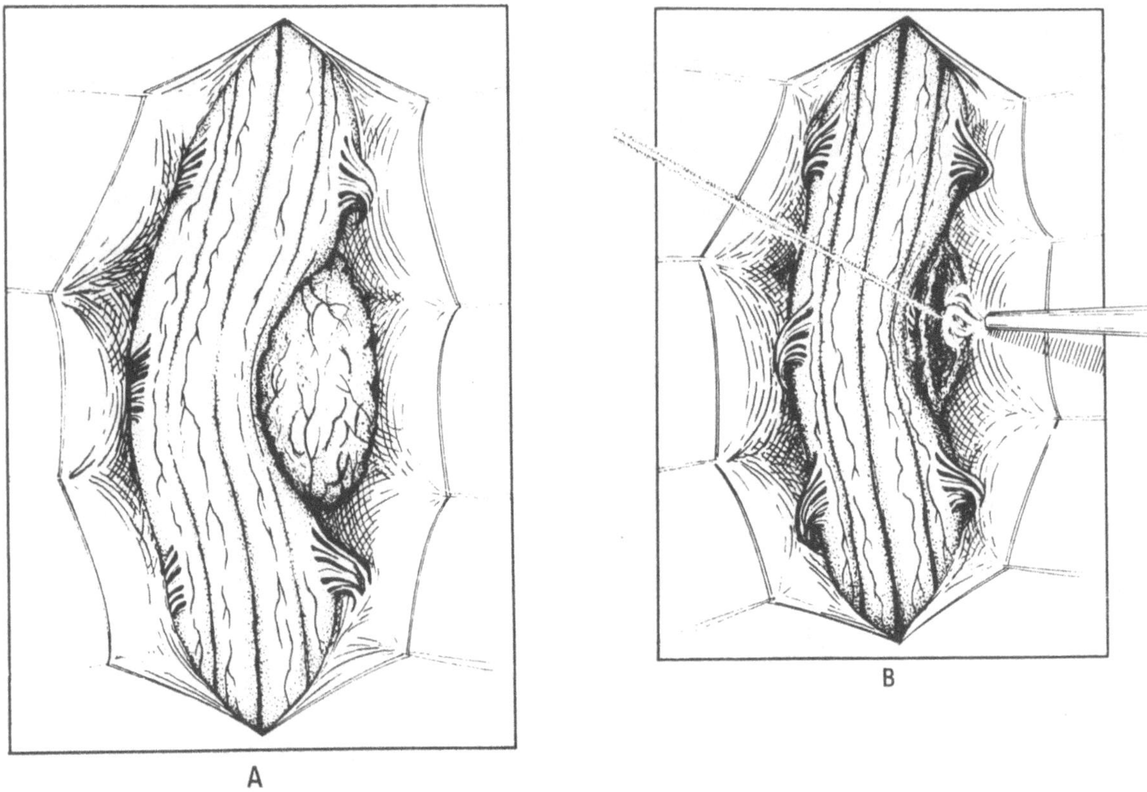

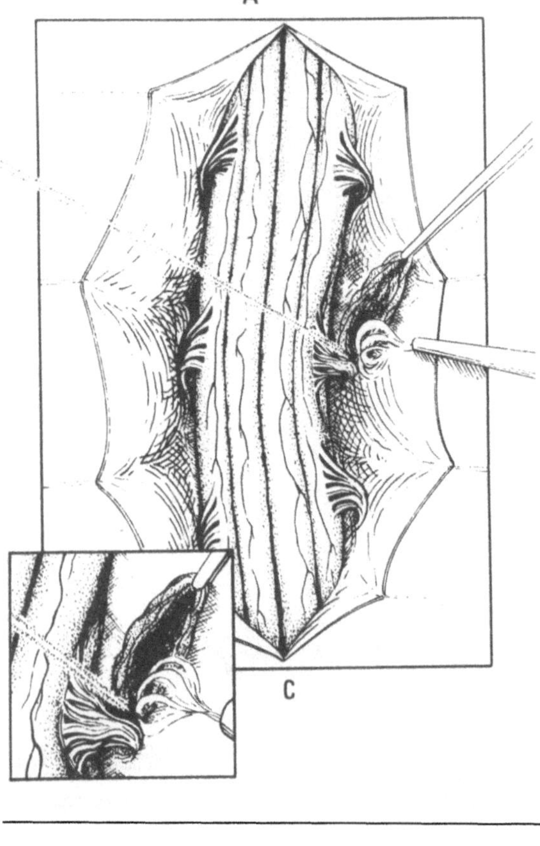

FIGURE 10-4. (A) Idealized illustration depicting the displacement of the spinal cord seen with thoracic meningiomas. (B) An internal decompression is performed on the tumor mass in order to allow all retraction and mechanical forces to be applied to the tumor rather than the spinal cord. (C) Once the tumor is removed along with the involved dural attachment, the cord is more relaxed.

improve the exposure. The spinal cord and nerve roots are then protected with cotton pledgets soaked in physiological solution. The laser is then used to effect an internal decompression of the tumor mass. This allows the operator to retract on the capsule to begin separating it from the cord without applying major distracting forces to the spinal cord itself. Once the capsule has been emptied, the volume of the mass is usually sufficiently decreased to allow removal of the entire capsule along with its dural attachment.

In meningiomas located anterior to the spinal cord, the tumor should be approached using an anterior or anterolateral approach as outlined earlier in the discussion of metastatic tumors. Once adequate operative exposure is achieved, the internal decompression and subsequent tumor removal is accomplished as with the other intraspinal meningiomas. After removal of the meningioma, a free graft of bank dura mater, synthetic dural substitute, or fascia lata is applied to the ventral surface of the cord and folded back on the dorsal surface like a hammock in an attempt to prevent a cerebrospinal fluid leak [23].

Neurinomas found within the dura are removed much like the meningiomas. The major difference is that removal of the meningiomas requires removal of the dural attachment, whereas in neurinomas it is often necessary to section the nerve roots from which the tumors arise if the tumor capsule cannot be isolated from the nerve roots.

Dumbbell neurinomas present a different set of technical problems. These tumors may present with their major bulk within the spinal canal, with only a small growth into the intravertebral foramen (i.e., the bottle neurinomas), or they may present with an accompanying paravertebral tumor mass connected by tumor that extends through the foramen. The bottle neurinomas present no particular difficulty, because the portion of the tumor within the foramen can be delivered into the spinal canal once the intraspinal portion has been removed. If a paravertebral mass is small, additional bone removal may be required, but its removal does not present any unique problems. In dumbbell neurinomas with a large paravertebral component, we have preferred a combined approach performed in cooperation with a thoracic surgeon because of the increased risk for pleural injury and pneumothorax in the postoperative period.

JUXTAMEDULLARY

Subdural lipomas represent a special class of tumors in adults in that they are not really either extramedullary or intramedullary, but instead are juxtamedullary subpial tumors. There is ample description of this entity in the literature [3, 12, 15, 34, 41], and only the surgical technique will be discussed here.

Unfortunately, there is rarely a sharp plane of cleavage between tumor and nerve tissue because of fibrous or fibrolipoid attachments that arise from the tumor capsule and plunge into the nervous parenchyma. It is these fibrolipomatous attachments that have complicated previous attempts to totally remove adult lipomas.

After opening the dura, which is usually adherent to the lipomatous mass, the laser is used to evaporate as much of the tumor as possible. This is performed quite easily as a result of the high water content of these tumors and the ability of the carbon dioxide laser to evaporate intracellular water [4, 33]. Once the juxtamedullary portion is removed, gentle traction is exerted on the tumor capsule to expose the fibrous attachments in the midline of the spinal cord. Bipolar coagulation and sharp dissection are used to interrupt these attachments as close to the tumor capsule as possible. The exposed spinal cord is protected with cotton pledgets soaked in physiological solution, and the fibrous attachments are then vaporized using the carbon dioxide laser set at about 20 W and applied in pulsed bursts. The last remnants of tumor are usually tightly adherent to the spinal cord and may be very difficult or impossible to remove without causing undue damage to the

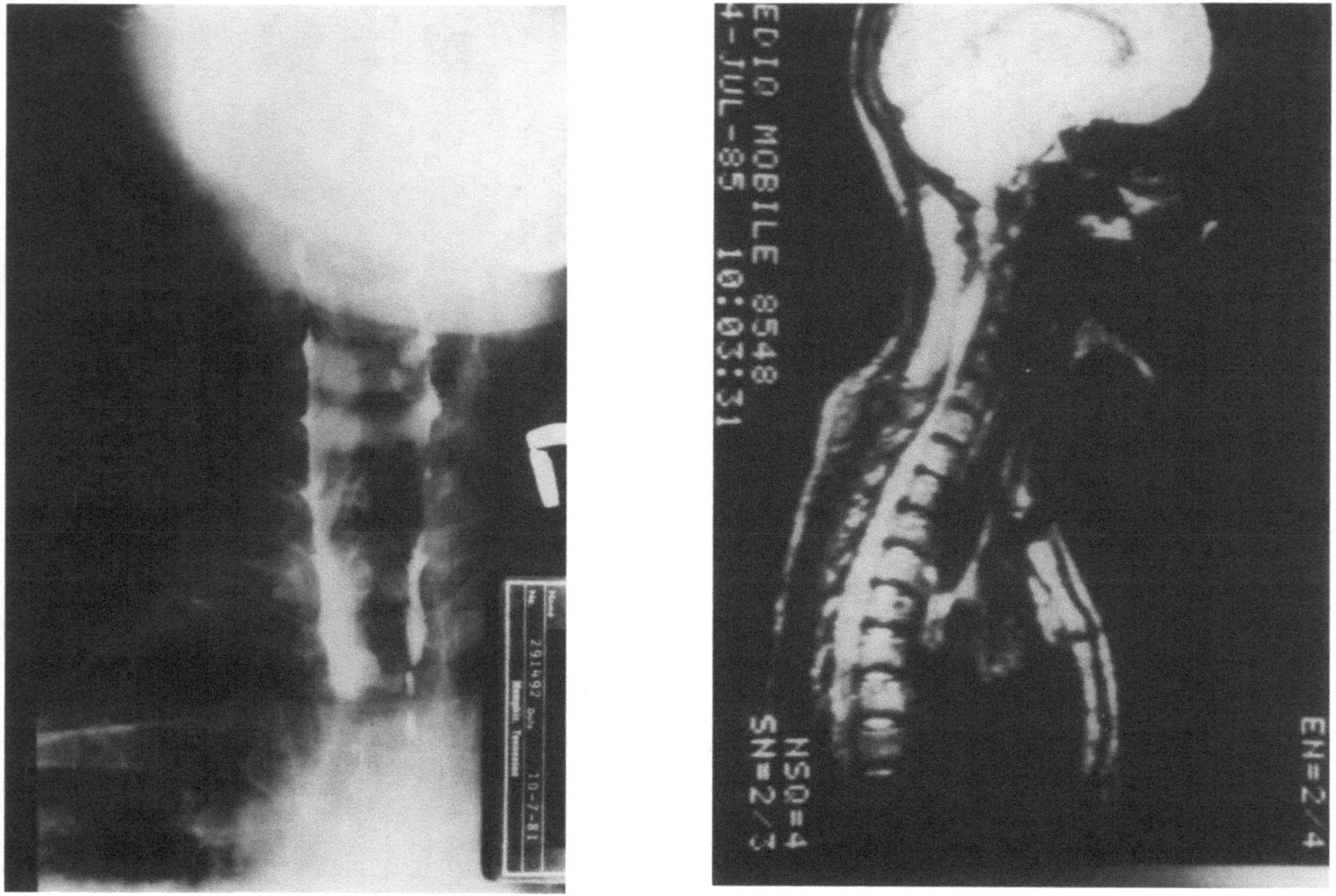

A B

FIGURE 10-5. (A) Cervical pantopaque myelogram showing widening of the cervical cord suggestive of an intramedullary lesion. (B) Sagittal MRI scan demonstrating an intramedullary astrocytoma of the cervical spinal cord.

cord. When these last remnants cannot be vaporized, we believe that it is best to suspend further attempts at removal and leave a few remnants of tumor rather than damage the cord by attempting a radical removal. Evoked potential monitoring may provide a good guide regarding how vigorous a dissection may be attempted without damaging the spinal cord.

INTRAMEDULLARY

Intramedullary tumors are the least common of the intraspinal tumors, with the reported incidence ranging from 14% to 30% [7, 9, 24, 30, 38]. The most frequently encountered tumors are ependymomas and astrocytomas [9, 19, 24, 27, 32, 38] (Figure 10-5). Ependymomas are seen most frequently in the region of the conus and the filum terminale, whereas astrocytomas occur more frequently in the cervical or cervicothoracic regions. Other intramedullary tumor types are generally benign, malignant tumors are rare.

With the exception of new hemostatic methods and microsurgical dissection, the basic surgical technique for removal of intramedullary tumors has changed little since Elsberg's description [9]. Greenwood outlined the use of bipolar coagulation and binocular loupe magnification for the total removal of intramedullary ependymomas [20]. It is generally felt that ependymomas can be totally removed [22, 30, 39], and the combination of the carbon dioxide laser with standard microsurgical technique facilitates these efforts. Currently we advocate the principles of (1) adequate exposure; (2) gentle, minimal traction on the spinal cord proper when necessary; (3) bipolar coagulation as an aid to maintaining hemostasis; (4) maintenance of a cleavage plane between the tumor and the spinal cord with the assistance of the operating microscope; and (5) use of the carbon dioxide laser for performing the myelotomy and internal decompression of the tumor mass.

A posterior exposure is performed in a conventional manner, with enough laminae removed to expose normal spinal cord both above and below the area suspected of containing tumor. The dura is opened widely and the spinal cord inspected for discoloration, abnormal vascularity, thinning of the cord, or other signs suggestive of an intramedullary neoplasm. Either a midline or paramedian myelotomy is performed, depending on the location of the mass. If an avascular area is not apparent in the selected line of incision, the laser is used with 5 W of power in a defocused fashion to produce an avascular line for incision. The power is then increased in the range of 10 to 20 W and the beam focused for cutting the myelotomy. This technique of performing the myelotomy does not require any manipulation of the spinal cord with instrumentation. Initially, motion artifact associated with respiration can be troublesome, but this is easily managed by short periods of apnea controlled by the anesthetist.

As the myelotomy is performed, the spinal cord falls open as a result of increased intramedullary pressure. In some cases, the tumor mass will actually partially extrude through the myelotomy as described by Elsberg [10]. The coagulation effect of the laser easily divides any vascular adhesions that may be present between the tumor and the spinal cord. In patients who have had previous operations, the problem of adhesions and distortion of the anatomical landmarks often creates problems, especially when the dura mater was not closed at the initial operation. As the myelotomy is completed over the extent of the intramedullary tumor mass, the pial edge is gently retracted with fine 7-0 sutures to expose the tumor mass and the interior of the spinal cord.

The carbon dioxide laser is then used to perform an internal decompression of the tumor with a higher energy, defocused beam. Once the decompression is complete, the beam is focused and, using approximately 10 W of power in conjunction with conventional microsurgical techniques, a cleavage plane is developed between the tumor mass and the spinal cord. The remaining edges of tumor are removed piecemeal using either conventional microsurgical

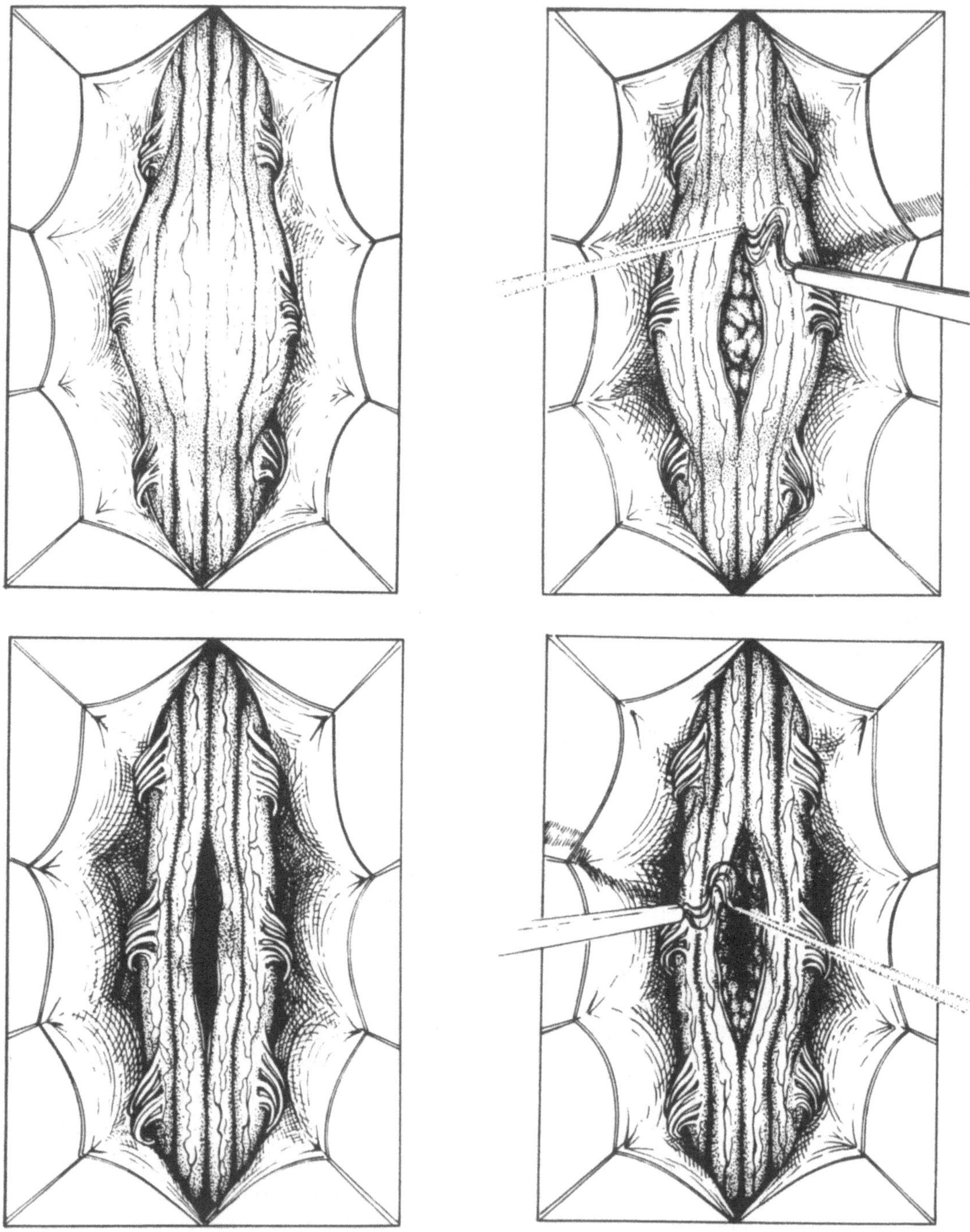

FIGURE 10-6. (A) With the dura opened and retracted, the widened spinal cord is inspected for signs suggestive of an intramedullary neoplasm. (See text). (B) As the laser is used to perform the midline myelotomy, the cord falls open as a result of the increased intramedullary pressure. (C) A defocused laser beam is used to perform an internal decompression of the tumor mass. (D) With the tumor removed, the spinal cord relaxes, and more normal intramedullary pressure is now evident.

technique or the laser to vaporize the remaining pieces. At the completion of the tumor removal, the tumor bed may be coagulated with a low-energy, defocused laser beam. This tends to sterilize remaining tumor cells and provides excellent hemostasis in the tumor bed (Figure 10-6).

Astrocytomas present a different problem—it may be quite difficult to define a distinct interface between tumor and the spinal cord. An intramedullary low-grade astrocytoma should be approached with the intention of total tumor removal; this has been reported [11, 39], but is believed to be rarely possible by others [24, 30]. The techniques described earlier for the removal of intramedullary ependymomas would likewise apply here, the exception being that when a plane of dissection cannot be appreciated, one must often accept a subtotal removal.

Throughout the tumor removal, standard microsurgical dissection techniques are used in conjunction with the carbon dioxide laser. Bipolar coagulation is required for tumor vessels greater than about 1.5 mm in diameter, because the carbon dioxide laser does not readily coagulate these larger vessels.

Conclusion

The techniques for removal of intraspinal tumors utilizing the carbon dioxide laser have been described. It is important that the laser be combined with microsurgical technique in order to achieve the full benefits of this technology.

References

1. Ammirati M, Sundaresan N, Lane JM: Technique of vertebral body resection and stabilization for the treatment of spinal metastases. *Surg Rounds* 8:21–34, 1985.
2. Brice J, McKissock W: Surgical treatment of malignant extradural spinal tumors. *Br Med J* 1:1341–1344, 1965.
3. Caram PC, Scarcella G, Carton CA: Intradural lipomas of the spinal cord. *J Neurosurg* 14:28–42, 1957.
4. Clark WC, Robertson JH, Gardner G: Selective absorption and control of thermal effects: A comparison of the laser systems used in otology and neurotology. *Otolaryngol Head Neck Surg* 92:73–79, 1984.
5. Cobb CA, Leavens ME, Eckles N: Indications for nonoperative treatment of spinal cord compression due to breast cancer. *J Neurosurg* 47:653–658, 1977.
6. Cook WA: Transthoracic vertebral surgery. *Ann Thorac Surg* 12:54–68, 1971.
7. DeSousa AL, Kalsbeck JE, Mealey JH, et al: Intraspinal tumors in children: A review of 81 cases. *J Neurosurg* 51:437–445, 1979.
8. Doppman JL, Girton M: Angiographic study of the effect of laminectomy in the presence of acute anterior epidural masses. *J Neurosurg* 45: 195–202, 1976.
9. Elsberg CA: Tumors of the vertebral column, spinal cord and membranes. In Elsberg CA (ed.): *Diagnosis and Treatment of Surgical Disease of the Spinal Cord and its Membranes* Philadelphia, Saunders, 1916, pp 236–281.
10. Elsberg CA, Beer E: The operability of intramedullary tumors of the spinal cord. *Am J Med Sci* 142:636–647, 1911.
11. Epstein F, Epstein N: Surgical treatment of spinal cord astrocytomas of childhood: A series of 19 patients. *J Neurosury* 57:685–689, 1982.
12. Fromm H, von Wild K: Clinical aspects, operative treatment, and rehabilitation of paraplegia caused by lipomas of the spinal cord: With particular emphasis of the intramedullary lipomas. *Paraplegia* 12:15–20, 1974.
13. Giannotta SL, Kindt GW: Metastatic spinal cord tumors. *Clin Neurosurg* 25:495–503, 1978.
14. Gilbert RW, Kim JH, Posner JB: Epidural spinal cord compression from metastatic tumor: Diagnosis and treatment. *Ann Neurol* 3:40–51, 1978.
15. Giuffré R, Gambacorta D: Lipoma of the spinal cord. *J Neurosurg* 35:335–337, 1971.
16. Gorter K: Results of laminectomy in spinal cord compression due to tumors. *Acta Neurochir* 42:177–187, 1978.
17. Grant FC: Surgical experiences with extramedullary tumors of the spinal cord. *Ann Surg* 128:679–684, 1948.
18. Greenberg HS, Kim JH, Posner JB: Epidural spinal cord compression from metastatic tumor: Results with a new treatment protocol. *Ann Neurol* 8:361–366, 1980.
19. Greenwood J: Intramedullary tumors of the spinal cord: A followup study after total surgical

removal. *J Neurosurg* 20:655–668, 1963.

20. Greenwood J: Surgical removal of intramedullary tumors. *J Neurosurg* 26:276–282, 1967.
21. Greenwood J: spinal cord tumors. In Youmans JR (ed): *Neurological Surgery*. Philadelphia, Saunders, 1973, pp 1514–1534.
22. Guidetti B: Intramedullary tumors of the spinal cord. *Acta Neurochir* 17:7–23, 1967.
23. Guidetti B: Removal of extramedullary benign spinal cord tumors. In Krayenbuhl H (ed): *Advances and Technical Standards in Neurosurgery*, Vol 1. New York, Springer-Verlag, 1974, pp 173–197.
24. Guidetti B, Mercuri S, Vagnozzi R: Long-term results of the surgical treatment of 129 intramedullary spinal gliomas. *J Neurosurg* 54:323–330, 1981.
25. Harrington KD: The use of methyl methacrylate for vertebral body replacement and anterior pathological fracture-dislocation of the spine due to metastatic malignant disease. *J Bone Joint Surg* 63A:36–46, 1981.
26. Johnson RM, Southwick WO: Surgical approaches to the spine. In Rothman RH, Simeone FA (eds): *The Spine*. Philadelphia, Saunders, 1975, pp 69–156.
27. Kopelson G, Linggood RM, Kleinman GM, et al: Management of intramedullary spinal cord tumors. *Radiology* 135:473–479, 1980.
28. Levy WJ, Bay J, Dohn D: Spinal cord meningioma. *J Neurosurg* 57:804–812, 1982.
29. Livingston KE, Perrin RG: The neurosurgical management of spinal metastases causing cord and cauda equina compression. *J Neurosurg* 49:839–843, 1978.
30. Malis LI: Intramedullary spinal cord tumors. *Clin Neurosurg* 25:512–539, 1978.
31. McGauley JL: Spine and spinal cord tumors. In Schneider RC, Kahn EA, Crosby EC, Taren JA (eds): *Correlative Neurosurgery*. Springfield, IL, Thomas, 1982, pp 975–1009.
32. Mork SJ, Loken AC: Ependymoma: A followup study of 101 cases. *Cancer* 40:907–915, 1977.
33. Robertson JH, Clark WC: Carbon dioxide laser in neurosurgery. *Contemp Neurosurg* 5:1–6, 1983.
34. Rogers HM, Long DM, Chou SN, French LA: Lipomas of the spinal cord and cauda equina. *J Neurosurg* 34:349–354, 1971.
35. Siegal T, Siegal T, Robin G, et al: Anterior decompression of the spine for metastatic epidural cord compression: A promising avenue of therapy? *Ann Neurol* 11:28–34, 1982.
36. Siegal T, Tiqva P, Siegal T: Vertebral body resection for epidural compression by malignant tumors. *J Bone Joint Surg* 67A:375–382, 1985.
37. Simeone FA: Intraspinal neoplasms, In Rothman RH, Simeone FA (eds): *The Spine*. Philadelphia, Saunders, 1975, pp 823–836.
38. Sloof JL, Kernohan JW, MacCarty CS: *Primary Intramedullary Tumors of the Spinal Cord and Filum Terminale*. Philadelphia, Saunders, 1964, pp 3–9.
39. Stein BM: Surgery of intramedullary spinal cord tumors. *Clin Neurosurg* 26:529–542, 1979.
40. Sundaresan N, Galicich JH, Bains MS, et al: Vertebral body resection in the treatment of cancer involving the spine. *Cancer* 53:1393–1396, 1984.
41. Thomas JE, Miller RH: Lipomatous tumors of the spinal canal. *Mayo Clin Proc* 46:393–400, 1973.
42. Tomaszek DE, Mahaley MS: Management of spinal epidural metastases. *Contemp Neurosurg* 5:1–6, 1983.
43. White WA, Patterson RH, Bergland RM: Role of surgery in the treatment of spinal cord compression by metastatic neoplasm. *Cancer* 27:558–561, 1971.
44. Winter RB, Moe JH, Wang JF: Congenital kyphosis: Its natural history and treatment as observed in a study of 130 patients. *J Bone Joint Surg* 55A:223–256. 1973.
45. Wright RL: Malignant tumors in the spinal extradural space: Results of surgical treatment. *Ann Surg* 157:227–231, 1963.

11. LASER IN PAIN MANAGEMENT

Clark Watts
Walter J. Levy

Over the past 20 years the laser has been introduced into the neurosurgical armamentarium and become widely accepted [4, 13]. As our understanding of the physics of lasers has improved, standard techniques for utilizing the properties of lasers to remove central nervous system tumors, excise scar tissue, and repair critical structures such as nerves and blood vessels have developed.

These techniques have recently been expanded to permit the use of lasers in controlled destruction of nervous tissue in the management of pain syndromes. The physical parameters for this controlled destruction are not unique to the managment of pain; rather, they are based upon an extension of our understanding of the biophysics of laser-tissue interactions. Our experience, and that recorded in the literature, has led us to conclude that the laser is a useful instrument for producing destructive lesions in the dorsal root entry zone (DREZ) for certain deafferentation pain syndromes, in myelotomies for pain of malignant and nonmalignant origin, and possibly in selected cases of rhizotomy for pain of peripheral origin.

DREZ Lesions

The experience of Nashold and others is that certain deafferentation pain syndromes, such as those that occur following brachial plexus avulsion injuries or traumatic paraplegia, may be effectively managed by the placement of radiofrequency lesions in the DREZ of the spinal cord [10]. A discussion of the neuroanatomical and neurophysiological concepts underlying this clinical experience is beyond the scope of this chapter. However, they have been well summarized in recent publications. [11].

An analysis of laboratory work using a cat model, and our clinical experience, allows us to conclude that the laser can be used to produce lesions in the DREZ with clinical results comparable to those seen following radiofrequency lesions with fewer complications [7, 8]. Edwards and associates, using both the carbon dioxide and the argon lasers, have achieved satisfactory results—characterized by at least a 50% reduction in pain intensity in over two-thirds of their patients with chronic benign painful states [4, 12]. The results were better in patients suffering painful syndromes associated with traumatic paraplegia and brachial plexus avulsion, post-rhizotomy dysesthetic pain, and phantom limb and amputation stump pain. Less satisfactory results were obtained in patients with pain of lumbar arachnoiditis and other chronic miscellaneous pain states. This was also the experience of Levy and his associates [8]. These results parallel those reported by Nashold and others with radiofrequency lesions. It can thus be anticipated that patients with pain following traumatic paraplegia or brachial plexus avulsion can receive excellent relief of pain for months to years following the appropriate placement of DREZ lesions with laser.

Robertson, J.H. and Clark, W.C. (eds), Lasers in Neurosurgery.

A review of published works suggests some disagreement as to the precise technique for the production of the lasered lesion. We prefer the carbon dioxide laser. It is the most widely used form of laser equipment because its major use is in the destruction of tissue, such as in the removal of brain tumors. In the DREZ lesion, one does not have to worry about hemostasis if the lesions are precisely placed under microscopic control. In the laboratory, we found that when the laser lesion was compared with the radiofrequency lesion, the latter was larger and three times more variable in size than the laser lesion [7]. The very brief period of the laser pulse, 0.1 second, means that the surgeon does not have to worry about movement of the spinal cord with respiration and heartbeat and, thus, movement of the surgical instrument while the lesion is being produced. This is a potential problem with the hand-held radiofrequency electrode.

The technique in humans is relatively simple. A standard laminectomy overlying the area of interest is performed with the patient in either the sitting or prone position. If the pain syndrome is associated with prior tissue destruction or injury, such as with a brachial plexus avulsion or traumatic paraplegia, the laminectomy should be extended a segment or two above and below the site of injury in order to identify the DREZ in normal spinal cord. Often, arachnoid and pial scarring that are found in the spinal cord itself will distort normal spinal cord architecture, making it necessary to extrapolate from the normal area of the spinal cord. The dura is opened in the midline and retracted laterally with sutures. If the procedure is performed with the carbon dioxide laser and is carried out in the prone position, it is important to keep the field dry of spinal fluid. It is helpful to have the respiratory rate slowed, but it is not absolutely necessary to have the patient apneic. The arachnoid is opened. Any arachnoidal scarring should be carefully dissected to avoid excessive manipulation of the spinal cord.

The lesions are made along the DREZ, separated by 1 to 2 mm at the dorsal base of each rootlet (Figure 11-1). The dentate ligaments are left intact and the spinal cord is not rotated. The

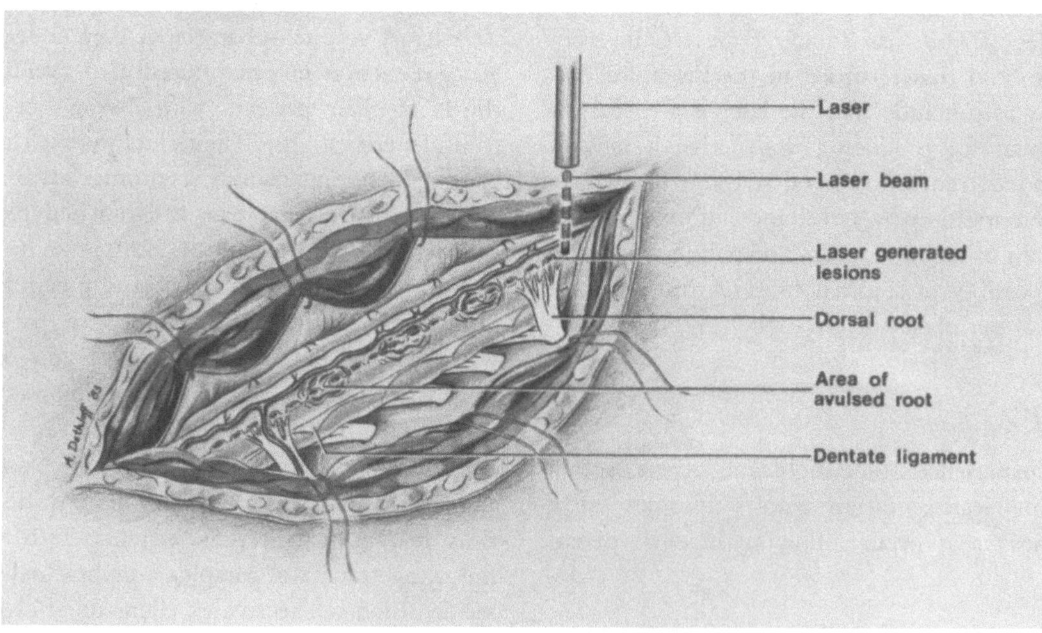

FIGURE 11-1. Laser generated dorsal root entry zone lesions.

beam is directed toward the cord at a 25-degree angle from the vertical midline of the cord. This should theoretically place the lesion directly under the point of entry of the rootlet. However, one must keep in mind that the anatomy of some patients with traumatic lesions is somewhat obscure or inexact. We use a pulse of 0.1 seconds with a power setting of approximately 10 to 20 W and a spot size of less than 0.4 mm. This lesioning is performed under direct microscopic control with the micromanipulator, with the parameters adjusted after observing the extent of the lesion produced by a single pulse. At these settings it is usually approximately 1 mm deep. A second pulse of laser energy is then directed at the initial lesion, increasing its depth to approximately 2 mm. This is initially measured by the tip of a small nerve hook. However, once several lesions have been made, the operator becomes accustomed to the depth, and an exact measurement need not be made each time. It is important to note that when making a lesion in scar, one has to first work through the pial scar into the cord. Therefore, the apparent depth will vary in these areas. Ordinarily it is not necessary to coagulate vessels on the surface of the cord which might be in the way. Instead, they may either be dissected so they may be retracted out of the way, or the lesion may be placed adjacent to the vessel.

There are several advantages to the use of the laser for this procedure. The size of the lesion is controlled by the surgeon under direct vision. Little if any manipulation of the spinal cord occurs. Those who report use of the radiofrequency lesion have noted significant ipsilateral long-tract injury, both to the spinothalamic and the corticospinal tracts in some patients. Neither Edwards' nor Levy's groups have reported these complications with the laser [4, 7, 8]. The lesions can be made rapidly once the geometry of the cord has been recognized.

The procedure does have some disadvantages that conceivably could, because of its deceptively easy approach, lead to problems. First the wound must be kept dry of cerebrospinal fluid. In animal experiments, we noted there was sometimes a discrepency between the location of the aiming beam and the location of the lesion produced by the laser beam. This seems to vary among units of equipment and usually occurs when the mirrors in the articulating arm of the carbon dioxide laser are not in proper alignment. It is an important point, however, because an error of a fraction of a millimeter may result in an inappropriate cord lesion, or injury to an important vessel. Therefore, we recommend that the equipment should receive regular preventive maintenance checkups and should first be evaluated in the laboratory so the surgeon can learn the extent of any variations that cannot be eliminated with realignment of the mirrors. In the operating room, this variation can be further evaluated by targeting a cottonoid patty or other material before lesions are actually produced in the spinal cord. Once the possibility of this variability is recognized it can be easily compensated for.

Intraoperative monitoring with sensory evoked potentials [6] or motor evoked potentials [9] is of interest, but we believe that the experience is not great enough to allow an understanding of the predictability of any changes that might occur with these monitoring techniques.

Commissural Myelotomy

One of the procedures in the surgical armamentarium of the neurosurgeon who treats pain of both malignant and benign origin is the commissural myelotomy. It was developed in an attempt to ablate pain sensation below the lesion without affecting touch sensation or motor function. However, using the standard knife technique, the development of significant motor, bowel, and bladder dysfunction below the level of the lesion limited the procedure primarily to the treatment of pain of malignant disease below the cervical area. With the development of microsurgical techniques, however, these risks have been lessened, and the procedure has been used increasingly for chronic benign pain. The standard indications for and technique of commissural myelotomy are well described elsewhere and are not the subject of this report [2, 3].

The introduction of the laser permits a further refinement of this technique such that major risks of the procedure may be reduced [5]. With the laser, the crossing pain fibers of the anterior white commissure may be cut with minimal manipulation of the spinal cord and interruption of small spinal cord blood vessels.

A standard bilateral laminectomy is performed, exposing the appropriate area of the spinal cord. The operating microscope is used with a 300-mm focal lens, the arachnoid is incised and dissected from the posterior surface of the spinal cord. It is necessary when using the carbon dioxide laser to keep the field dry of cerebrospinal fluid. An incision is made in the midline of the spinal cord with the laser between the fasciculi gracili. It is begun with the smallest beam spot size, no greater than 0.4 mm. The laser can be used in the continuous or pulsed mode with an output of approximately 10 W. The power output and spot size are varied, based upon the results noted under microscopic vision.

The laser incision is carried into the spinal cord superior to inferior with a total length of approximately 4.0 cm, bisecting the desired cord level. The crossing fibers in the anterior white commissure can be easily identified under the microscope, and minimum retraction is necessary. The myelotomy is continued anteriorly until the dura mater is identified. Careful observation is necessary to identify and avoid the anterior spinal artery should it reside in the midline.

Hemostasis can be obtained by defocusing the laser beam or by the use of small pledgets of gelfoam. Once hemostasis is obtained, the wound is thoroughly irrigated and the dura is closed in the usual fashion. No special restrictions are noted postoperatively.

As with the DREZ lesions, intraoperative monitoring is of interest, but its value is not proven.

Rhizotomy

Early studies on the effect of the carbon dioxide laser on nervous system tissue revealed an inhibition of axonal regrowth [4]. This led to the belief that carbon dioxide transection of peripheral nerves might be useful for both painful peripheral nerve lesions, such as neuromas, and as a treatment for other painful conditions for which rhizotomy has been advocated in the past [1]. However, long-term observations have not indicated that this method of peripheral transection results in any greater period of relief than standard surgical rhizotomy [4]. This has certainly been our experience with pain syndromes following chest surgery or injury. Because of the delay in operative time caused by the use of the laser instrument, and because results seem to be no better than for standard surgical incision and excision of peripheral nerve lesions, we currently believe that the laser should not be used routinely in these cases, but should rather be reserved for selected cases in which the particular advantages of laser technology may be maximally utilized.

References

1. Ascher PW: The use of CO_2 laser in neurosurgery. In Kaplan I (ed): *Laser Surgery II*. Jerusalem, Academic Press, 1978, pp 8–30.
2. Broager B: Commissural myelotomy. *Surg Neurol* 2:71–74, 1974.
3. Cook AW, Kawakami Y: Commissural myelotomy. *J Neurosurg* 47:1–6, 1977.
4. Edwards MSD, Boggan JE, Fuller, TA: The laser in neurological surgery. *J Neurosurg* 59: 555–566, 1983.
5. Fink FA: Neurosurgical treatment of nonmalignant intractable rectal pain: Microsurgical commissural myelotomy with carbon dioxide laser. *Neurosurgery* 14:64–654, 1984.
6. Grundy, BL: Monitoring of sensory evoked potentials during neurological operations: Methods and applications. *Neurosurgery* 11:556–575, 1982.
7. Levy WJ, Gallo C, Watts C: Comparison of laser and radiofrequency dorsal root entry zone lesions in cats. *Neurosurgery* 16:327–330, 1985.
8. Levy WJ, Nutkiewicz A, Ditmore QM, Watts C: Laser-induced dorsal entry zone lesions for

pain control. *J Neurosurg* 59:884–886, 1983.
9. Levy WJ, York DH, McCaffrey M, Tanzer F: Motor evoked potentials from transcranial stimulation in the motor cortex in humans. *Neurosurgery* 15:287–302, 1984.
10. Nashold BS, Jr: Current status of the DREZ operation. *Neurosurgery* 15:932–944, 1984.
11. Nashold BS Jr (ed): Proceedings of the First World Conference on Dorsal Root Entry Zone (DREZ), Mainz, West Germany, March 10–11, 1984. *Neurosurgery* 15:887–970, 1984.
12. Powers SK, Adams JE, Edwards MSD, et al: Pain relief from dorsal root entry zone lesions made with argon and carbon dioxide microsurgical lasers. *J Neurosurg* 61:841–847, 1984.
13. Saunders MA, Young HS, Becker DE, et al: The use of the laser in neurological surgery. *Surg Neurol* 14:1–10, 1980.

IV. OTHER USES

12. LASER SURGERY IN CONGENTIAL ABNORMALITIES

Hector E. James

Laser Surgery in Spinal Dysraphism

Spinal dysraphia is a term that encompasses certain variable congenital anomalies that result from errors in formation of the fetus during and after the closure of the neural tube in the early weeks of gestation [6, 7, 12, 21]. It represents a syndrome that is characteristically slow and insidious in its clinical presentation due to progressive denervation. There may be a slow and progressive deformity of one or both lower extremities [6, 21] or urinary symptoms with a recurrent or unexplained infection due to denervation, at times associated with continence that may evolve to incontinence in later life [4, 6, 7, 14]. Cutaneous changes may accompany spinal dysraphism with or without symptoms of the disease [6, 19].

Neuroimaging will confirm the location of the underlying pathology [7]. In the newborn period and up to approximately 1 year of age the spinal contents may be readily visualized by high-resolution spinal ultrasonography [17], and this may be the only study needed. At a later age the dorsal elements of the spinal canal thicken and ossify, and ultrasonography will no longer be of value. In these cases, magnetic resonance imaging (MRI) is the procedure of choice. Computed tomography (CT) with or without contrast enhancement will delineate the pathology in detail when MRI is not available [7].

Robertson, J.H. and Clark, W.C. (eds), Lasers in Neurosurgery.

CLINICAL INDICATIONS

When spinal dysraphia is detected, many authors recommend early operation to prevent the progressive crippling effects of this condition [4, 6, 7, 14, 21]. With modern neuroimaging, early diagnosis of the disease is feasible [7, 17]. The objective of the operation is to remove the underlying pathology whenever possible [7, 20, 21]. The underlying pathophysiology will then be corrected. If there is a mass that is compressing neural elements, which may occur with lipomas involving the conus, removal of the mass will halt further deterioration [4, 14]. On the other hand, if the problem is to restrict cranial migration of the neural elements, which may be seen with a thickened filum terminale, release of the filum will have the same effect [6]. On occasion the operative correction of the underlying pathology may be accompanied by improved neurological function [2, 4, 8, 14]. However, because the central nervous system axons and neurons do not regenerate, the deficits that occurred prior to surgery are most often not reversible.

INDICATIONS FOR LASER SURGERY

The concern about creating further damage to the neural elements involved in the dysraphic state has discouraged surgery for this disease process. Often a child is seen with occult dysraphism and has minimal neurological findings.

TABLE 12-1. Advantages of Laser Surgery in Spinal Dysraphia

1.	Reduces blood loss.
2.	Minimizes damage to normal neural tissues.
3.	Does not interfere with electrosphysiological monitoring systems.

This, added to the tender age of the child, is often used by the physician to withhold surgery and justify "observation progression." Unfortunately, the progression is often insidious and therefore not detected until irreversible damage has occurred [6].

The advent of microsurgical technology has allowed neurosurgical interventions to be performed with meticulous preservation of key structures. Consequently, interventions that were previously performed with difficulty and morbidity are now performed with less morbidity and better long-term results. Carbon dioxide laser surgery has added a new tool to the armamentarium of the neurological surgeon. In spinal dysraphia, the three major advnatages of carbon dioxide laser surgery are: (1) reduction of blood loss [14], (2) microdissection with an instrument that minimizes tissue manipulation [11], and (3) noninterference with electrophysiological monitoring [11] (Table 12-1).

1. *Reduction of blood loss.* One of the concerns in performing surgery in children, especially in infants, is that of blood loss. For the most part, acute operative hemorrhages are not well tolerated in small children, and immediate blood replacement is needed. With the concerns of hepatitis and the acquired immune deficiency syndrome, an operative procedure in an infant that would require transfusions would not only disconcert parents, but the primary care physician as well.

   Spinal surgery in any age group will be accompanied by some degree of hemorrhage. Recently, McLone and colleagues [14], reported operating on 50 successive spinal lipomas using the carbon dioxide laser, and in none of the 50 were operative or postoperative transfusions required. This is a significant achievement in that the carbon dioxide laser eliminated the potential transfusion complications mentioned above, plus the additional complication of the development of antibodies in the child's blood and their effect on future transfusions and pregnancies.

2. *Microdissection with minimal tissue manipulation.* The presence of neural elements adjacent to the pathology, be it in the form of a mass such as a lipoma involving the conus or arachnoidal bands adhering to the nerve roots or the cord [21], makes microdissection important in minimizing harm to the neural structures. Using the carbon dioxide laser under microscopic control allows the dissection to be performed by vaporizing the pathology, with minimal instrumentation to the surrounding normal tissues. Consequently, there is none of the traction or distraction of these elements that may occur even with the best of microinstruments. Residual pathology adherent to normal structures can be delicately vaporized with a focused beam at 1 to 3 W, with minimal risk of harming adjacent structures. In spinal lipomas the microlaser dissection permits a clear visualization of the liponeural interface, minimizing damage to the neural structures [11].

3. *Laser surgery and monitoring systems.* Monitoring of evoked responses or rectal electromyogram (EMG) with urodynamic equipment adds an additional factor of safety to the operative procedure in spinal surgery [7]. The carbon dioxide laser does not interfere with electrophysiological monitoring or create artifactual changes during the dissection. Actual recording time is enhanced due to the fact that there is less need to use the bipolar cautery because of the sealing of small vessels by the defocused laser beam.

TECHNICAL ASPECTS

Patients are prepared in the prone position and the operation is directed to the appropriate spinal level resulting from the clinical evaluation. Infants have a small roll placed under the pelvic-lower abdominal junction to allow for free diaphragmatic movements, because they primarily employ their diaphragm for respiration. In older children, the placement of rolls to primarily support the shoulders and the iliac crests as in the adult not only allows for diaphragmatic and abdominal movements, but those of the rib cage as well.

In patients who are primarily undergoing surgery of the conus and cauda equina, I prefer to monitor them during surgery with the rectal electromyogram (EMG) portion of a urodynamic monitoring system [7]. For that purpose, electrode wires are placed on each side of the midline in the external rectal sphincter with a 27-gauge needle, which is then connected to the bladder diagnostic unit (Life Tech Instruments, Houston, Texas). The oscillations of the recording stylus are continuously analyzed by the urology technician during the operative intervention. In lesions that involve higher levels of the spinal cord, evoked potentials may be monitored from a peripheral nerve in a lower extremity.

A standard midline approach to the spinal canal is then performed. If one wishes to reduce blood loss, the carbon dioxide laser is perpared and draped for free-hand use [14]. The scalpel is employed for the skin incision, and the remainder of the dissection is performed with the handheld laser in a continuous energy beam, set at 10 W, with beam focusing for cutting and beam defocusing for vaporization [14]. If malformed lamina are present, they are removed with rongeurs, and the opening is extended into the area of normal anatomy. This allows the different tissue planes to be identified. The normal dura is then opened. The neural elements can best be followed from normal to abnormal surgical anatomy. If neural elements are believed to be present and need to be identified, a disposable Nerve-Locator stimulator is employed (Edward Weck & Company, Inc., Long Island City, New York), with 3 volts at 0.5 to 2 ma. This will permit the surgeon to identify the conus and the S2, S3 and S4 nerve roots that may be intermingled with the pathology [1].

According to the degree of abnormalities present, the operative procedure may proceed with loop magnification and hand-held laser [14] or with the carbon dioxide laser connected to the operating microscope [11]. We prefer the latter due to the advantage of the magnification offered by the microscope and the improved precision offered by the micromanipulator.

The objectives of the operative procedure relate to the underlying pathophysiology. Lipomas involving the neural elements such as lipomeningoceles or leptomyelolipomas can be carefully followed into the lipoma-neural interface and vaporized with 1 to 5 W, with focused beam, with precision and good visualization of structures [2, 4, 14]. Carbonized residue should be cleared with gentle scraping and irrigation, using microsuction. Arachnoidal bands and adhesions to the conus or nerve roots can be freed from the surrounding structures with the same technique; allowing the neural elements to be released [6, 20, 21]. Dermoids or related tumors can likewise be vaporized and removed from the neural elements. If the underlying pathology is a thickened filum terminale that impairs the normal upward migration of the cord, this may be sectioned either with sharp instrumentation or the laser. In the nonossified diastematomyelia, microlaser vaporization of the pathology can be readily achieved with minimal minipulation of the surrounding cord by using a focused laser beam at 2 to 4 W. When the diastematomyelia is ossified, sharp rongeurs are necessary.

The result of the operative procedure should be the removal of any pressure from the nerual structures, with an accompanying release of these structures from any pathology that would restrict the normal upward migration of the spinal cord [6, 20, 21].

Following the above, the neural tube should be reformed when necessary [14], and the dura closed with artificial dura if needed. This is to ensure a slack dura and a capacious subarachnoid space surrounding the spinal cord. When properly performed, this dural reconstruction reduces the risk of retethering of the neural elements secondary to scar formation [14]. A water-tight, layer-by-layer closure of the wound should be performed, and the cutaneous sutures should remain for a minimum period of ten postoperative days to prevent a cerebrospinal fluid (CSF) fistula. CSF fistulas will always have a tendency to occur in those disorders of closure of the midline because of varying degrees of malformation of the mesoderm of the area and the consequent poor connective tissue support.

COMPLICATIONS

The complications that may ensue following laser spinal surgery relate to similar complications that follow any surgery in this area, in any age group. CSF fistulas may occur due to leakage into the muscle layers and consequent skin dehiscence. At times, the CSF may be contained and a pseudomeningocele may result, with local discomfort and cosmetic deformity. This does not necessarily result from the use of the laser [11], but from the lack of adequate formation of the mesodermal structures. It is of utmost importance to repair these wounds with meticulous detail to minimize this risk. McLone and coworkers [14], employing the hand-held laser and dissecting the subcutaneous as well as the spinal component of local lipomas, had the problem of CSF subcutaneous pockets recollecting in ten of 50 patients. On the other hand, I have not employed the laser in that fashion, but used it only for the microdissection of the intraspinal component in 15 spinal lipomas. Of this number, four patients developed CSF fistulas that required another operative intervention.

In my experience, the incidence of wound infection in those patients with laser operations for spinal dysraphia was the same as with those that were performed prior to laser availability.

The prime concern in performing operative procedures of this type in patients that have minimal or no significant neurological abnormality is the risk of creating further neurological impairment with operative intervention. This may occur with or without laser surgery. Till [20] reported a worsening after operation in four patients in a series of 204 patients that underwent an operation for spinal dysraphia without the benefit of the operating microscope or the laser. It is important to note that in his series, the worsening in two patients was due to the failure to recongize a second pathological condition. In the specific situation of spinal lipomas, several series now demonstrate that the operative correction can be performed both with [14] and without the laser [2, 4, 21] with no neurological worsening and with actual neurological improvement in some. My experience with this disease and the complications that ensued, are listed in Table 12-2 and 12-3.

RESULTS AND PROGNOSIS

Spinal lipomas constitute a category of their own in spinal dysraphia, and reports of operative procedures with and without the laser exist. McLone and associates [14] reviewed 50 successive laser interventions for spinal lipomas. In the group that had surgery as infants, an improvement in motor function was noted postoperatively in two of the three infants with preoperative motor dysfunction. Seventeen of 18 infants operated on had normal postoperative motor function. Twelve of 15 patients operated upon initially as adolescents had normal motor function. Two of the five children with abnormal motor function preoperatively showed improvement following the operation. Likewise, one of the nine children with preoperative incontinence acquired continence following surgery. Seventeen patients had had previous incomplete operations, and following laser surgery nine were found to have normal motor function when seen in long-term followup [14]. No patient was made worse by the operation in that series [14]. In another series of ten patients with spinal lipomas operated on with laser microsurgery, one was made worse with surgery, two had dramatic neurological improvement, and seven remained unchanged.

Other conditions that required laser microneurosurgery are listed in Table 12-3. In all of these, the laser made the dissection easier and more meticulous for the previously stated reasons. Removal of dermoid tumors was accomplished by vaporization of the fatty mass, even in that portion inside the conus medullaris. Arachnoidal bands restricting rostral migration of the cord, and banding and scarring that presented in a previously repaired myelomeningocele in adolescence were incised without difficulty with a focused beam with 1 to 2 W of power.

TABLE 12-2. Spinal Laser Operative Procedures: Technical Aspects

Patient No.	Age at operation	Diagnosis	Operative Procedure
1	11 days	Lipomeningocele	Microlaser resection of lipoma into the conus; release of tethered cord
2	7 years	Thoracic syringomyelia	Microlaser midline myelotomy for decompression and exploration; placement of syringoperitoneal shunt
3	6 weeks	Lipomeningocele; tethered conus	Microlaser resection of lipoma into conus; release of tethered cord
4	5 months	Lipomeningocele; tethered conus	Same as above
5	13 years	Tethered cord at myelomeningocele repair	Microlaser release of scar tissue on conus and cauda equina
6	6 years	Lipomeningocele; tethered conus	Microlaser resection of lipoma into conus; release of tethered cord
7	6 weeks	Lipomeningocele; tethered conus	Same as above
8	4 years	Tethered conus; syringomyelia of conus	Microlaser release of arachnoidal bands; midline myelotomy and placement of syringoperitoneal shunt
9	4 weeks	Lipomeningocele; tethered conus	Microlaser resection of lipoma into conus; release of tethered cord
10	22 months	Thoracic dermoid	Microlaser resection of dermoid tumor
11	5 months	Intraspinal (conus) lipoma	Microlaser resection of lipoma into conus
12	3 months	Lipomeningocele; tethered conus	Microlaser resection of lipoma into conus; release of tethered cord
13	8 years	Lipomeningocele; tethered conus	As above
14	2 years	Spinal lipoma	Microlaser resection of lipoma into spinal cord.
15	18 years	Intraspinal lipoma; tethered conus	As above; release of tethered conus
16	15 months	Intraspinal lipoma	Microlaser resection of extensive lipoma compressing spinal cord.
17	13 months	Lipomeningocele; syringocele; tethered conus	Microlaser resection of lipoma; release of tethered cord; midline microlaser myelotomy and fenestration of conus syringocele
18	2 months	Lipomeningocele; Tethered conus	Microlaser resection of lipoma into conus; release of tethered cord
19	4 weeks	Lipomeningocele; tethered conus	As above
20	7 years	Conus lipoma	Microlaser resection by midline myelotomy of conus (intrinsic) lipoma

TABLE 12-3. Laser Operative Procedures for Congenital Spinal Disorders

Patient No.	Age at Operation	Diagnosis	Presentation	Result	Complications	Follow-up and Comments
1	11 days	Lipomeningocele; tethered conus	Lumbar mass; neurologically normal	Transient weakness right leg	None	At 2 years, concern of progressive right leg weakness, reoperated: arachnoidal bands and lipoma encountered
2	7 years	Syringomyelia	Gait disturbance	Gait normalized	None	10 months
3	6 weeks	Lipomeningocele; tethered conus	Lumbar mass Neurologically normal	No change	None	4 years
4	5 months	Lipomeningocele; tethered conus	Spinal aplasia cutis Neurologically normal	No change	None	2 years
5	13 years	Tethered cord at myelomeningocele repair	Urinary retention; scoliosis	Transient urinary retention	Subcutaneous CSF Fistula	3 years Treated with subcutaneous-peritoneal shunt
6	6 years	Lipomeningocele; tethered conus	Orthopedic syndrome [5]	Transient urinary retention; improved.	None	3 years
7	2 years	Intraspinal lipoma	Absent spinous process at multiple levels	Persistent postoperative	Neurological deterioration	3 years; gradual incomplete improvement
8	18 years	Intraspinal lipoma; tethered cord	Orthopedic syndrome [6] Skin (gluteal) dimple	Transient urinary retention No motor change	Urinary reflexes malfunctioning, but improving.	4 months; still requires intermittent catheterization
9	13 months	Intraspinal lipoma; trenauney-Weber syndrome	CT finding; inability to walk	Acquired gait 3 weeks after operation	Subcutaneous CSF fistula	2 years; treated with subcutaneous peritoneal shunt

10	13 months	Lipomeningocele; conus syringocele; tethered conus	Lumbar mass; neurologically normal	No change	Subcutaneous CSF fistula	3 years; treated with subcutaneous peritoneal shunt
11	2 months	Lipomeningocele; tethered conus	Lumbar mass; neurologically normal	Transient urinary frequency	None	2 years
12	4 weeks	Lipomeningocele; tethered conus	Lumbar mass; neurologicallynormal	Transient incontinence of feces	Wound infection	4 years; requires intermittent catheterization
13	7 years	Conus lipoma	Orthopedic syndrome [5]	Transient urinary retention	None	3 years
14	6 weeks	Lipomeningocele	Lumbar mass	No change	Wound infection	4 years; incontinent of feces
15	4 years	Tethered conus; syringomyelia of conus	Back pain; inability to walk	Improved Gait normalized	None	2 years
16	4 weeks	Lipomeningocele; tethered conus	Lumbar mass Neurologically normal	No change	None	3 years
17	22 months	Thoracic dermoid	Draining sinus tract; neurologically normal	No change	None	1 year
18	5 months	Intraspinal (conus) lipoma	Urinary tract	Improved	None	6 years—4 years after operation had urological deterioration and underwent reoperation adhesions were found
19	3 months	Lipomeningocele; tethered conus	Lumbar mass Aplasia cutis; Neurolomproved	None	3 years	

CONCLUSIONS

I believe that the carbon dioxide laser has added a new technical option for the neurological surgeon in the treatment of spinal dysraphia due to its highly precise dissection, minimal traction and harm to the surrounding tissues, reduction of hemorrhage, reduction in the instrumentation in the operative field, and enhancement of monitoring time by eliminating interference with electrophysiological recordings. Other laser wavelengths should now be explored and evaluated as adjuvants in spinal cord surgery.

Laser Surgery in Craniosynostosis and Craniofacial Dysostosis

Operations for craniosynostosis are for the most part straightforward, and have been extensively described in the literature. When the carbon dioxide laser arrived at University of California, San Diego, I employed this instrument in various reconstructive procedures for the osteotomies in an attempt to identify benefits from this technology from the standpoint of technical advantages over conventional instrumentation, and in reference to calvarial bone healing [5]. These aspects will be discussed in the ensuing sections.

EXPERIMENTAL BASIS FOR CARBON DIOXIDE LASER SURGERY

At times the reossification process following craniosynostosis surgery can lead to a restriction of the growth of the calvaria and recurrence of the synostosis [13, 16]. This is of particular concern in the more advanced forms of the disease, such as craniofacial dysostosis [13, 16]. There is currently no precise manner of determining when a particular operation is going to be followed by early reossification. Various materials have been advocated to be interposed or placed on the osteotomy site to avoid the early ossification following operation [1, 13]. Such foreign materials may lead to complications of their own and at times fail to halt the reossification and premature reclosure of sutures [13].

One of the theoretical considerations in the use of the carbon dioxide laser in craniosynostosis surgery is that, when applied to the calvaria, it may delay bone healing. To study that aspect, carbon dioxide laser osteotomies were performed on 4-week-old rabbits, and these osteotomies were compared histologically to contralateral osteotomies performed with the high-speed drill [10]. Histological cross-sections of the calvaria were performed at 2, 4 and 6 weeks following the osteotomies. As early as 2 weeks following the high-speed-drill osteotomy, connective tissue bridged the bone edges. By 4 weeks, this bridge was thickened and endowed with numerous blood vessels. At 6 weeks numerous osteoblasts lined the bone edges and the connective tissue bridge [10]. Following laser osteotomy (10 W, focused beam, handheld), the carbonized edges interrupted the connective tissue from bridging the defect at 2 and 4 weeks. By 6 weeks, connective tissue had grown incompletely past the carbonized residue, and the healing process proceeding with osteoblast proliferation from points beyond the carbonized residue [10].

It thus seems reasonable to state that the carbon dioxide laser osteotomy does indeed interfere and delay calvarial reossification. To what extent this applies to human calvarial healing in infants, is yet to be determined in a large series with adequate long-term followup.

CLINICAL INDICATIONS

In a previous preliminary report, I discussed the results of carbon dioxide laser osteotomies in craniosynostosis and craniofacial surgery [5]. The osteotomies were performed in a wide variety of syndromes [5]. It then became obvious that this technique did not add much to the conventional instrumentation from the technical standpoint in some of the syndromes, whereas it helped in others. A list of operative procedures in which it has proven useful is presented in Table 12-4.

From the standpoint of the general advantages of carbon dioxide laser osteotomies, the hand-held, defocused carbon dioxide osteotomy can seal diploic channels in the calvaria, minimizing hemorrhage at the osteotomy site. In infants it effectively replaces the high-speed drill in those situations where the latter is needed, as long as the bone is only a few millimeters thick. The bone of the older child and the adult has a 43.9% to 55% water content [18], and therefore does not readily absorb the radiating carbon dioxide laser energy. Infant bone is not only thinner, but also has a higher water content. As a result, it will permit the carbon dioxide laser to act as an incising instrument. I have found this to be true until approximately 1 year of age, when the bone not only thickens but may also lose a significant amount of its water content. An added advantage in carbon dioxide laser osteotomy over other osteotomies performed with other techniques is the potential delay of reossification of the cal-

TABLE 12-4. Operative Procedures for Craniosynostosis

Patient No.	Age at Operation	Diagnosis	Procedure	Energy
1	3 months	Unilateral coronal synostosis	Left lateral canthal advancement; straight beam and 45°-angle mirrors employed	40–80 W, superpulse
2	2 months	Unilateral coronal synostosis	Same as above	40–60 W
3	2 months	Crouzon's disease	Monoblock supraorbital release and advancement; straight beam and angled mirrors employed	40–60 W and superpulse
4	5 months	Severe metopic synostosis	Synostectomy Bilateral canthal advancement; straight beam and angled mirrors	40–60 W and superpulse
5	2 months	Apert's syndrome	Monoblock supraorbital release and advancement; straight beam and angled mirrors	40–60 W and superpulse
6	6 months	Severe metopic synostosis	Synostectomy; bilateral canthal advancement; straight beam and angled mirrors	60 W and superpulse
7	1 month	Apert's syndrome	Craniectomy, supra and lateral orbital release; straight beam and angled mirrors	40–60 W
8	2 months	Severe metopic	Synostectomy; bilateral canthal advancement; straight beam and angled mirrors	60 W and superpulse
9	11 months	Unilateral coronal synostosis	Unilateral canthal advancement and frontal reconstruction Straight beam and angled mirrors	20–40 W and superpulse
10	11 months	Unilateral coronal synostosis	As above	40 W and superpulse
11	6 months	Unilateral coronal synostosis	As above	40 W and superpulse

varia, with its attendant minimization of the risk of recurrence of the synostosis (see previous section).

Disadvantages of the carbon dioxide laser in craniosynostosis work are the cumbersome aspect of setting up the laser for what is commonly a short operative procedure in simple synostosis, as well as the cost effectiveness of employing advanced technology of this nature.

As a consequence of the previous considerations and the experience I have acquired with carbon dioxide laser osteotomies in craniosynostosis over the past few years, I employ the laser in specific situations, primarily in those patients under 12 months of age where it is predicted that the high-speed drill will be needed. In this group of patients, the carbon dioxide laser will be an effective tool and will supplant the need for the high-speed-drill system. The rationale for these statements is as follows:

1. The carbon dioxide laser osteotomies do not generate the bone dust that is created by the high-speed-drill systems.
2. The "end point" of the completion of the osteotomy can readiy be seen by the surgeon as the HeNe beam is visualized past the osteotomy.
3. The reduced instrumentation in the operative site enhances the surgeons visibility of the area.
4. With mirrors of 45- and 90-degree angles on the hand-held laser, the osteotomy can be performed in corners and angles not readily accessible by drill systems, for example, the lateral canthal incision in the lateral canthal advancement step for coronal synostosis [3].
5. In osteotomies at the skull base, such as those that are performed with lateral canthal advancement, or related procedures for coronal synostosis, early reossification is a major concern. This is especially true in the genetic syndromes such as Crouzon's disease and Apert is syndrome. Carbonization with high-energy carbon dioxide laser radiation can readily create a barrier for the normal connective tissue bridge that leads to the reossification process [10], and the delay in bone healing will permit a better subsequent forward migration of the supraorbital structures. A better correction of the underlying deformity will then follow [15].

INDICATIONS FOR LASER SURGERY

Currently I employ the laser only in infants under 12 months of age with unilateral or bilateral coronal synostosis and in syndromes that require osteotomies at the skull base. These, or combinations of these disorders, may be seen in simple coronal synostosis or in the craniofacial syndromes such as Saethre-Chotzen, Apert, Crouzon, Pfeiffer, and related syndromes. In certain situations of severe metopic synostosis, the lateral portions of the supraorbital rims recede. In these situations I perform not only a removal of the metopic suture with rongeurs, but a bilateral canthal advancement as well. For the latter procedure, the supraorbital and lateral canthal osteotomies are performed with the carbon dioxide laser. Before laser surgery, this step was performed with a high-speed drill.

TECHNICAL ASPECTS

For the conditions previously described, I employ the carbon dioxide laser almost exclusively for the osteotomy portion of the operation. Although the use of the laser for the skin incision and muscle incision has been previously described, this is now seldom done due to the amount of time involved. However, in those situations where blood loss is a serious concern, the necessary additional time is clearly justified and the muscle incisions should be performed with the laser.

The laser unit employed during the past years can deliver 1 to 80 W of carbon dioxide radiating energy and is also equipped with a superpulse option (Sharplan Model 743, Sharplan Laser Industries Limited, Israel). It is employed hand-held with the 50-mm lens. A straight beam as well as stainless steel angled mirrors (45

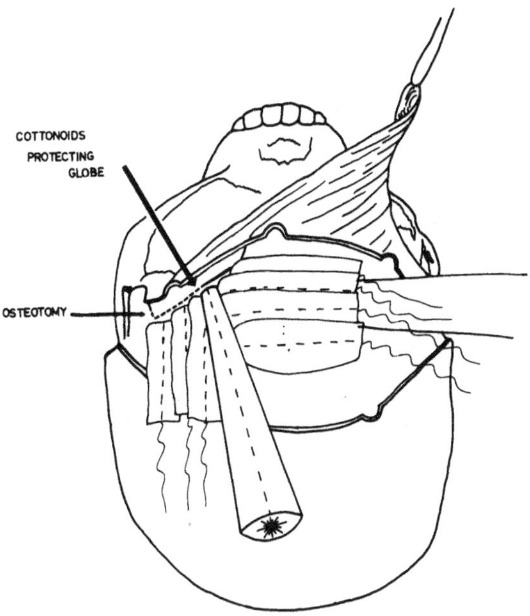

FIGURE 12-1. Carbon dioxide laser osteotomy with hand-held straight beam in the supraorbital region. Note that the dura and the globe are protected at all times by moistened cottonoids.

or 90 degrees) should be available. The angled beams are useful for locations where the beam cannot be aimed directly to the desired spot of the calvaria. Following elevation of the skin and galeal flaps, the 50-mm straight laser beam is very useful in dissecting the tissues surrounding the lateral canthus of the orbit in a tangential fashion (defocused form, 20–40 W). The insertion of the temporal muscle as well as local fat can be readily incised with minimal hemorrhage, and all tissue cleaned from the bone [5]. Standard burr holes are then performed with the D'Errico drill. Cottonoids soaked in saline are then passed from burr hole to burr hole, or from burr hole to the desired area of the osteotomy, to protect the underlying dura from the radiating energy.

The osteotomies can then be performed with a defocused beam at 40 to 80 W, or better still with the superpulse mode. The latter permits some dissipation of the thermal effect between each high-energy impact. The osteotomy need not be completely through the bone. The laser incision can then be readily completed with Mayo scissors. The underlying cottonoids will absorb the thermal energy as well as any carbon dioxide radiation that passes through the osteotomy site. When orbital osteotomies are performed, it is most important to protect the globe by inserting moistened cottonoids between the orbital capsule and the osteotomy site (Figure 12-1). This is done by dissecting the pericranium off the supraorbital rim, and this continues in the orbit as the orbital capsule. Flat metal brain retractors are interposed in the space, and cottonoids soaked in saline are then placed on these, thus absorbing the radiating energy traversing the laser osteotomy site. The orbital roof behind the supraorbital rim is usually thin in the infant, and 10 to 20 W of energy is more than sufficient for the osteotomy. The lateral canthus however is commonly much thicker, and 40 to 80 W is often needed. If available, the superpulse mode should be used for the previously discussed reasons. This is performed with the angled mirrors (45–90 degrees) as shown in Figure 12-2. Upon completion of the osteotomies the laser is withdrawn, the site is thoroughly irrigated, hemostasis is ensured, and the galea and scalp repaired.

Table 12-4 describes the patient population operated upon to date as well as the technical aspects of laser surgery.

COMPLICATIONS

No complications to date can be directly attributed to laser surgery. Two infections were noted shortly after discharge. These presented with swelling and redness in the area of the incision, with underlying purulent collections that were caused by *Staphylococcus aureus*. These were notably the result of instrumental contamination at time of operation. No CSF fistulas have occurred. In one child the scalp incision dehisced 18 days after operation, but the underlying tissues were under tension from supporting remodeling bone struts that then had to be removed. There has been no mortality from craniosynostosis or craniofacial surgery to date.

RESULTS AND PROGNOSIS

In all operations there has been uniformly good cranial reconstructive results. In two patients, a significant delay in bone healing in a localized area of the calvaria has been noted. However, I have observed such a finding, and it has been reported by others, in children who have had osteotomies without the laser. It appears to be a consequence of changes in the external layers of the dura that impair the normal ability for the generation of membranous bone. This ability is normally present in infant bone and permits the prompt reossification that usually follows craniosynostosis surgery.

Table 12-4 shows the diagnosis, procedure performed, and the amount of laser energy used in my craniosynostosis cases. The series is too small to allow a determination of whether laser surgery was of benefit for these patients when compared to conventional surgical interventions. A larger series followed up for sufficient time will be needed to document the advantages of this technology.

CONCLUSIONS

The carbon dioxide laser has, in my experience, been demonstrated to be of definite technical applicability in certain procedures for craniosynostosis and craniofacial surgery. The operative procedures can certainly be performed without the laser, and one should not consider acquiring a carbon dioxide laser for this limited application. However, it reduces hemorrhage at the osteotomy sites, performs osteotomies in infants under 12 months of age quite well, aids in the dissection of soft tissues in certain areas (such as around the bony orbit) very effectively, and may delay the reossification process. In children under 1 year of age, it does replace the high-speed drill in certain steps of the reconstructive process.

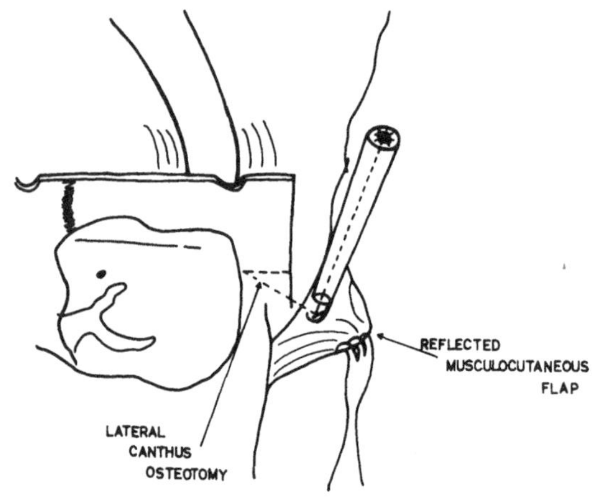

FIGURE 12-2. Carbon dioxide laser osteotomy with hand-held angled mirrors for the lateral canthal osteotomy. This procedure follows that described in Figure 12-1.

Acknowledgments

I extend my gratitude to Miss Sylvia Schneider for the excellent secretarial assistance in the preparation of this manuscript. This work was supported in part by research funds from the Division of Neurosurgery of the University of California San Diego School of Medicine, and by the Foundation for Pediatric and Laser Neurosurgery, Inc., San Diego, California.

References

1. Anderson FM, Gieger L: Craniosynostosis: Survery of 204 cases. *J Neurosurg* 22:229–240, 1965.
2. Bruce DA, Schut L: Spinal lipomas in infancy and childhood. *Childs Brain* 5:192–203, 1979.
3. Hoffman HJ, Mohr G: Lateral canthal advancement of the supraorbital margin: A new corrective technique in the treatment of craniosynostosis. *J Neurosurg* 45:376–381, 1976.
4. Hoffman HJ, Taecholarn C, Hendrick ED, et al: Management of lipomyelomeningoceles. *J Neurosurg* 62:1–8, 1985.
5. James HE: The role of the carbon dioxide laser in craniosynostosis and craniofacial dysostosis.

Concepts Ped Neurosurg 3:202–204, 1983.

6. James CCM, Lassman LP: Spinal dysraphism: An orthopedic syndrome in children accompanying occult forms. *Arch Dis Child* 35:315–327, 1960.
7. James HE, Walsh JW: Spinal dysraphism. *Curr Probl Pediatr* 9:1–25, 1981.
8. James HE, McLaurin RL, Watkins WT: Remission of pes cavus in surgically treated spinal dysraphism. *J Bone Joint Surg* 61A:1096–1098, 1979.
9. James HE, Mulcahy JJ, Walsh JW, et al: Use of anal spyncter electromyography during operations on the conus medullaris and sacral nerve roots. *Neurosurgery* 4:521–523, 1979.
10. James HE, Wiley CA, Schneider A: The effect of carbon dioxide laser irradiation on cranial bone healing: An experimental study. In Press.
11. James HE, Williams J, Brock W, et al: Radical removal of lipomas of the conus and cauda equina with laser microneurosurgery. *Neurosurgery* 15:340–343, 1984.
12. Lichtenstein BW: "Spinal dysraphism": Spinal dysraphism and myelodysplasia. *Arch Neurol Psychiatry* 44:792–810, 1940.
13. Matson DD: *Neurosurgery of Infancy and Children*, 2nd ed. Springfield, IL, Thomas, 1969.
14. McLone DG, Naidich TP: Laser resection of fifty spinal lipomas. *Neurosurgery* 18:611–615, 1986.
15. Mohr H, Hoffman HJ, Munro I, et al: Surgical management of unilateral and bilateral coronal synostosis: 21 years of experience. *Neurosurgery* 2:83–92, 1978.
16. Norwood CW, Alexander E, Davis CH, et al: Recurrent and multiple suture closures after craniectomy for craniosynostosis. *J Neurosurg* 41:715–719, 1974.
17. Scheible W, James HE, Leopold G, et al: Occult spinal dysraphism in infants: Screening with high-resolution real-time ultrasound. *Radiology* 146:743–746, 1983.
18. Sohl AT: *Mineral Metabolism.* New York, Rheinbold Press, 1940.
19. Tavafoghi V, Ghandchi A, Hambrick GW, et al: Cutaneous signs of spinal dysraphism. *Arch Dermatol* 114:573–577, 1978.
20. Till K: Occult spinal dysraphism: The value of prophylactic surgical treatment. *Excerpta Medica Int Congr Series* 293:3, 1969.
21. Till K: Spinal dysraphism: A study of congenital malformations of the lower back. *J Bone Joint Surg* 51B:415–422, 1969.

13. NEUROSURGICAL APPLICATIONS OF THE ND:YAG LASER FOR VASCULAR LESIONS

Robert E. Wharen, Jr.
Robert E. Anderson,
Thoralf M. Sundt, Jr.

Since the original prediction of laser light by Albert Einstein and the invention of the first ruby laser in 1959 [16], laser technology and our understanding of the application of this technology with biological tissue have advanced considerably. The use of a continuous-wave Nd: YAG (neodymium: yttrium-aluminum-garnet), near-infrared laser and its potential applications in neurosurgery have been under investigation now for approximately 6 years, and the capabilities and limitations of this laser are beginning to be better defined.

Beck [2], in 1980, reported on the effectiveness of the Nd:YAG laser for deep coagulation of brain tissue. Further clinical reports described the effectiveness of the Nd:YAG laser for coagulation and hemostasis during the removal of vascular tumors [2, 4, 6, 9, 11, 12, 14, 18], arteriovenous malformations [2, 9, 12, 18, 21], and arterial aneurysms [9, 12].

More recent studies have attempted to define the response of neural tissue [7, 19, 20, 22, 23] and blood vessels [15, 19, 20] to Nd:YAG laser energy to determine the safety of this instrument in neurosurgery. In comparison to the carbon dioxide laser, the thermal effects of the Nd:YAG laser penetrate brain tissue to a much greater extent, and this fact must always be of concern in any clinical application of this laser. This chapter will review the current understanding of the interaction of Nd:YAG energy with brain tissue and the clinical investigations in the use of this laser for the treatment of vascular lesions.

Laboratory Studies

The response of brain tissue to Nd:YAG monochromatic coherent light is a function of three parameters: (1) the energy delivered to the tissue; (2) the inherent interactions of brain tissue for light of 1.06 μ wavelength; and (3) the ability of the tissue to dissipate an applied energy. The energy delivered includes considerations of incident power, duration of exposure, and the spatial profile of the laser beam. The inherent interactions include the absorption, reflection, and scattering of brain tissue for Nd: YAG light. The ability of tissue to dissipate energy is largely dependent upon the flow volume and flow velocity of blood in the local blood vessels.

Robertson, J.H. and Clark, W.C. (eds), Lasers in Neurosurgery.

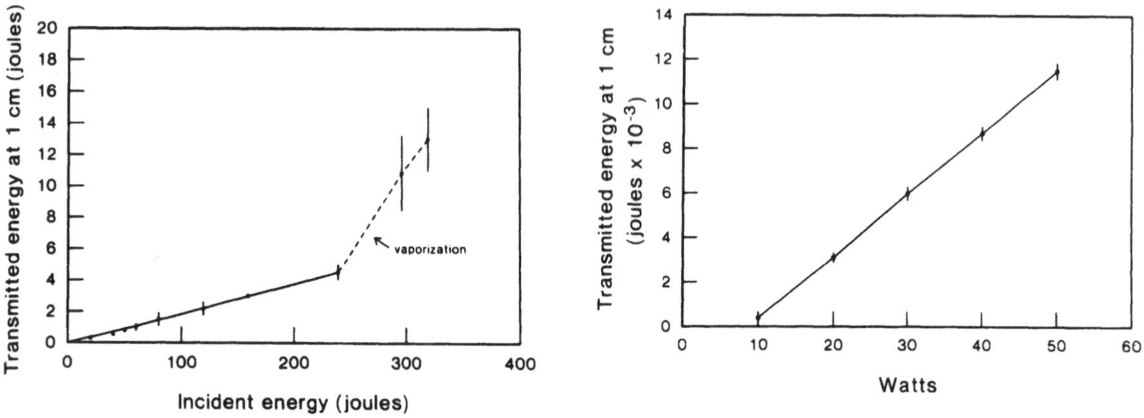

FIGURE 13-1. (Left) Transmitted versus incident engery for Nd:YAG light through 1-cm-thick section of cat brain. A linear relationship is evident except at high incident energies where vaporization occurred. Each point is the mean and standard deviation of five independent measurements. (Right) Transmission of Nd:YAG light through 1 cm of heparinized arterial cat blood.

The parameters of the response of normal brain tissue and of tumor tissue to the Nd:YAG laser from both animals and humans have been investigated thus far by three methods: (1) determination of the absorption coefficients of various tissues; (2) determination of the thermal profiles of brain upon application of laser energy; and (3) pathological evaluation of laser-induced lesions.

In contrast to the carbon dioxide laser, which is strongly absorbed by water, the Nd:YAG laser is poorly absorbed by water and thus is absorbed rather poorly by tissue [13]. As a result of this decreased absorption, Nd:YAG light has an increased scatter within the tissue compared to carbon dioxide, and this difference in tissue reaction to the different wavelengths contributes to the coagulation ability of the Nd:YAG laser.

The in vitro transmission of Nd:YAG light through 1-cm sections of cat brain (Figure 13-1A) reveals a linear relationship between incident energy versus transmitted energy at levels between 240 joules with an absorption value $A = 1.08$ [20]. At levels greater than 240 joules, vaporization of the tissue occurred resulting in increased transmission. Similar transmission studies through 1 cm of heparinized arterial cat blood using incident energies of 10 to 50 joules demonstrated an absorption value of $A = 3.8$ (Figure 13-1B). Although absorption coefficients can be inadequate in predicting the interaction of laser light in tissue [3], the in-vitro absorption values of 1.8 and 3.8 for brain and blood do indicate that blood has a 100-fold greater absorption for 1.06 μm wavelength light compared to brain. This differential absorption enables Nd:YAG light to selectively heat blood vessels compared to brain tissue.

In addition to the absorption values, the calculated penetration depth, which is the thickness of brain that absorbs 90% of the incident energy, is 5.5 mm for in vitro brain. This is a rather significant penetration of energy, particularly in many neurosurgical applications. However, the penetration depth in vivo should be much smaller because of the preferential absorption by hemoglobin. In-vivo absorption values for brain tissue are more difficult to determine and have not yet been reported.

This differential heating of blood and brain tissue can be demonstrated through temperature profiles obtained following the application of Nd:YAG light to the cortical surface. Continuous temperature recordings have been obtained in anesthetized cats from thermocouples positioned 5 to 10 mm below the cortical surface, while Nd:YAG laser light was applied to the

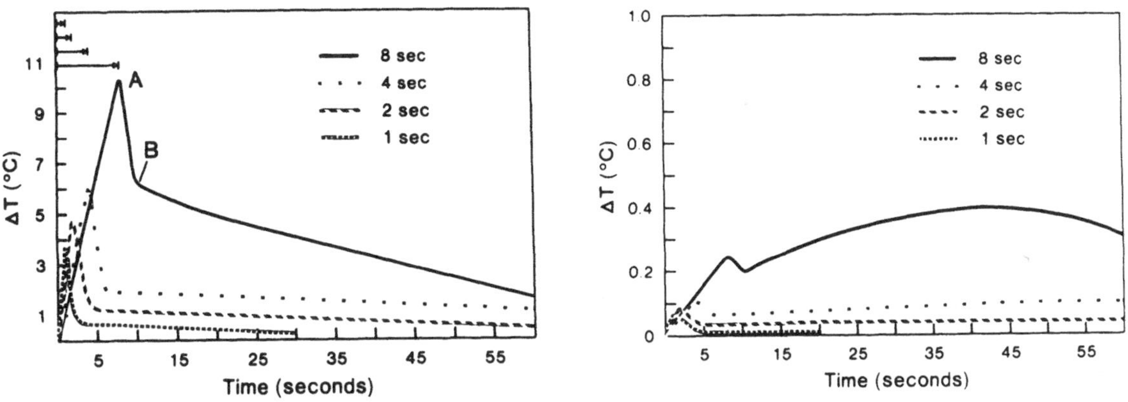

FIGURE 13-2. Temperature recordings following 10 W of Nd:YAG light applied for 1 to 8 seconds to the cat cortex in vivo at 5 mm (*left*) and 10 mm (*right*) from the cortical surface. ΔT represents the rise in temperature above baseline. Point A represents the maximum temperature rise of the blood, and Point B represents the maximum temperature rise of the brain. Indicators at the top represent the duration of the laser pulse.

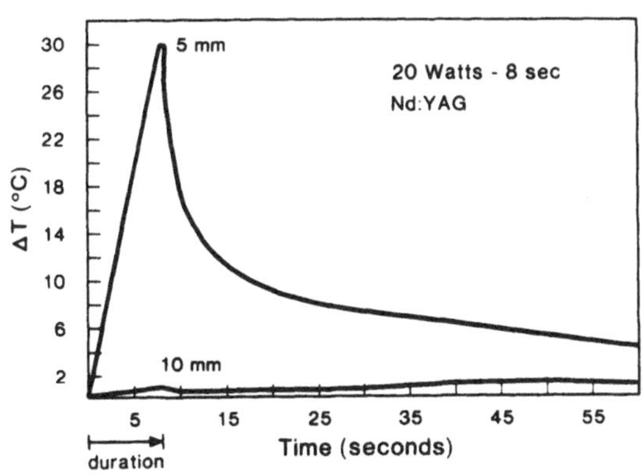

FIGURE 13-3. Temperature changes at depths of 5 mm and 10 mm following 20 W of Nd:YAG light applied for 8 seconds to the cortical surface. ΔT represents the rise in temperature above baseline.

cortical surface at various powers and durations [20]. Temperature recordings at depths of 5 mm to 10 mm with 10 W applied for 1 to 8 seconds (Figure 13-2) demonstrate an immediate temperature rise during the application of the laser, which peaked at point A, the maximum temperature to which the blood was heated, corresponding to the end of the laser pulse. At 5 mm this was followed by an immediate rapid decline in temperature to point B following cessation of the laser. From point B, the maximum temperature to which the brain tissue was heated, the temperature fell at a much slower rate and gradually returned to baseline in 30 to 90 seconds depending upon the applied energy. At 10 mm, the temperature again declined rapidly following the end of the laser pulse. However, instead of showing a gradual decline toward baseline as at 5 mm, the temperature showed a small but definite late rise at 30 to 45 seconds, particularly following high incident powers. This was followed by a gradual decline to baseline over the next 50 seconds. A comparison of the magnitudes of the temperature rise at 5 mm and 10 mm demonstrates (Figure 13-3) that significant temperature rises of 30°C occurred at 5 mm following the application of 20 W of Nd:YAG light for 8 seconds to the cortical surface, whereas at 10 mm the temperature rise was minimal. The maximum rise in brain temperature at a depth of 5 mm for various powers and durations (Figure 13-4, left) demonstrates a linear relationship between the brain temperature rise and the duration of the laser pulse for incident powers of 5 to 30 W. The maximum temperature rise of the blood at a depth of 5 mm demonstrates that approximately 90% of the maximum temperature rise of the blood occurs within the first 2 to 3 seconds. The heating curves for brain and blood are thus quite

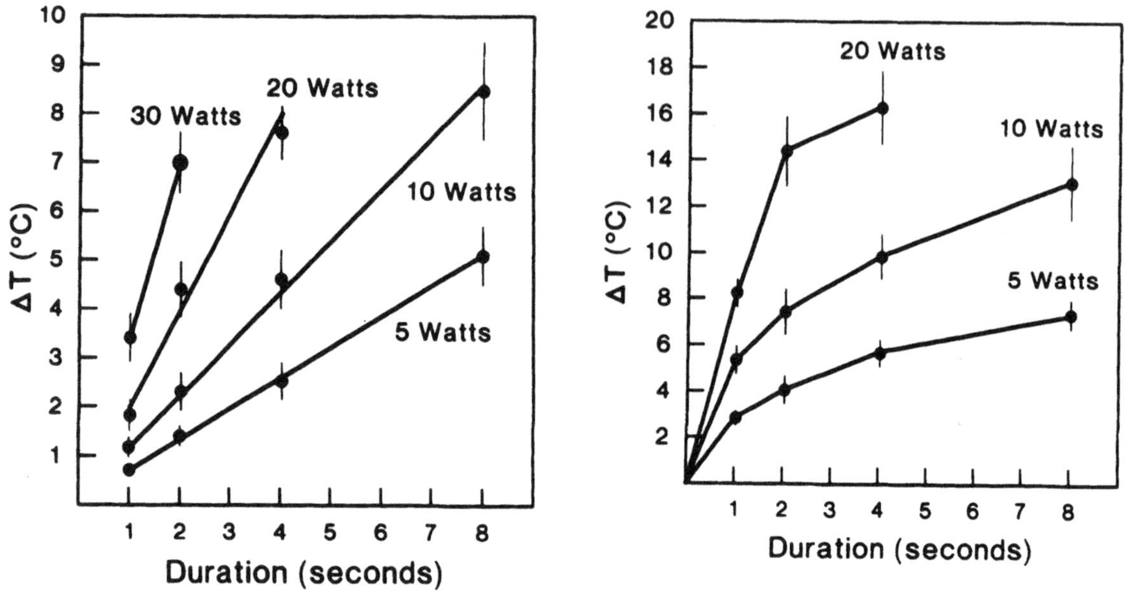

FIGURE 13-4. Maximum temperature rise for brain (*left*) and blood (*right*) at a depth of 5 mm following Nd:YAG light applied to the cortical surface at various powers and durations. ΔT is the rise in temperature above baseline. Each point is the mean and standard deviation of five independent measurements.

distinct since blood rapidly approaches its maximum temperature within 2 to 3 seconds while the brain temperature increases at a linear rate with prolonged durations.

The thermal response curves reveal a number of important practical considerations regarding the use of the Nd:YAG laser for coagulation. Because the brain temperature increases linearly while the blood temperature rises rapidly, attempts at vessel coagulation should consist of brief durations of Nd:YAG energy. If coagulation has not been achieved within approximately 3 seconds, further prolongation of the applied energy is not likely to be successful in coagulating the vessel and will serve only to increase the brain temperature further. If coagulation has not occurred within 2 to 3 seconds, it is better to increase the power rather than prolong the duration of the laser energy.

Secondly, the temperature rise of both brain and blood decreases rapidly. Because of this rapid cooling, repeated pulses of shorter duration with a brief cooling period between the pulses should result in less tissue damage than an equivalent energy delivered continuously over a prolonged duration. A similar effect has been noted when the Nd:YAG laser has been applied to bleeding gastric ulcers [17] where short pulses of energy at high power were more effective at coagulation with a decreased risk of gastric performation compared to continuous pulses at low power when the total energies were equivalent.

It must be emphasized that the thermal profiles were obtained from laser energy focused upon the cortical surface. As such, the pial blood flow is able to act as a heat dissipater. Once the pial surface has been penetrated, the thermal parameters will change depending on the local blood flow. Thus, thermal profiles within the white matter of the deep parenchyma or within tumors will vary considerably from those obtained from gray matter, depending on the local blood-flow characteristics of the tissue being irradiated.

Pathological effects of Nd:YAG laser–induced

lesions on cerebral cortex [7, 13, 20], cerebellar cortex [22], cerebral blood vessels [8, 15], and human brain tumors [23] have now been well described for both acute and chronic lesions. The dimensions of the lesions vary with the applied power and duration as well as the size of the incident beam and whether the laser probe is focused or defocused on the target. Acute lesions result in a central zone of carbonization or vaporization depending on the energy density of the incident light. Immediately adjacent is a zone of coagulation. According to Fasano [7], this consists of an area of coagulation underneath the carbonization zone, containing honeycombing and an area of coagulation in which the tissue remains homogenous and retains its original form. Surrounding the zone of coagulation is a zone of edema with rather ill-defined margins in which there is no recognizable tissue destruction. The edematous zone consists of perivascular and interstitial edema with associated microvascular congestion, although interstitial hemorrhage is rare. The appearance of these histological zones is dependent on the applied energy: low energies produce only a zone of edema, whereas higher energies result in coagulation and eventually carbonization and vaporization.

The application of Nd:YAG energy to brain tissue also results in a defect of the blood-brain barrier which can be demonstrated by Evans blue staining [8, 15, 20]. The region of blood-brain barrier breakdown appears to coincide well with the edematous layer [15].

Kuroiwa and coworkers [15] have studied the effect of Nd:YAG energy on the cerebral microvasculature of rabbits using microangiography, which demonstrated an oligovascular and avascular area corresponding to the edematous and coagulation zones, respectively. Vessels within the edematous zone were thinner and irregular in shape and arched toward the avascular coagulation zone. There was no extravasation of contrast medium. The finding of shrunken and tapered vessels with rare hemorrhages following Nd:YAG exposure was strikingly different from the microvascular dilation and congestion with frequent hemorrhages observed following carbon dioxide exposure. These studies again demonstrate the selective effect of Nd:YAG energy on blood vessels, which is the basis for its superior ability to produce coagulation compared to carbon dioxide, which evaporates tissue through selective absorption by water.

TABLE 13-1. Size of Lesions on Histological Section*

Power for 8 Seconds	Acute (diameter × depth)	Chronic (diameter × depth)
5 W	1 mm × 1 mm	1.5 mm × 1.5 mm
10 W	2 mm × 1.5 mm	3 mm × 2 mm
40 W	2.5 mm × 2 mm	4 mm × 3.5 mm

* Acute measurements were taken 20 minutes after the laser lesion was placed, and chronic measurements were taken 2 weeks after lesioning.

A major concern with the use of the Nd:YAG laser has been that because of the penetration and scattering of Nd:YAG energy in brain tissue, the resultant damage may be much greater than is immediately discernible at the time of laser application. Indeed, it has been well demonstrated that chronic lesions are always slightly larger than the acute lesions, with an increasing discrepancy noted at higher incident energies [20]. Using a focused beam with a diameter of 1.2 mm, the size of chronic lesions on histological section varied from 1.5 mm (diameter × depth) to 4 mm × 3.5 mm at powers of 5 to 40 W applied for 8 seconds (Table 13-1). Yamagami and colleagues [23], using a diverging probe positioned 2 mm from the cerebellar cortex, noted chronic lesions varying in depth from 1 mm to 3 mm following 30 to 60 W applied for 1 second. Yamagami and associates [23] have also studied the extent of thermal penetration of the Nd:YAG laser on various types of both intracranial and extracranial tumors during surgery and found that with the use of a diverging probe held 2 mm above the tumor surface, the thermal effect ranged from a depth of 6 to 10 mm following irradiation with four applications of 90 W for 2 seconds.

The thermal effects of the Nd:YAG laser are thus significant but have been characterized and are consistent and predictable depending upon the incident power density, length of exposure, and the vascularity and blood flow of the tissue being irradiated. By using short, intermittent pulses of light focused upon blood vessels, damage to the surrounding brain can be minimized. The safety of this laser must thus be carefully scrutinized, depending upon the characteristics of each individual case as to whether this degree of thermal penetration and destruction is desirable, acceptable, or prohibitive.

Clinical Applications

Beck [2], in 1980 reported the initial clinical applications of the Nd:YAG laser as a coagulation instrument during the removal of vascular tumors. Since then experience with this laser has expanded considerably and recently the Nd:YAG laser has been approved for use in neurosurgery by the Food and Drug Administration (FDA). Because of the ability of the Nd:YAG laser to selectively coagulate blood vessels, our initial interests focused on the use of the Nd:YAG laser as an adjunctive measure for hemostasis in the resection of arteriovenous malformations (AVM's). We hoped that this laser would be effective in coagulating the multiple thin-walled vessels feeding the deep portion of the AVM.

A Molectron 8000 Nd:YAG laser has thus far been used in the resection of 21 AVM's. The laser light was delivered via a 50-mm focused handpiece, which has a beam diameter of 1.2 mm at its focal point and a beam profile that approximates a square wave. Short intermittent pulses of less than 4 seconds duration at incident powers of 5 to 25 W and corresponding to power densities of 350 to 1740 W/cm were used for coagulation. The laser was used at its focal point for small vessels (less than 1 mm in diameter), but for larger vessels the beam was defocused until the beam size was at least as large as the vessel being coagulated. All the resections were performed under the operative microscope to which a KG3 filter was attached for eye protection. All operating room personnel wore protective eyewear while the laser was in use. Hypotension was induced by sodium nitroprusside as required at selected times, and all patients received propranolol (60 mg/day) orally both preoperatively and postoperatively to decrease cerebral blood flow following surgery [5].

A complete resection was verified in all cases by postoperative angiography.

CASE 1

This 23-year-old, right-handed female nursing student presented in 1980 with severe episodic headaches associated with transitory right-sided weakness and numbness. Angiography demonstrated a large left parietal AVM with multiple feeding vessels from the left middle, anterior, and posterior cerebral arteries. The malformation drained by multiple cortical veins into the sagittal sinus and the superficial middle cerebral veins and extended from the cortical surface to the roof of the lateral ventricle. In November 1980, she was referred for proton-beam radiation therapy. There was no improvement in her symptoms nor any change in the size of the AVM. She returned in December 1982 with a 2-month history of increasing frequency of her headaches and associated right-sided sensorimotor phenomena. Angiography (Figure 13-5) demonstrated a large AVM essentially unchanged from the angiogram taken in 1980. The AVM was subsequently resected through a left parasagittal parietal craniotomy. After ligating the large feeding vessels, the Nd:YAG laser was used to define the plane between the brain and the AVM. As the AVM shrank away from the brain, the small feeding vessels were coagulated. The laser was helpful in coagulating the thin-walled vessels feeding the deep portion of the lesion, but it was not superior to bipolar coagulation under water, nor was it faster.

Postoperatively, the patient developed right-sided focal seizures which required the use of intravenous thiopental sodium for 24 hours.

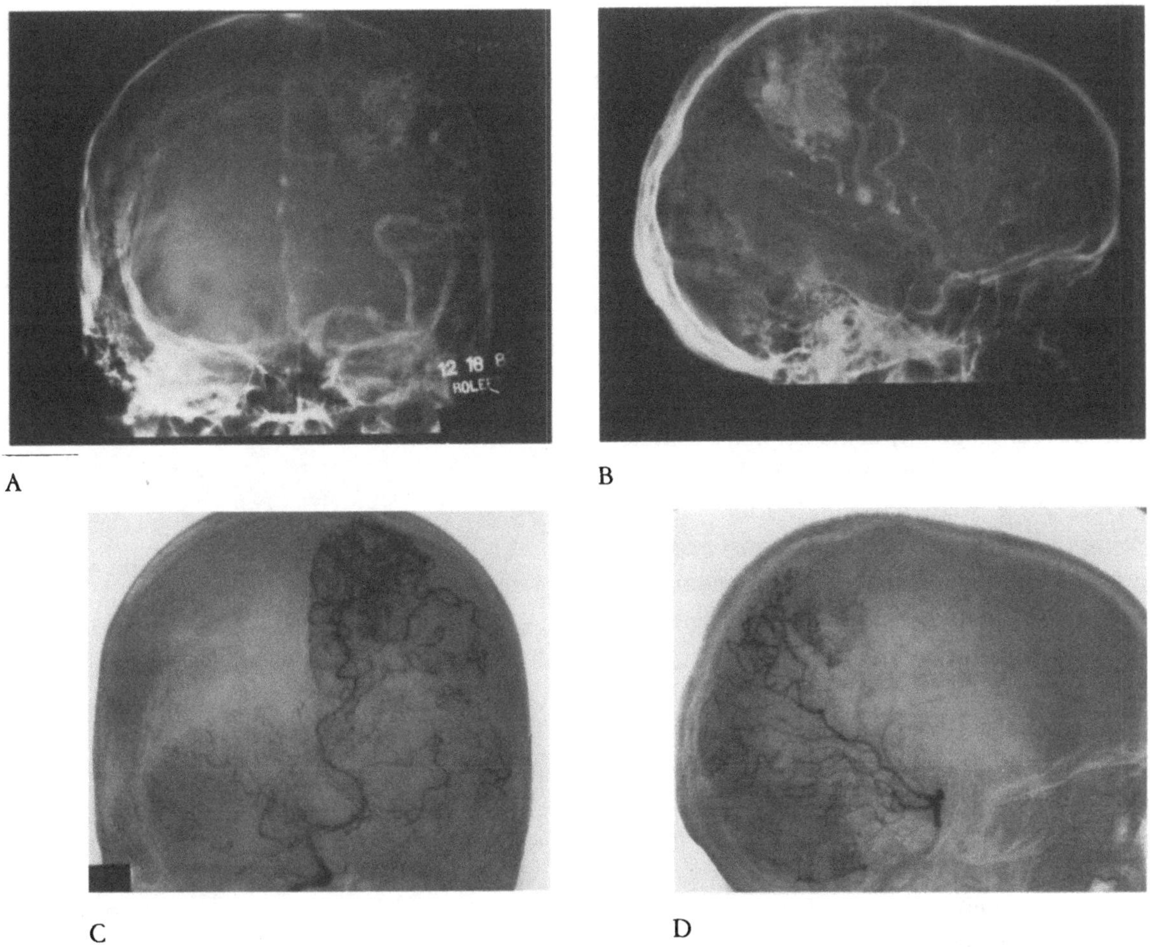

FIGURE 13-5. Anteroposterior and lateral views of left carotid (A and B) and right vertebral (C and D) angiograms demonstrating a large left parietal AVM with multiple feeding vessels from the left anterior, middle, and posterior cerebral arteries.

The seizures were eventually controlled, however, and the patient was discharged 14 days postoperatively with normal speech and strength, but with decreased facility in her right hand and foot. Postoperative angiography (Figure 13-6) demonstrated the complete removal of the AVM. Followup neurological examination 2 months postoperatively was normal.

Pathological examination of the resected specimen demonstrated nonspecific changes of focal mural thickening and focal endothelial cell proliferation which were rather nonspecific but could have been caused by previous radiation therapy. These changes were not prominent.

CASE 2

This 35-year-old, right-handed woman presented with a 10-month history of frequent incapacitating right temporal headaches and temporal lobe seizures that were poorly controlled despite treatment with phenytoin (Dilantin). She was found to have a large left temporo-occipital AVM on a computed tomographic (CT) scan at an outside hospital and was referred for further treatment. Neurological examination was entirely normal. An electroencephalogram (EEG) revealed sleep activation of left temporal spike and sharp waves. Angiography (Figure 13-7) demonstrated a mixed dural and pial AVM of the right temporal lobe fed by branches of the right-middle and posterior cerebral arteries and branches of the right ascending pharyngeal artery. Venous drainage was predominately into the right basal vein of Rosenthal. The malformation was resected through a right temporo-occipital craniotomy with the use of the Nd:YAG laser after first ligating multiple feeding vessels from the right-middle and then posterior cerebral arteries. The laser was remarkably useful for the coagulation of the dural portion of the AVM. Following resection, angiography demonstrated a complete removal of the lesion (Figure 13-8). Postoperatively, there were no complications and her neurological examination was normal except for a left upper homonymous quadrantanopia. The patient was maintained on Dilantin, and there were no postoperative seizures.

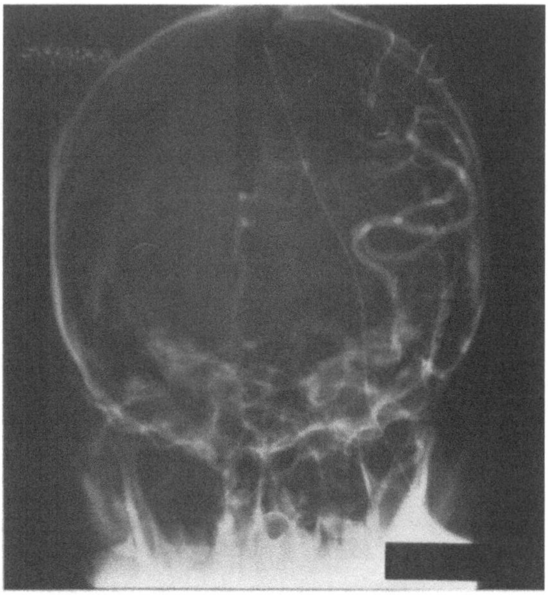

A

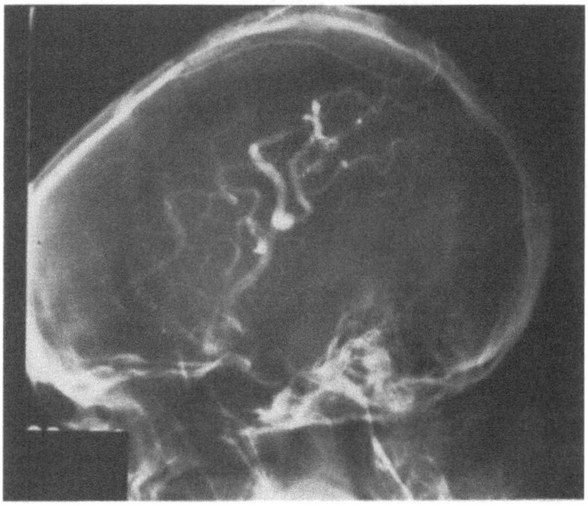

B

FIGURE 13-6. Postoperative anteroposterior (A) and lateral (B) left carotid angiograms demonstrating a complete removal of the AVM.

The Nd:YAG laser has now been used in the resection of 21 cases of AVM's. The cumulative Nd:YAG energy for each case has ranged from 4050 to 21,818 joules. Thus far, there have been no neurological deficits considered secondary to the use of the laser. The Nd:YAG laser has been helpful in the removal of these cerebral AVM's, but it has not reduced appreciably the operating time nor the blood loss. One of the most difficult problems in the resection of AVM's is the control of the small high-flow vessels on the deep surface of the malformation, which have extraordinarily thin walls and are hidden from view by normal-appearing white matter. As stated before, the primary purpose in our evaluation of this instrument was the possibility of discovering a better method of managing these vessels. The laser has not solved this problem to our satisfaction. Although these vessels can sometimes be coagulated after the application of a small aneurysm clip, the advantages of this are small, if any, and in most instances, these vessels would only be controlled with bipolar coagulation.

Nevertheless, the Nd:YAG laser was helpful for: (1) defining the plane between the AVM and the brain; (2) coagulating any dural component of the AVM; and (3) achieving hemostasis in the bed following resection of the lesion. Hemostasis in the bed is effectively achieved

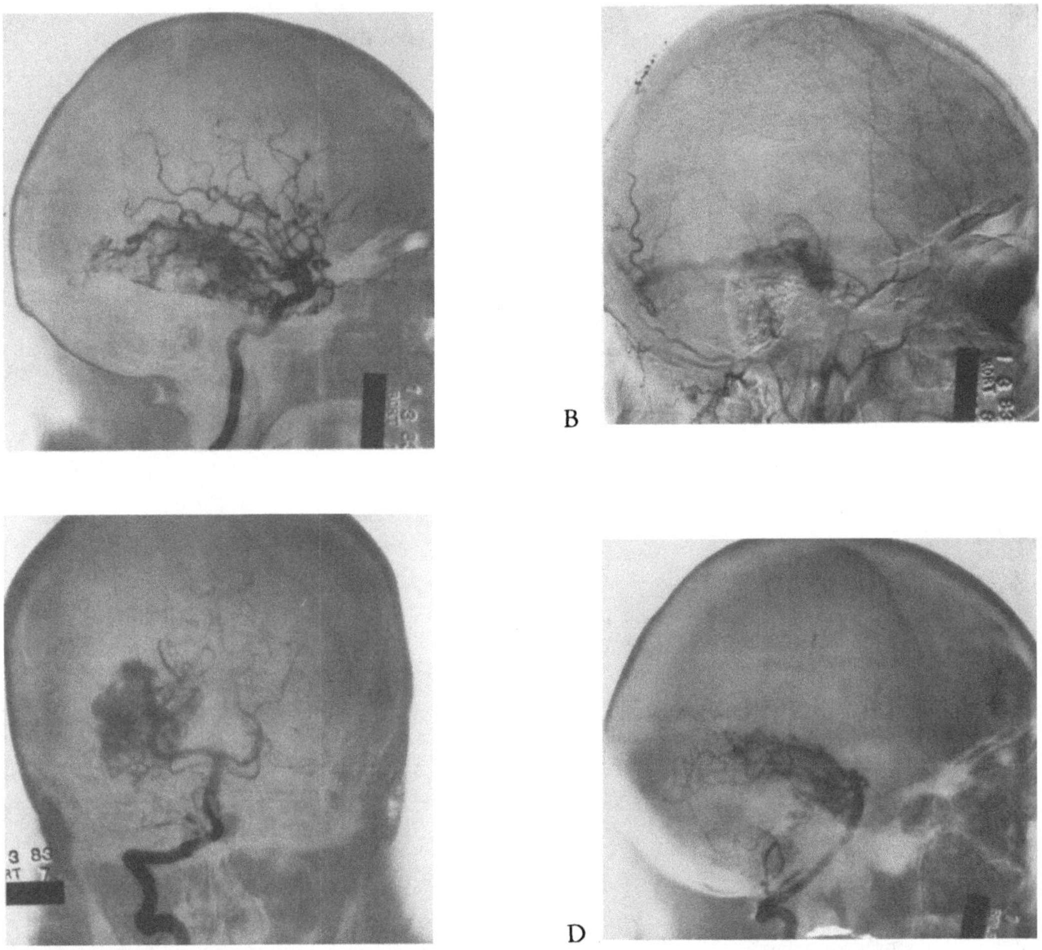

FIGURE 13-7. Lateral right internal (A) and external (B) carotid angiograms and anteroposterior (C) and lateral (D) views of the right vertebral angiogram, demonstrating a mixed dural and pial AVM of the right temporal lobe. The AVM is supplied by branches of the right-middle and posterior cerebral arteries and branches of the right ascending pharyngeal artery.

following resection of the malformation by using lower power outputs of 5 W with a focused beam. In this matter, the multiple tiny vessels along the surface can be coagulated. If too heavy a power setting is used for this purpose, a layer of coagulum develops which interferes with penetration of the beam into the area of bleeding.

As was discussed earlier, the heating of tissue with a Nd:YAG laser is largely dependent on the local blood flow which functions as a heat-sink. Because of the difference in blood flow, arteries are more difficult and require higher energies to coagulate than veins, which, despite their size, are usually easily coagulated in low energies.

Experience with the use of the Nd:YAG laser in the resection of AVM's has demonstrated that this laser can be used safely even in delicate areas of the brain. Case 1 involved a large high-flow AVM in the region of the motor strip, which was resected completely with the use of the Nd:YAG laser without a permanent neurological deficit. However, this laser does have the

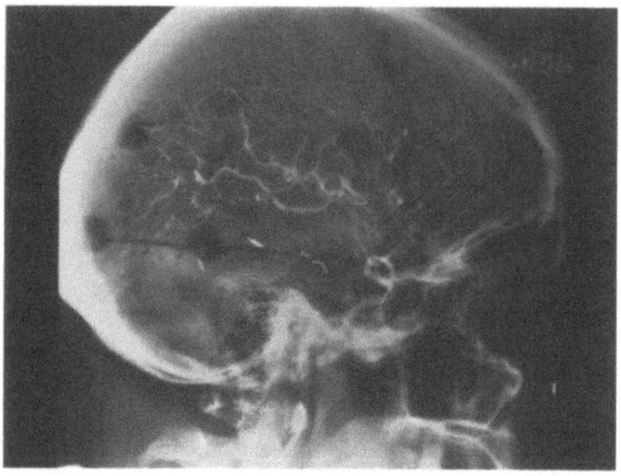

A

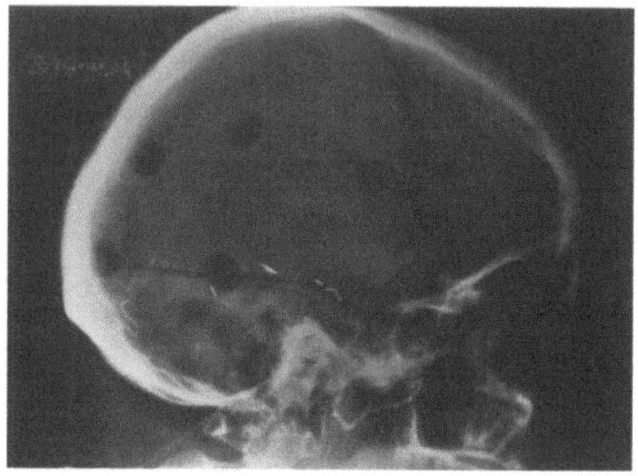

B

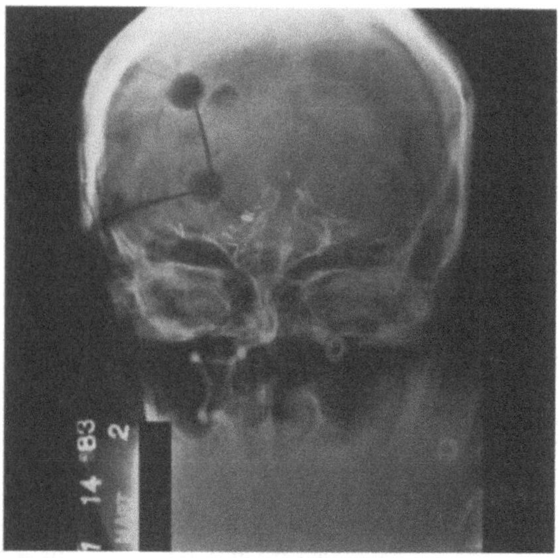

C

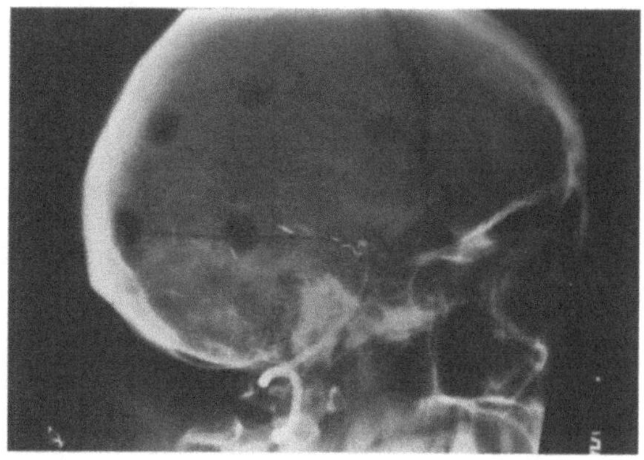

D

FIGURE 13-8. Postoperative angiograms. Lateral right internal (A) and external (B) carotid angiograms and anteroposterior (C) and lateral (D) views of the right vertebral angiogram demonstrating the complete removal of the arteriovenous malformation.

potential to spread heat and possibly damage surrounding tissue. The decision to use this instrument and the parameters invoked must be carefully considered in each case.

Although the Nd:YAG laser can be used safely, its overall benefit in the resection of AVM's remains to be determined. The most difficult problem in the resection of many of these lesions relates to the high-flow, thin-walled feeding vessels on the deep surface of the AVM, and in the our hands, the laser has been disappointing for the coagulation of these vessels. The greatest benefit in the use of this laser in the resection of AVM's has been to coagulate any dural component of the malformation as demonstrated in Case 2. The laser has been extremely effective in this regard and at present this is really the main indication to consider its

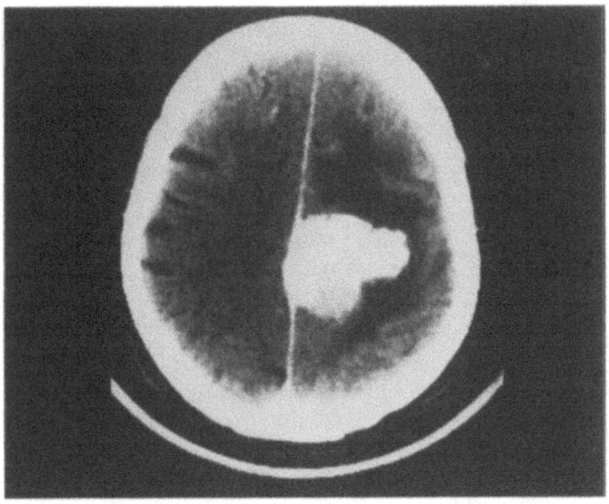

FIGURE 13-9. CT scan with contrast demonstrating a large, enhancing left parietal lesion with surrounding edema.

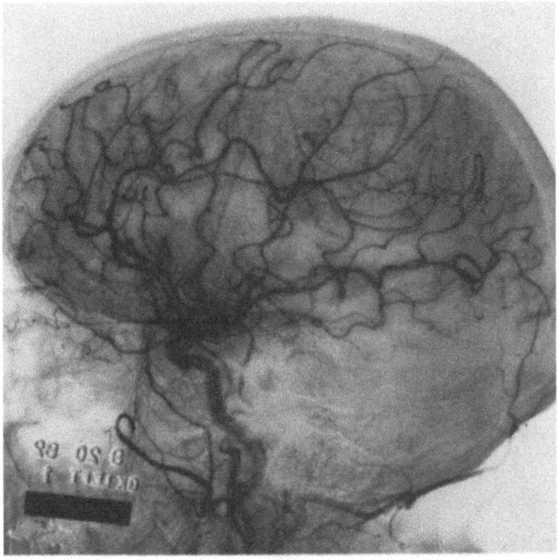

FIGURE 13-10. Left lateral common carotid angiogram demonstrating a left parietal mass with tumor vascularity supplied by the external carotid system consistent with a meningioma.

use in AVM surgery. The development of better instrumentation and techniques may increase the use of this instrument for these types of lesions. We have no experience thus far with the new sapphire-tip contact Nd:YAG laser, and it remains to be seen whether this will be of any

TABLE 13-2. Operative Cases the Using Nd: YAG Laser

Arteriovenous malformations	21
Tumors	20
Glioma(9)	
Neurlemoma(1) Meningioma(5)	
Hemangioblastoma(3)	
Metastasis(1)	
Choroid plexus papilloma(1)	
Transsphenoidals	26
Stereotactic biopsies	7
Total	74

benefit for the resection of AVM's.

The major application of the Nd:YAG laser has been its use as an adjunctive measure for hemostasis in the resection of vascular tumors, especially extraaxial tumors [1, 4, 9, 14]. Our experience with the Nd:YAG laser now consists of 74 cases (Table 13-2), including 20 cases of vascular tumors and 26 transsphenoidal approaches for pituitary tumors.

CASE 3

This 78-year-old, right-handed woman presented with a 2-year history of progressive right hemiparesis and episodic vertigo. Neurological examination revealed a severe right hemiparesis with moderate left leg weakness as well. CT scan (Figure 13-9) demonstrated a large left parasagittal lesion with surrounding edema, and angiography (Figure 13-10) demonstrated a tumor vascularity with supply from the external carotid system consistent with a meningioma.

At surgery, a left frontoparietal falx meningioma was removed, including a portion of the falx that had been perforated by the tumor and extended into the middle of the right parietal lobe. The Nd:YAG laser was used to very effectively cauterize the small feeding vessels on the surface of the tumor and for maintaining effective hemostasis during the gutting of the lesion. Postoperatively, her right hemiparesis and left leg weakness improved. There has been no tumor recurrence on CT scan 3 years later.

CASE 4

This 58-year-old, right-handed man presented with a 6-week history of headaches and gait ataxia. There was no family history of von Hipple-Lindau disease. Neurological examination revealed a mild abnormality of tendem gait. Fundus exam was normal. CT scan (Figure 13-11) demonstrated a densely enhancing right cerebellar mass with compression and shift of the fourth ventricle to the left. The remainder of the CT scan showed moderate hydrocephalus. Angiography (Figure 13-12) demonstrated a highly vascular lesion supplied by branches of the superior cerebellar and posterior inferior cerebellar arteries. A CT scan of the abdomen was negative. The hematocrit was 49.1%.

At surgery, a right cerebellar hemangioblastoma was removed in a circumferential fashion. The tumor was densely adherent to the lateral sinus and tentorium. The Nd:YAG laser was used effectively in coagulating the multiple feeding vessels particularly at the superior aspect of the tumor where it was adherent to dura. The laser was also useful in obtaining hemostasis of the tumor bed.

Postoperatively, the headaches and gait dysfunction resolved. A repeat CT scan 2 years later demonstrated a 0.5-cm enhancing nodule near the torcula suggestive of a tumor recurrence. He subsequently received radiation therapy (6000 rads) to a localized field encompassing the recurrence.

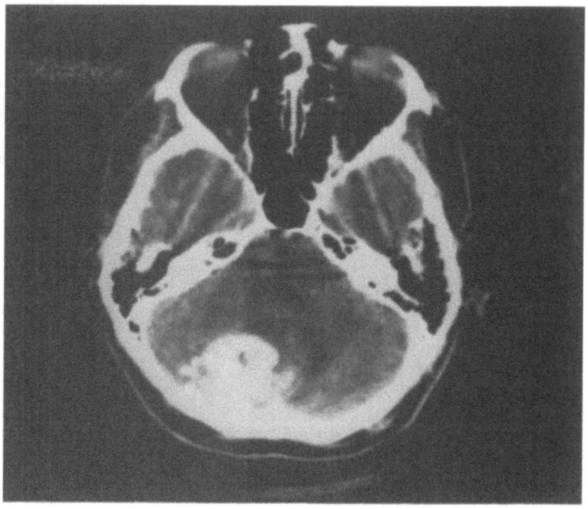

FIGURE 13-11. CT scan with contrast demonstrates a densely enhancing right cerebellar mass with compression and shift of the fourth ventricle to the left.

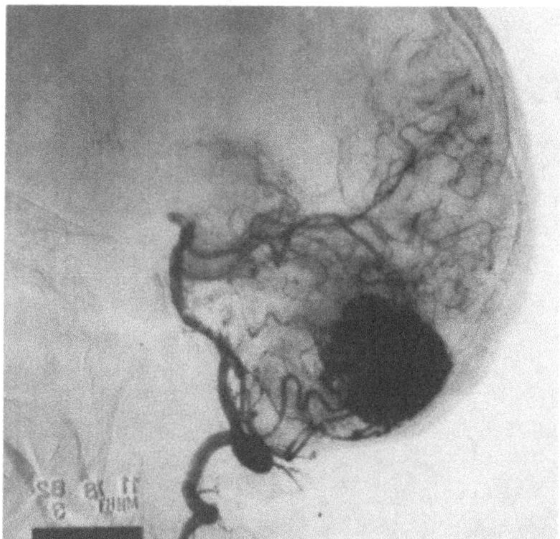

FIGURE 13-12. Right lateral vertebral angiogram demonstrates a highly vascular right cerebellar lesion supplied by branches of the superior cerebellar and posterior inferior cerebellar arteries.

The primary use of the Nd:YAG laser appears to be in the removal of extraaxial lesions, for devascularization during debulking, and for hemostasis of the vascular pedicle. The laser was very expeditious in maintaining hemostasis during the debulking of the large parasagittal meningioma in Case 3. Powers of 10 to 40 W for less than 3 seconds were delivered using a focused handpiece. Similarly, the laser was useful for coagulation of the tumor bed and the vascular pedicle in the removal of the cerebellar hemangioblastoma in Case 4. Powers of 5 to 20 W for less than 3 seconds duration were used in this case. In neither case did we feel that the laser was accomplishing anything that could not have been done using other techniques, such as a bipolar coagulator, but at least in these two cases the use of the laser was certainly efficacious. However, when using the Nd:YAG laser, the degree of tissue penetration and the temperature profiles must always be kept in mind as the interface between tumor and normal structures is approached. Intermittent applications of short duration at the lowest power possible to achieve coagulation should be used. The Nd:YAG laser should be used very cautiously near critical structures, if it is used at all.

Beck [1] has recommended that the Nd:YAG laser be used to devascularize tumor extending into the dural venous sinuses. We have no experience with this technique but would support the opinion of others [4, 10] that this technique of transdural denaturation has some theoretical dangers, particularly the risk of hemorrhage from tumor that has been rendered necrotic but not excised.

Using the Nd:YAG laser in transsphenoidal surgery can best be considered a convenience. The laser can be used to open the sphenoid and sellar floor and is quite effective in achieving hemostasis from the bone. This was found to be most helpful in achieving a dry operative field in patients with Cushing's disease where the sellar floor has not been thinned or in patients where the sphenoid sinus is not well pneumatized. In addition, the laser can be used to coagulate any anterior transcavernous dural venous sinuses prior to opening the dura. However, the laser has not been of use in the removal of the adenoma itself, which is best done by conventional techniques.

Overall, the use of the Nd:YAG laser for intraaxial tumors, in particular gliomas, has not been effective. The laser will assist in coagulation of the tumor bed but this has not been more effective than bipolar coagulation in our hands.

A few other selected cases in which the Nd:YAG has been effective merit mentioning. Occasionally the laser is very helpful in obtaining hemostasis following a stereotactic biopsy through the use of a quartz fiber, which can be inserted through a biposy probe. The majority of the time, however, this is not necessary. The laser was also quite effective in the removal of a choroid plexus papilloma of the right lateral ventricle, and in this particular case may have decreased the operating time slightly. However, the papilloma could certainly have been removed with the use of bipolar cautery.

Conclusion

The Nd:YAG laser has been an effective tool in selected cases, particularly for dural AVM's and vascular extraaxial tumors. Given an understanding of the inherent properties of the laser and its interaction with tissue, it can be used safely. Because of its greater penetration through tissue, however, there is always an inherent danger of damage to normal structures if used indiscriminately. There have been few, if any, cases in which we believed that the laser had accomplished something that was not possible by other techniques. However, in many cases, it was efficacious or convenient. As the technology improves and experience expands, its overall utility may increase.

Acknowledgments

We are grateful to Miss Jill Nicklas for her assistance in the preparation of this manuscript. Portions of this manuscript and its accompanying tables and illustrations have been published elsewhere [20, 21].

References

1. Beck OJ: Clinical use of the Nd:YAG laser in neurosurgery. *Neurosurg Rev* 7:151–158, 1984.
2. Beck OJ: The Use of the Nd:YAG and the CO_2 laser in neurosurgery. *Neurosurg Rev* 3:261–266, 1980.
3. Boggan JE, Edward MSB, Davis RL, et al: Comparison of the brain tissue response of rats to injury by argon and carbon dioxide lasers. *Neurosurgery* 11:609–616, 1982.
4. Cerullo LJ: Laser in the removal of extraaxial tumors of the brain and spinal cord. In Fasano VA (ed): *Advanced Intraoperative Techniques in Neurosurgery*. Wien/New York, Springer-Verlag, 1986, pp 154–161.
5. Davis DH, Sundt TM Jr: Relationships of

cerebral blood flow to cardiac output, mean arterial pressure, blood volume, and alpha and beta blockade in cats. *J Neurosurg* 52:745–754, 1980.

6. Fasano VA: Contact laser. In Fasano VA (ed): *Advanced Intraoperative Techniques in Neurosurgery*. Wien/New York, Spinger-Verlag, 1986, pp 140–144.
7. Fasano VA: Laser effect on normal nervous tissue (CO_2-Nd:YAG). Histological data. In Fasano VA (ed): *Advanced Intraoperative Techniques in Neurosurgery*. Wien/New York, Springer-Verlag, 1986, pp 72–84.
8. Fasano VA: Laser effect on normal vessels (CO_2-Nd:YAG-Argon) histological data. In Fasano VA (ed): *Advanced Intraoperative Techniques in Neurosurgery*. Wien/New York, Springer-Verlag, 1986, pp 85–92.
9. Fasano VA: Laser neurosurgical techniques. In Fasano VA (ed): *Advanced Intraoperative Techniques in Neurosurgery*. Wien/New York, Spring-Verlag, 1986, pp 107–139.
10. Fasano Va: The role of laser in neurosurgery. In Fasano VA (ed): *Advanced Intraoperative Techniques in Neurosurgery*. Wien/New York, Springer-Verlag, 1986, pp 251–253.
11. Fasano VA, Lomnard GF, Ponzio RM: Preliminary experiences with the use of three lasers (CO_2, Nd:YAG, argon) in some posterior fossa tumors in childhood. *Childs Brain* 10:26–38, 1983.
12. Fasano VA, Urciuoli R, Ponzio RM: Photocoagulation of aneurysms with the neodymium: ytrrium-aluminum-garnet or argon laser: Preliminary results in twelve patients. *Neurosurgery* 11:754–760, 1982.
13. Frank F: Biophysical basis and technical requisites for the use of Nd:YAG laser in neurosurgery. *Neurosurg Rev* 145–150, 1984.
14. Handa H, Takeuchi J, Yamagami T: Nd:YAG laser as a surgical tool. *Neurosurg Rev* 7:159–163, 1984.
15. Kuroiwa T, Tsuyuma M, Takei H, Inaba Y: Effects of Nd:YAG and CO_2 lasers on cerebral microvasculature. *J Neurosurg* 64:128–133, 1986.
16. Maiman TH: Stimulated optical radiation in ruby. *Nature* 187:493–494, 1960 (letter).
17. Rutgeerts P, Vantrappen G, Geboes K: Safety and efficacy of neodymium-YAG laser photocoagulation: An experimental study in dogs. *Gut* 22:38–44, 1981.
18. Takeuchi J, Handa H, Taki W, et al: The Nd:YAG laser in neurological surgery. *Surg Neurol* 18:140–142, 1982.
19. Walter GF, Ascher PW, Ingolitsch E: The effect of carbon dioxide and neodymium YAG lasers on the central and peripheral nervous systems, and cerebral blood vessels. *J Neurol Neurosurg Psychiatry* 47:745–749, 1984.
20. Wharen RE, Anderson RE, Sundt TM: The Nd:YAG laser in neurosurgery Part 1. Laboratory investigations: dose-related biological response of neural tissue. *J Neurosurg* 60:531–539, 1984.
21. Wharen RE, Anderson RE, Sundt TM: The Nd:YAG laser in neurosurgery Part 2. Clinical studies: an adjunctive measure for hemostasis in resection of arteriovenous malformations. *J Neurosurg* 60:540–547, 1984.
22. Yamagami T, Handa H, Hashimoto N, et al: Histological changes in rat brain tissue caused by neodymium–yttrium aluminium garnet laser irradiation II. Cerebellum. *Surg Neurol* 24:421–427, 1985.
23. Yamagami T, Handa H, Takeuchi J, et al: Extent of thermal penetration of Nd:YAG laser-histological considerations. *Neurosurg Rev* 7: 165–170, 1984.

V. EXPERIMENTAL TECHNIQUES

14. INVESTIGATIONAL APPLICATIONS

W. Craig Clark

To date, the laser has been used almost exclusively as an ablative tool. The majority of uses of this technology in medicine and surgery have involved the application of thermal energy to tissues, resulting in some permanent alteration of the tissues.

Of great interest are several adaptations of this technology where low amounts of power are used to weld tissues, cause certain poorly defined biostimulatory effects, activate cytotoxic compounds, or allow the intraluminal removal of atherosclerotic plaques. Although these potential uses are still being investigated, they will be briefly discussed because we believe that these applications and other similar uses currently under investigation may represent one of the major directions in which laser use and experimentation will be directed in the future.

Photodynamic Therapy

Photodynamic therapy (PDT) is an exciting modality that has been demonstrated to be remarkably effective in treating early superficial cancers of the skin, bladder, and lungs [5, 6, 7, 51]. This type of treatment depends upon the light activation of a photoreactive drug, or photosensitizer, that has been taken up and retained by tumor cells.

Robertson, J.H. and Clark, W.C. (eds), Lasers in Neurosurgery.

Ideally, a patient with a malignant tumor is given a photosensitive tumor sensitizer that is nontoxic and either selectively taken up or retained by malignant tissues, resulting in a high tumor/normal tissue concentration. The photosensitizer is then activated by a wavelength of light that penetrates deeply into tissues to produce a high level of photochemical activity. Theoretically, this allows tumor destruction with minimal or no damage to adjacent normal tissues [7].

Photosensitizers that have been used in cancer therapy include fluorescein, eosin, tetracycline, acridine orange, and the porphyrins [13, 17, 29, 37, 45, 46, 48]. Of these, the porphyrins, especially hematoporphyrin derivative (HpD), have been the most widely investigated agents to date. Hematoporphyrin derivative was first produced and used in the early 1960s for the identification of malignant tumors and for therapy. Basically, when HpD is administered to an organism harboring a neoplasm, it is selectively concentrated at a higher level in malignant tumors than in the surrounding tissues, with the exception of the kidney, spleen, and liver [25].

Hematoporphyrin does not accumulate in normal brain tissue [40]. It is rejected by the intact blood-brain barrier as a result of its molecular structure and protein binding. Studies have shown that the most effective brain-tumor concentrations are reached when the HpD is injected directly into the tumor [30]. HpD can be activated effectively by light with wavelengths that extend from the near ultraviolet to red (6, 7, 14, 24). With activation by blue light at 405 nm, the HpD fluoresces, and this property has been used successfully for the localization of pulmonary cancers, pituitary tumors [32], and gliomas [38, 50]. When exposed to light of longer wavelengths (e.g., red light at 630 nm), activation and cytotoxicity result, albeit less pronounced than at the shorter wavelengths. Regardless, longer wavelengths must be used to achieve good penetration into solid tumors [26]. The cytotoxicity that is produced is probably the result of the release of singlet oxygen, hydroxyl radicals, or superoxide radicals [29, 49], and has been demonstrated in an experimental glioma model [30, 38], in cell culture [26], and in patients with glial-derived brain tumors [32, 50].

Much work remains before HpD will be a useful photochemotherapeutic agent for brain tumors because of its inconsistency of tumor staining [50] and the questionable efficacy of this agent for the photochemotherapy of malignant brain tumors [32]. As a result, other sensitizers are being investigated, including rhodamine [40] and uroporphyrin I [15], but it will probably be a while longer before any of these agents are developed to the point of widespread clinical trials.

Laser Angioplasty

Atheroma and thrombus can be vaporized with laser energy [20], and a number of investigators have shown that this can be accomplished in both in vitro and in vivo models in animals [2, 3, 9, 11, 21, 33]. There have been a small number of clinical trials in humans, with most attempts at revascularization being tried in the coronary or peripheral arteries [1, 12, 22, 23, 36]. There is one report of percutaneous laser recanalization of carotid arteries in seven cadavers and one living patient [11], but there is no wide experience reported for this particular application.

The lasers that have been discussed most frequently include the argon, Nd:YAGs carbon dioxide, and excimer lasers. The technique used involves one of several approaches: (1) manipulating the optical fiber in a fluoroscopically directed attempt at recanalization (angioplasty); (2) using an angioscope to visually identify the site of occlusion (angioscopy); or (3) performing an open endarterectomy using standard surgical techniques supplemented by laser removal of the atherosclerotic plaque under direct visualization (open endarterectomy).

The argon laser has been used most often in the laser irradiation of atherosclerotic plaques. It is readily absorbed by the oxygenated hemoglobin of blood and can be converted to thermal energy to debulk the plaque. It has the obvious advantage of the capability of being directed through an optical fiber that allows its use in angioplasty and angioscopy applications as well as open endarterectomies. Clinical experience with percutaneous laser angioplasty has shown vessel wall perforations in two of 15 and three of 16 patients in two separate reports [12]. Occasionally, these perforations are the result of a mechanical disruption of the vessel by the catheter itself, rather than the result of laser vaporization.

When used in conjunction with an angioscope, the argon laser was successful in recanalizing ten of 11 totally occluded superficial femoral arteries. Although calcific plaque was readily vaporized in this study, fresh thrombus was not adequately vaporized due to a "gel effect" and the high water and fibrin content of fresh thrombus that may allow much of the laser energy to pass through without being absorbed [2].

An adaptation of the argon laser to open endarterectomy has also been described. In this approach the vessel is exposed and a longitudinal arteriotomy is performed in a conventional fashion. The argon laser is then used to create a line of small confluent craters at either end of the plaque that extend into the media. The craters are then connected using about 1.0 W of continuous argon energy, and the plaque is elevated away from the vessel by developing a cleavage plane within the media to dissect the plaque out of the artery. Once the plaque is removed, the end points of the endarterectomy are sealed to the media to prevent a possible intimal flap that might be thrombogenic [16].

The Nd:YAG laser may also be directed through a fiber optic and can, at least theoretically, be adapted for use in angioplasty. Attempts at using this device intravascularly initially resulted in an unacceptably high incidence of vessel wall perforations [21], and most investigators no longer use the Nd:YAG laser for this application. Its use has also been reported for open endarterectomy, but due to its volumetric, tissue necrosis effects, it would not seem to be the most desirable device for this application either.

The carbon dioxide laser cannot currently be passed down a commercially available fiber optic and cannot be used for angioplasty techniques. However, it should be noted that a variety of halide and other fibers capable of transmitting the carbon dioxide beam are being investigated and may be available soon. Only then will it be determined if this device will be useful for percutaneous angioplasty. It can be used in conjunction with an angioscope, but its intravascular use is severely limited by the necessity for a dry environment to ensure controlled tissue absorption of the beam. On the other hand, because of the purely surface effect of the carbon dioxide beam, and the ability to deliver a superbly controlled lesion, the carbon dioxide laser is ideal for removing atherosclerotic plaque cleanly without causing abrasion, perforation, or thermal damage to the artery itself [36]. As a result, trials are underway where the carbon dioxide laser will be used to perform open endarterectomies in patients whose coronary occlusion is in the distal part of the artery and otherwise inoperable.

A new xenon chloride excimer laser has created much excitement among cardiologists committed to the development of a percutaneous laser angioplasty technique. The excimer laser's beam can be directed through catheters via an optical fiber. The beam is emitted in slow, pulsing bursts that allow the area being treated to dissipate heat, thus avoiding tissue damage. Unlike any of the other laser devices mentioned, the excimer laser does not rely on heat to achieve its effects. Rather, it destroys the plaque by breaking the material's intramolecular bonds. Further, the excimer laser's pulsation can be controlled with great precision in bursts of 10 to 200 nsec, presumably reducing the danger of vessel wall perforation [34]. Although the excimer laser presently is primarily a laboratory device, it should be subjected to clinical trials in the near future.

Although perforation of vessels has been a major stumbling block to the routine use of laser angioplasty, a new technique called laser-induced fluorescence (LIF) may provide a breakthrough. Shining a low-powered or attenuated laser on both atheroma and normal arterial wall results in differing patterns of fluorescence for the two materials. The low-powered laser is transmitted through a flexible fiber to the area to be vaporized. The fluorescence is picked up and transmitted through another fiber back to a computer than can discriminate between atheroma and the arterial wall.

Regardless of the wavelength of laser light or delivery system used, vessel wall perforation [10, 12, 23] and postlaser reocclusion [9] remain significant unsolved problems. Although distal embolization has not proven a problem to date [8], fiber burnback, catheter guidance, and dosimetry will all require further work before laser angioplasty will be widely used clinically [10].

Laser-Assisted Microsurgical Anastomosis

Recent reports indicate that it may be feasible to perform microsurgical anastomoses of muscular arteries and peripheral nerves using either the argon, Nd:YAG, or carbon dioxide laser [4, 18, 19, 27, 43].

Various authors have described their particular techniques and the associated histological changes associated with the thermal coaptation of small muscular arteries. Both Quigley and associates [42–44] and Pribil [41] describe the use of a milliwatt carbon dioxide and argon laser, respectively, to seal the everted edges of small vessels that have been approximated with small sutures. Jain [27] has described a smiliar technique that is sutureless and uses a Nd:YAG laser.

Regardless of the laser system used, independently conducted vessel-welding studies have reported that the basic mechanism and light microscopic changes are quite similar [47]. With the argon and Nd:YAG lasers, the changes consisted of a localized swelling and homogenization of the adventitia as well as a coagulation necrosis of smooth muscle cells in the underlying media [27, 41]. Vascular bonding with the carbon dioxide laser principally involved the adventitia and outer muscular layer [19, 43]. Light and electron microscopy have shown the sealing to be due to changes seen in the collagen present. Collagen fibrils had lost their periodicity, were greatly increased in caliber, and were split into fine fibrillary substructures with a roughly concentric arrangement on cross-section. The fibrils were closely interdigitated, and this interdigitation seemed to be the basis for the laser-induced welding effect [47].

While elucidation of the exact mechanism may require further investigation, what is clear is that this technique has not yet found any wide acceptance clinically. Investigators using the milliwatt carbon dioxide laser reported a 10% rate of pseudoaneurysm formation at the site of anastomosis, and significant intimal proliferation that might contribute to late occlusion of the graft [42, 44]. Likewise, a study with the argon device showed that, with increasing time after anastomosis, there was a trend toward increasing angiographically-proven stenosis of the anastomotic segment and histologically demonstrated pseudoaneurysm formation of the vessel wall at the bonded site [41]. Based on the data presently available it would appear that further investigation and experience are needed before laser-assisted microvascular anastomosis can be accepted as an alternative to conventional microvascular suture technique [41, 42].

Laser Acupuncture

During recent years a number of investigators have studied the proposed mechanisms of the biological action of low-energy laser radiation. As early as 1973 Plog began his first experiments with the application of laser irradiation to the acupuncture points [39] and by 1978 the first prototype helium-neon (He:Ne) laser acupuncture device was undergoing trials in Europe [31].

Various effects of these laser acupuncture treatments have been observed in both the laboratory and clinic, but they remain poorly understood. Theoretically, laser irradiation acts much like the needle stimulation of acupuncture at trigger points to somehow block the pain gate and decrease the perception of certain types of pain [28]. However, no studies have shown measurable evidence of how this laser effect is supposed to work, nor have any specific, measurable physiological parameters been delineated.

As a result of the well-recognized placebo effects seen in the treatment of both acute and chronic pain disorders, any reported application of laser acupuncture for the relief of pain should be greeted by a fairly healthy degree of skepticism unless it is substantiated by a well-designed, controlled study.

Conclusion

Exciting advances are occurring almost weekly with regard to the use of laser technology in medicine and surgery. Some of the applications just discussed, although they are at present under investigation, may become established modes of therapy for the physician and surgeon in the near future. As our knowledge of lasers and various methods of delivering and controlling them continues to grow, we will see new, interesting, and exciting applications of this technology.

References

1. Abela GS: Laser angioplasty: Progressing, but opinious, forecasts vary (medical news). *JAMA* 253:1525–1533, 1985.
2. Abela GS: Laser recanalization shows promise for occlusive vascular disease. *Microsurg Pract* 3:2, 1986.
3. Abela GS, Normann SJ, Cohen DM, et al: Laser recanalization of occluded atherosclerotic arteries in vivo and in vitro. *Circulation* 71:403–411, 1985.
4. Beggs JL, Fischer DW, Shetter AG: Comparative study of microepineural anastomoses made with carbon dioxide laser and suture techniques. Part 2. *Neurosurgery* 18:266–269, 1986.
5. Benson RC, Farrow GM, Kinsey JH, et al: Detection and localization of in situ carcinoma of the bladder with hematoporphyrin derivative. *Mayo Clin Proc* 57:548–555, 1982.
6. Carruth JAS: Photodynamic therapy: The state of the art. *Lasers Surg Med* 6:404–407, 1986.
7. Carruth JAS, McKenzie AL: Pilot study on photoradiation therapy in the treatment of superficial tumors of the skin and head and neck. *Clin Oncol* 11:47–50, 1985.
8. Case RB, Choy DSJ, Dwyer EM, Silvernail PJ: Absence of distal emboli during in vivo laser recanalization. *Lasers Surg Med* 5:281–289, 1985.
9. Choy DSJ: Laser-opened coronary arteries close again within months, *JAMA* (medical news) 253:1525–1533, 1985.
10. Choy DSJ: Laser revascularization: State of the art. *Laser Surg Med* 6:408–411, 1986.
11. Choy DSJ, Stertzer SH, Rotterdam HZ, et al: Transluminal laser catheter angioplasty. *Am J Cardiol* 50:1206–1208, 1982.
12. Cumberland DC, Sanborn TA, Tayler DI, et al: Percutaneous laser thermal angioplasty: Initial clinical results with a laser probe in total peripheral artery occlusions. *Lancet* 1: 1457–1459, 1986.
13. Dougherty TJ, Grindy GB, Fiel B, et al: Cure of animal tumors with hematoporphyrin and light. *J Natl Cancer Inst* 55:115–119, 1975.
14. Dougherty TJ, Kaufman JE, Goldfarb A, et al: Photoradiation therapy for the treatment of malignant tumors. *Cancer Res* 38:2628–2635, 1978.
15. El-Far MA, Pimstone NR: Superiority of uroporphyrin I over other porphyrins in selective tumor localization. In *Proceedings of Clayton Foundation Symposium on Porphyrin Localization and Treatment of Tumors*, New York, Plenum, 1983.
16. Eugene J, McColgan SJ, Hammer-Wilson M, Berns MW: Laser endarterectomy. *Lasers Surg Med* 5:265–274, 1985.
17. Figge FHJ, Weiland GS, Manganiello LOJ: Cancer detection and therapy: Affinity of neoplastic, embryonic, and traumatized regenerating tissues for porphyrins and metalloporphyrins. *Proc Soc Exp Biol Med* 68:640–641, 1948.
18. Fischer DW, Beggs JL, Kenshalo DL, Shetter AG: Comparative Study of microepineural anastomoses with the use of CO_2 laser and suture techniques in rat sciatic nerves. Part 1. *Neurosurgery* 17:300–308, 1985.
19. Frazier OH, Painvin GA, Morris JR, et al: Laser-assisted microvascular anastomoses: Angiographic and antomopathologic studies on growing microvascular anastomoses. *Surgery* 97: 585–589, 1985.
20. Gerrity RG, Loop FD, Golding LAR, et al: Arterial response to laser operation for removal of atherosclerotic plaques. *J Thorac Cardiovasc Surg* 85:409–421, 1983.
21. Geschwind HJ, Boussignac G, Teisseire B, et al: Conditions for effective Nd:YAG laser angioplasty. *Br Heart J* 52:484–489, 1984.
22. Ginsburg R, Kim DS, Cuthener D, et al: Salvage of an ischemic limb by laser angioplasty: Description of a new technique. *Clin Cardiol* 7:54–58, 1984.
23. Ginsburg R, Wexler L, Mitchell RS, Proffit D: Percutaneous transluminal laser angioplasty for treatment of peripheral vascular disease: Clinical experience with 16 patients. *Radiology* 156:619–624, 1985.
24. Gluckman JL, Waver M, Shumick K, Peerless S: Photodynamic therapy: A viable alternative to conventional therapy for early lesions of the upper aerodigestive tract. *Arch Otolaryngol Head Neck Surg* 112:949–952, 1986.
25. Gomer CJ, Dougherty TJ: Determination of (3H) and (14C) hematoporphyrin derivative distribution in malignant and normal tissue. *Cancer Res* 39:146–151, 1979.
26. Hamilton D, McKean JDS, Tulip J, et al: In vitro photoradiation therapy of the rat 9L gliosarcoma. *J Neurosurg* 64:775–779, 1986.
27. Jain KK: Sutureless end-to-side microvascular anastomosis using Nd:YAG laser. *Vasc Surg*

17:240–243, 1983.

28. Kamikawa K, Ohnishi T, Suzuki M, Kanaya M: Development of laser acupuncture system. In Atsumi K, Nimsakul N (eds): *Proceedings of the IV Congress of the International Society for Laser Surgery*, Ch. 21, 1981, pp 5–6.
29. Kochevar IE: Phototoxicity mechanisms: Chlorpromazine photosensitized damage to DNA and cell membranes. *J Invest Dermatol* 77:59–64, 1981.
30. Kostron H, Bellnier DA, Lin CW, et al: Distribution, retention, and phototoxicity of hematoporphyrin derivative in a rat glioma. *J Neurosurg* 64:768–774, 1986.
31. Kroetlinger M: On the use of laser in acupuncture. *Acupuncture Elecrother* 5:297–311, 1980.
32. Laws ER, Cortese DA, Kinsey JH, et al: Photoradiation therapy in the treatment of malignant brain tumors. *Neurosurgery* 9:672–678, 1981.
33. Lee G, Ikeda RM, Dwyer RM, et al: Feasibility of intravascular laser irradiation for in vivo visualization and therapy of cardiocirculatory diseases. *Am Heart J* 103:1076–1077, 1982.
34. Litvak F: Laser angioplasty (medical news) *JAMA* 253:1525–1533, 1985.
35. Livesay JJ: Laser angioplasty (medical news). *JAMA* 253:1525–1533, 1985.
36. Livesay JJ, Cooley DA: Laser coronary endarterectomy: Proposed treatment for diffuse coronary atherosclerosis. *Texas Heart Inst J* 11:276–279, 1984.
37. Moore GE: Fluorescein as an agent in the differentiation of normal and malignant tissues. *Science* 106:130–131, 1947.
38. Perria C: Photodynamic therapy of human gliomas by hematoporphyrin and He-Ne laser. *IRCS Med Sci* (Cancer) 9:57–58, 1981.
39. Plog FMW: Laser acupuncture. In Koebner HK (ed): *Lasers in Medicine*. New York, John Wiley, 1980, p 21.
40. Powers SK, Pribil S, Gillespie Y, Watkins PJ: Laser photochemotherapy of rhodamine-123 sensitized human glioma cells in vitro. *J Neurosurg* 64:918–923, 1986.
41. Pribil S, Powers SK: Carotid artery end-to-end anastomosis in the rat using the argon laser. *J Neurosurg* 63:771–775, 1985.
42. Quigley MR, Bailes JE, Kwaan HC, Cerullo LJ: Laser-assisted vascular anastomosis (letter). *Lancet* 1:334, 1985.
43. Quigley MR, Bailes JE, Kwaan HC, et al: Microvascular anastomosis using the milliwatt CO_2 laser. *Lasers Surg Med* 5:357–365, 1985.
44. Quigley MR, Bailes JE, Kwaan HC, et al: Aneurysm formation after low power carbon dioxide laser-assisted vascular anastomosis. *Neurosurgery* 18:292–299, 1986.
45. Rall DD, Loo TL, Lane M, et al: Appearance and persistence of fluorescent material in tumor tissue after tetracycline administration. *J Natl Cancer Inst* 19:79–86, 1957.
46. Rasmussen-Taxdall DS, Ward GE, Figge FHJ: Fluorescence of human lymphatic and cancer tissue following high doses of intravenous hematoporphyrin. *Cancer* 8:78–81, 1955.
47. Schober R, Ulrich F, Sander T, et al: Laser-induced alteration of collagen substructure allows microsurgical tissue welding. *Science* 232:1421–1422, 1986.
48. Tomson SH, Emmett EA, Fox SH: Photodestruction of mouse epithelial tumors after acridine orange and argon laser. *Cancer Res* 34: 3124–3127, 1974.
49. Weishaupt KR, Gomer CJ, Dougherty TJ: Identification of singlet oxygen as the cytotoxic agent in photoactivation of a murine tumor. *Cancer Res* 36:2326–2329, 1976.
50. Wharen RE, Anderson RE, Laws ER: Quantitation of hematoporphyrin derivative in human gliomas, experimental central nervous system tumors, and normal tissues. *Neurosurgery* 12: 446–450, 1983.
51. Wile AG, Dahlman A, Burns RG: Laser photoradiation therapy of cancer following hematoporphyrin sensitization. *Lasers Surg Med* 2:163–168, 1982.

INDEX

FSC
www.fsc.org
MIX
Papier | Fördert
gute Waldnutzung
FSC® C083411

Kolibri 360 GmbH
Ferdinand-Jühlke-Straße 7
99095 Erfurt, Deutschland
produktsicherheit@kolibri360.de